Realities of Nutrition

Third Edition

Judi S. Morrill, Ph.D.
Ronald M. Deutsch

Interior Design/Production: Ann Reisenauer
Illustrations: Ann Reisenauer, Ken Miller
Index: Roy P. Basler
Cover: George Willett
Technical Support: Jean Shiota
Printer: Entire Printing, Santa Clara, CA

Orange Grove Publishing
1239 Bellair Way
Menlo Park, CA 94025-6612

www.orangegrovepub.com

Preface

Nutrition knowledge continues to grow in volume and complexity. The 1989 edition of the Recommended Dietary Allowances (RDAs), for example, was published in one thin book. These reference values have expanded to Dietary Reference Intakes (DRIs), published in several thick volumes (totaling thousands of pages) over several years, and accessible for free online (www. nap.edu).

The vast amount of nutrition information, particularly online, is both overwhelming and wonderful. But in the mix, there's a vast amount of misinformation, making it all the more important for consumers to be armed with the basics to meet the challenge of separating fact from fiction.

David Bull died soon after the second edition of this book was published. Though he was "simply" the editor and publisher, he became a cherished friend during the three years that we worked together. My hope is that this edition does what he did so well—keep the focus on what is both informative and interesting to those without a background in science.

Nutrition textbooks continue to grow in detail, size, and cost, with even more bells and whistles —linked websites, PowerPoint presentations, test banks. This book keeps its modest size and cost, and its goal of teaching basic scientific principles and the fundamentals of nutrition simply, clearly, and interestingly.

Judi Sakimoto Morrill

Preface to the 1993 edition

Ronald Deutsch died in 1988, soon after beginning this edition. He had long been a favorite author of mine—I loved the way he explained complex material clearly and creatively. He knew how to shape and sugar the pill to get it down. In fact, I learned to my surprise only recently that the first edition of this book was used successfully as a college textbook—it certainly was unlike any textbook I ever had as a student!

Although nutrition science has grown a lot since that first edition 17 years ago, some things haven't really changed. For one, people are still looking for "nutrition magic"—a vitamin pill perhaps to take care of that "tired feeling"—and there are still plenty of marketers anxious to sell it to them. For another, textbooks still tend to be dry and crammed with details.

So the goal of this second edition is the same as the first-to teach basic scientific principles and the fundamentals of nutrition simply, clearly, and interestingly. And the target audience is the same—people with an interest in nutrition but without a background in science. My hope is that this edition continues Ronald Deutsch's tradition.

I've also tried to uphold Bull Publishing Company's tradition of excellence—I've long told my students that they can depend on Bull publications to be reliable sources of information, something that cannot be said of many companies that publish books on diet and health. It has been a privilege and a pleasure to work with David Bull on this edition.

Judi Sakimoto Morrill

Contents

Part 8 From Farm to Table

Appendices

Chapter 1

Nutrition Myths and Tests of Reality

Do You Sometimes Wonder...?

Do you wonder about food advertisements that say Cholesterol Free...or All Natural!...or Only 2% Fat? *Do you wonder whether you should take supplements, or whether you are getting enough protein? When you hear one thing on the radio and read the opposite on the Internet, do you wonder which is right? If you do, you are wondering about nutrition reality, and how to separate it from myth. As you will see in this chapter, you are not alone. And you can learn ways to separate reality and myth—and save your wondering for harder questions.*

Through the ages, man has wondered about the connection between food and human health and performance. In ancient times, many theories emerged, but there was no systematic method to test them. Myths developed and were handed down in every culture, some of which survive in modern forms today.

Nutrition as a science is little more than 200 years old, and most nutrients have been discovered within the last century. But recently, as the scientific method has been used more and more to seek new information, the body of knowledge in nutrition science has grown rapidly.

In this chapter, we look at some ancient myths, long since dispelled by the scientific method. Categories of nutrients are introduced, along with an explanation of why some are "essential" and some are not. The scientific method itself is described, as distinguished from reliance on anecdotal evidence. Examples show how myths can survive in today's world, and how they can be proved false by science-based knowledge.

The Mysterious Link Between Food and Life

From earliest history, people have understood that food is the primary physical source of life. Beginning with the Stone Age, even the most primitive tribes seem to have arrived at the same fundamental conclusion: Food isn't only the sustainer of life—and a key to its quality—it provides the very physical substance from which life is made.

What is remarkable and almost unique in the history of human thought is that all of modern science confirms this ancient perception of nutrition. From witch doctor to the present-day biochemist, those who have sought to explain the relationship between life and food would probably agree on a single definition of human nutrition as *the study of foods and their effects on a person's development, health, and performance.* One might say that the study of nutrition unravels the mystery of how food becomes you.

For some 10,000 years, virtually every culture has sought to understand the mystery of how

these phenomena of nutrition take place. Each culture has developed systems of choosing food for health, performance, and longevity. In the oldest records of humanity, we find an awareness of a relationship between what we eat and what we are. We find in some form the idea that food supplies the energy of life, that food can become a part of us and change us.[1-4]

Some facts of nutrition are obvious. It takes little science to learn that in general we feel good when we eat, and bad when we go hungry. People learned early that those who have enough food are less likely to get sick.

Up to a point, the study of foods by various cultures is a very realistic business. The first problem is to identify the potential sources of food and to learn what is safely edible and what isn't. One finds truth by experiment. If a person finds that the blueberry is good and satisfying food, it may be tempting to try the lethal berries of the neighboring nightshade—but probably not a second time.

It becomes important to know which mushroom is safe, which leaf, which root. Guessing in the world of food can easily go wrong. If one knows that the tuber of the potato plant is safe and nourishing, one would not have any way to guess that the leaves can be toxic. Or if one knows that the leaves of rhubarb are unsafe to eat, one might not guess that the stalks provide good food.

But even as such knowledge has accumulated, it has contributed little to a more basic understanding of how foods nurture. There's almost a magical quality to the relationship between food and life. Indeed, even for the modern scientist, nutrition is so close to the miracle of life itself that understanding it can evoke a sense of awe.

The Search for Nutrition Magic

Consider some of the essential questions posed by the very definition of nutrition. How do you change such commonplace things as roots and stems, leaves and seeds, eggs and milk, water and air, and the meats of birds, animals, and fish into the wonder of a new child? How do these bits of food turn a helpless infant into an active child who can read and run? In children and adults alike, how do they make the difference between weakness and strength, disease and health, lassitude and energy?

Small wonder that primitive people endow foods with magical power and believe that qualities of the food may be transmitted to the eaters.[5] The people of the Aru and Buru Islands of the Pacific believed that a good way to become more nimble was to eat a dog.

In this light, we can see the logic of the Bakalai of Africa's Guinea Coast, who held that each man had his own special taboo food. We can understand the thinking of those Moroccan tribesmen who, thinking the hyena to be stupid, believed that a woman who wanted to rebel against her husband had only to feed him a stew with a sauce made from hyena brains, and she would forever dominate the marriage.

Often such ideas are confirmed repeatedly by the psychological effects of belief. Certain African tribes believed that to eat the flesh of the lion was to become brave and strong, but to dine on rabbit meant weakness and timidity. It doesn't take much imagination to see why the system worked, and what happened to the warrior who went into battle believing he would be weak and timid after eating rabbit. One can also understand why there have been those who would go hungry rather than risk the threat of the taboo.

This seeming magic of food and life was for long given mystical explanations. Indeed, when the Liberty Bell first rang in Philadelphia, there was still little difference between the nutrition thinking of the witch doctors and that of the best physicians of the time. For the mystery of how food affects life remained intact, like an unbroken code, a puzzle with many clues but not much hint of solution. There was, as there always had been, plenty of nutrition advice and superstitious taboo—but there was no nutrition science.

The Search for the Science of Nutrition

For well over 2,000 years, nutrition has been viewed as a dominant force in medicine. Yet, medical science was slow to learn the realities of nutrition. For centuries, two schools of thought

dominated medical teaching. In both, nutrition was seen to be at the foundation of health and disease.

One school of thinking arose in China of the 6th century B.C. and is credited to Ho the Physician. He adapted to medicine the philosophic concept of two opposite yet mysteriously complementary forces as the core powers of the universe—yin and yang.

Yin is the female principle, typifying coolness and moistness. *Yang* is the male principle, standing for such qualities as warmth and expansion. These forces were seen to account for the occult characteristics of food, which supposedly influenced health by heightening the yin and yang of the body.

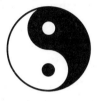
Yin-Yang Symbol

In the 3rd and 4th century B.C., another school of thought was represented by Hippocrates, the famed physician of Greece's golden age. Aristotle reports Hippocrates' theory of disease and his concern with the physical qualities of foods:

Either because of the quantity of things taken [eaten] or through their diversity or because the things taken happen to be strong and difficult of digestion, residues are thereby produced...And when the things that have been taken are of many kinds, they quarrel with one another in the belly, and...there is a change into residues...From the residues arise gases, which having arisen, bring on disease.[6]

There was also special emphasis on such attributes of food as its temperature, hardness, and color. For example, the Greek Regimen in Health gave this Hippocratic advice on eating in warm weather:

In summer the barley-cake [a staple of the ancient Greek dietary] is to be soft, the drink diluted and copious, and the meats in all cases boiled. For one must use these in summer, that the body may be cold and soft.[6]

Eventually, the Oriental teaching entered the Arab world, and through it, the Greek. By the time of the first Crusades—and partly because of them—the concept was brought into northern Europe. The Oriental and Greek nutrition traditions blended well. Both related to the observable physical properties of foods. And whatever could not be explained in any other way could be attributed to the mystical balance or imbalance of yin and yang.

For many centuries thereafter, nutrition science progressed little. "Civilized" people—despite their advanced knowledge of astronomy, architecture, and so forth—lived with a nutrition understanding which was really not a great deal different from that of "primitive" people. Nutrition—as it would have been known to Columbus, Elizabeth the First, Sir Francis Drake, Isaac Newton, or young Benjamin Franklin—is typified by a segment of a poem, the *Regimen sanitatis Salernitanum* [Health Regimen of Salerno (Italy)], probably dating from the 1200s:

Peaches, apples, pears, milk, cheese, and salted
   meat,
Deer, hare, goat and veal,
These engender black bile and are enemies of
   the sick.
Fresh eggs, red wines, fat broth,
Together with fine pure flour, strengthen nature.
Wheat, milk, young cheese,
Testicles, pork, brain marrow,
Sweet wine, food pleasant to the taste,
Soft-boiled eggs, ripe figs, and fresh grapes,
Nourish as well as make fat.[6]

However, in the late 18th century, the discoveries of oxygen and some of the first ideas of true chemistry at last began to open the way for understanding the life-giving qualities of food. In the period 1780 to 1794, the French chemist Antoine Lavoisier showed that oxygen was taken into the body and used in a "burning" process which yielded heat. From this, came the first insights into food's work as fuel. In one famous line, Lavoisier forged the key to all true nutrition science—*La vie est une fonction chimique* (Life is a chemical function). Lamentably, Lavoisier's pioneering was cut off by a stroke of the French Revolution's guillotine. But slowly others developed his basic concept.

Life as a Chemical Matter

There developed the understanding that foods are merely the raw materials which provide the "chemicals" for the chemistry of life. But it took more than a century of work by thousands of scientists before we acquired more than the most superficial information about the composition of foods and how that composition affects us. Only relatively recently have we acquired a scientific understanding of food and nutrition.

Today, we understand that each person is a kind of chemical factory. We grow, think, feel, see, heal our wounds, walk, breathe, reproduce ourselves—perform virtually every act of living—by making life chemicals. And like any other factory, all forms of life—from the simplest single-celled bacterium to the humblest blade of grass, from the tiniest insect to the largest elephant—require certain raw ingredients for this chemical manufacture.

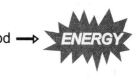

The raw material for our chemical "factory" includes water, protein, fat, carbohydrate, vitamins, and minerals. Using these nutrients, the human body produces more than 100,000 biochemicals (life chemicals) with which to grow, function, and maintain itself. The fact that these ingredients of biochemistry come from the food we eat is the basis of nutrition science.

The Science of Nutrition

The optimal support of life's chemistry depends upon balancing the foods which supply life-supporting chemicals with life's needs for these chemical ingredients. Thus, the realities of nutrition are based on a knowledge of two main bodies of information:
• The kind and quantity of nutrients contained in each food.
• The kind and quantity of nutrients required to carry out the chemical reactions needed for a healthful life.

Timeline of Some Discoveries in Nutrition Science	
1750	Oranges and lemons can cure scurvy
1800	Animals use oxygen to burn fuel, emitting heat and carbon dioxide
1850	Cod liver oil used successfully to treat rickets
	Four nutrients known carbohydrate, fat, protein, "ash"
1900	Beriberi is a dietary deficiency disease
	Discovery of "5th nutrient" (vital amines/vitamins)
	First vitamin discovered (thiamin)
	Liver-rich diet cures pernicious anemia
	Vitamin A plays a role in vision
1950	Last vitamin discovered (vitamin B-12)
	Dietary fat related to heart disease
	High-fat diet associated with certain cancers
	Heavy alcohol intake associated with high blood pressure
	Leptin hormone helps regulate appetite and metabolism
2000	Ghrelin hormone stimulates appetite
	Obestatin hormone lessens appetite

Although Lavoisier had revealed the basic chemical principle of nutrition before the close of the 18th century, nutrition science was still extremely simplistic at the end of the 19th century. Only four nutrients were known: carbohydrate, fat, protein, and "ash."

The first three are the energy-providing nutrients—suppliers of energy and building materials. And ash is the sum of all the minerals in foods—literally, the material which remains when food has been thoroughly burned. Carbohydrate was not clearly identified or named until the middle of the 19th century. Fats were chemically identified at about the same time. And protein was known only by its characteristic of coagulating when heated or dried, as in egg white or blood.

But when young experimental animals were fed purified diets of only the four known nutrients, they stopped growing. It was clear that there must be a fifth nutrient. Around 1906, English scientist Frederick Hopkins found that just a bit of milk added to a purified diet got his young rats growing again. For his work in characterizing this "fifth nutrient"—which we now know as the vitamins (*vital amines*)—Hopkins was awarded the Nobel Prize in 1929.

The first of the vitamins was isolated in 1926. The last and 13th vitamin was discovered in 1948. For their discoveries relating to vitamins, scientists were awarded a cluster of Nobel Prizes in 1928, 1929, 1934, 1937, 1938, 1943. The early part of that century marked the golden age of nutrition. The rapid acquisition of knowledge of vitamins and the use of this knowledge to cure nutritional deficiency diseases generated great excitement among scientists—much like the excitement of scientists in today's golden age of biotechnology and neurobiology.

It's sad to note, however, that despite the discovery of "simple cures" for nutritional deficiency diseases, these diseases are still widespread throughout the world. We know that many people die from a simple lack of calories (starvation). But few of us know, for example, that in many parts of the world, vitamin A deficiency is still a major cause of blindness in children. Barriers such as poverty and politics still lie between what is scientifically possible and what is, in fact, achieved in preventing these diseases.

Modern Challenges

Ironically, we don't need science to point out a truly modern nutrition challenge; we only need to people-watch at our local shopping mall. Obesity has risen dramatically and steadily over the past 25 years to where two of every three adults are overweight or obese (see Fig. 1-1).

For all the hoopla surrounding scientific discoveries of related hormones and genes, the stark

Figure 1-1: Increase in Obesity in the U.S.[7]

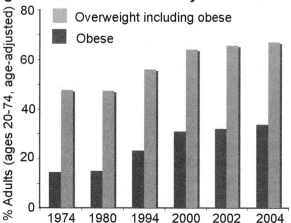

Figure 1-2: Increase in Diabetes[13]

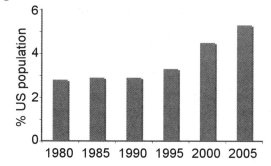

reality is simply that if we take in more calories than we burn, we become fat. Excess calories is a problem in many developing countries as well. The world's overfed (~1.2 billion) now outnumber the underfed (~800 million). The realities of energy balance are discussed in Chapters 2 and 3.

Obesity raises the risk of many diseases, including diabetes, heart disease, and some cancers. As expected, the age-adjusted prevalence of diabetes is going up (Fig. 1-2).

Science's exploration in nutrition goes deep—and wide. Such discoveries as hormones that regulate appetite, and insulin receptors that resist insulin action, provide insight into how obesity and diabetes might be prevented and treated.

Looking deep into cells and molecules, scientists discover the workings of individual atoms of minerals, and the exact roles of vitamins in chemical reactions. One then understands in precise detail why vitamins and certain minerals are needed for good health. Scientists explore how different dietary fats act to cause—or prevent—the narrowing of an artery, and work to pinpoint the dietary factors that may promote or prevent cancer.

Echoes of the Past

Despite the advances of nutrition science, nutrition myths persist. Many people today ascribe the health values of nutrients to factors inconsistent with chemical science—not entirely unlike some of the ancient myths. Yesterday's warrior ate the flesh of the lion to become brave and strong. Today's athlete gulps a myriad of dietary supple-

ments for a "winning edge." The ancient words of Ho the Physician and Hippocrates—clothed in modern language—still echo in today's best-selling health books.

We hear of such things as toxic products formed by eating certain foods in combination, and of obesity resulting from incomplete digestion of foods—ancient theories that scientists disproved long ago. Ancient and obscure voices? Hardly. Search the web by keying in toxic food combinations and get millions of hits.

Just as fashions cycle, so do these unscientific ideas of food and health. The words shift to accommodate present-day jargon, but the basic themes come back time and time again. Science moves on while the unscientific hits a responsive chord and stays put. In fact, if one updates the language, it's hard to distinguish the same unscientific ideas that appear even centuries apart.

These ideas have a ready audience because people have so many misconceptions about nutrition. For example, many falsely believe that a deficiency of vitamins and minerals is the most common cause of feeling tired and run down. Another common false belief is that man-made vitamins are inherently inferior to natural vitamins. In more subtle areas of nutrition—such as separating fact from advertising hype when choosing foods, the balancing of the diet, or attempts to lose weight—the misconceptions are even more widespread.

Fortunately, most of these nostrums and such are quite harmless. Some do, in fact, make one healthier—sometimes because, despite the false theory, poor diets are made better, and sometimes because of the power of believing. The diets most likely to be dangerous are those that severely limit the variety of food.

Cold Science vs. Eating Pleasure

For all of the progress made in the science of nutrition, it's ironic that many people still don't accept science's answers to some of nutrition's earlier mysteries. Myths and misconceptions often persist because the ideas seem reasonable, logical, and more appealing. There is still something cold and mechanical about the word "science" that seems incompatible with nutrition.

Each of us tends to have strong feelings about foods, about what's "good" for us and what's "bad." Psychologists explain that we learn about food and love at the same time—as infants, when the world is no bigger than a mother's encircling arms. Ever after, food is an emotional issue.

But science is no "colder" than the physical realities of life. It's no more, or less, than a systematic way of arriving at what's real. As the dictionary defines it, *science is a state or fact of knowing; knowledge, often opposed to intuition, belief.*

Perhaps the newness of so much of our scientific understanding helps to account for the fact that so few seem to accept fully the concept of nutrition as chemistry. "Natural" appeals. "Chemical" repels. But, in fact, what's "natural" is also "chemical."

When it comes to food and health, it's important to be able to separate reality from myth, fact from illusion, and scientific principles from quackery. Nutrition doesn't have to be a mystery. The central question is, how do we separate myth from reality?

Tests of Reality

In 1973, Dr. Henry Bieler announced that he had discovered the true cause of the common cold, measles, and polio—and he could cure them all. Of course, medicine had long been confident that all of these illnesses were caused by specific viruses. But Dr. Bieler explained that medicine had been fooled. True, the viruses actually were in the bodies of the sick, but they were merely feeding on *"stagnating waste products,"* which were the real cause of the trouble. He stated that *"germs do not cause disease...Improper foods cause disease; proper foods cure disease."*

Dr. Bieler gave examples: the common cold occurs more in winter because people overeat during the holidays and are less active, thus building up body wastes. Polio can come from a number of foods, but especially *"...from the putrefaction of ice cream in the bowels. Polio strikes most viciously at children who eat large quantities of ice cream. One indication of this is that the majority of cases occur during the peak of the summer ice-cream season."*

These ideas seem patently absurd. Yet until his death, Dr. Bieler was physician to many of the Hollywood famous. His book, *Food is Your Best Medicine,*[8] was bought by hundreds of thousands of Americans. Evidently, his ideas about food chemistry and its effect on health seemed reasonable to a lot of people.

We can easily test the medical realities of these ideas by referring to the scientific evidence on the viral cause of these diseases. But what if—as commonly happens—certain foods are proposed as causes or cures for diseases that do not have such clear causes? For instance, Dr. Bieler identified certain foods as the cause or cure of cancer. How can we test claims that threaten or promise so much in the name of nutrition?

Food Composition as a Testing Device

Perhaps the most worn volumes on a nutritionist's bookshelf are the handbooks of food composition. A nutritionist's first interest in food is its nutrient composition. Food composition tables tell us which nutrients are present in foods and to what extent. A quick look is often enough to determine the sense or nonsense of a nutritional claim. The nutrient content of a food is a basic reality determined by chemical analysis.

If we look closely at Dr. Bieler's statements about foods and weigh them against tables of food composition, we quickly find that his chemistry was sadly lacking. He especially touted zucchini as medicine. Why zucchini? Because, he said, sodium is so important in treating the toxicities which cause disease, and zucchini is *"especially rich in sodium."*

At this point, we have a specific statement to which we can apply a test of reality. The U.S.

Department of Agriculture puts out volumes of food composition tables which are used by nutritionists world-wide. Others put out food composition tables based on this information, and food companies provide food composition information for their specific products.

Looking up zucchini, we find that a cup contains 3 mg of sodium.[9] Is this a lot of sodium? Looking further, we find that a cup of carrots contains 103 mg of sodium, and a cup of macaroni and cheese contains 749 mg. Plainly, the amount of sodium in Dr. Bieler's "sodium-rich zucchini" is trivial. His chemical information was wrong in the most obvious way without even considering the added fact that most American diets contain too much sodium (1 teaspoon table salt = 2130 mg sodium).

Do these realities disprove Dr. Bieler's theories of disease? To some extent they do. They suggest that his information about nutrients was grossly in error, and show that the rationale for his "food cures" was spurious. Scientists do make mistakes, of course, but not such basic ones, and they are protected by peer review—that is, letting colleagues review and criticize their work before publishing it.

Let us use food composition to test some other ideas. It is a common misconception that foods grown with chemical fertilizers are less nutritious than those grown with natural fertilizers. But when scientists analyze and compare the nutrient content of foods grown both ways, they can't tell one from the other.

Some popular authors tell us that we must get our vitamins from fresh foods, and that frozen and canned foods are inferior. Again, food composition tables tell us differently. In fact, frozen foods can be higher in vitamins than those purchased "fresh"

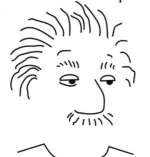

"The whole of science is nothing more than a refinement of everyday thinking."
Albert Einstein

because the time between harvest and freezer is usually much shorter than the time between harvest and grocery-store purchase.

In other words, frozen fish, vegetables, fruit, and such, are often "fresher than fresh." Canned foods can be lower in vitamins because they are heated, but when fresh food is cooked, there's not much difference.

There are, of course, sensory differences, which is why many people prefer fresh to frozen or canned. Also, salt is typically added to vegetables before they are canned, making canned vegetables higher in sodium.

The Test of Science

What support did Dr. Bieler have for his claim that improper foods cause disease and proper foods cure them? A lot—in terms of the number of enthusiastic testimonials from those who took his dietary advice. Dr. Bieler would call this documented evidence of his claims. Scientists, however, would call this *anecdotal evidence* which, in science, is the flimsiest kind of evidence.

However, scientists can—and sometimes do—form hypotheses based on anecdotal evidence. A basic difference between mythmakers and scientists is that mythmakers draw conclusions based on this kind of evidence, whereas scientists would only use it as a starting point for investigation. Your favorite uncle claims that vitamin E heals burns faster; he says he knows because he has tried it himself. For him, this is evidence enough.

Science uses a formal method to examine such claims. *The Scientific Method* is an orderly and objective way to test theories:

1. Scientist states the hypothesis.
2. Does a controlled experiment to test the hypothesis.
3. Reports the results and conclusion.
4. Other scientists evaluate the experiment and verify its conclusion.

This is a time-honored method used by scientists throughout the world. Lavoisier, for example, postulated that oxygen was necessary for animal life. He performed controlled experiments to test his theory and concluded that he was correct.

He presented the details to his fellow scientists, who critically examined his data and performed experiments themselves to confirm his conclusion. Then, and only then, was the necessity of oxygen for animal life accepted into the body of scientific fact.

Epidemiology, the study of the factors linked with diseases in a population, is a starting point for many theories. Breast cancer, for example, is more common in countries with high-fat diets. Scientists went on to test the hypothesis that this is a cause-and-effect relationship, not just an association.

Let us consider how the scientific method might be applied to Dr. Bieler's claim that zucchini can cure disease. The hypothesis is that zucchini is effective in curing disease.

To test it, it is necessary to compare patients given zucchini (*experimental group)* with those who are not (*control group*). Sick patients are randomly divided into two groups that are given the same nutritionally adequate diet—except that the experimental group has zucchini hidden in their muffins. Because the patients do not know if they are getting zucchini, the psychological effect *(placebo effect)* is neutralized: patients won't be affected by believing in zucchini if they don't know whether they are eating it or not.

Placebo effect: An effect that results from, but is not caused by the test substance or procedure, e.g., feeling better simply because you expect to.

After a time, Dr. Bieler examines everyone and compares their health at the start and the end of the experiment. He is not told who had zucchini, so that he, like the patients, will not be biased by his belief in zucchini into seeing those getting zucchini as healthier (*double-blind study:* neither the subjects nor the experimenter knows which group the subjects are in). The results are then statistically analyzed to see if the zucchini group is now healthier than the control group.

If, in fact, the results support Dr. Bieler's claim for zucchini, his experiment would still have to undergo the scrutiny of other scientists (*peer review*). If subsequent experiments by other scientists come to similar conclusions, Dr. Bieler could

rightly say that there is scientific evidence that zucchini can cure disease. The question to ask of an "amazing claim" is whether or not it has met the test of scientific validity.

The Food and Nutrition Science Alliance, a partnership that includes the American Dietetic Association, lists some things that should make us suspicious:

Ten Red Flags of Junk Science

- Recommendations that promise a quick fix.
- Dire warnings of danger from a single product or regimen.
- Claims that sound too good to be true.
- Simplistic conclusions drawn from a complex study.
- Recommendations based on a single study.
- Dramatic statements that are refuted by reputable scientific organizations.
- Lists of "good" and "bad" foods.
- Recommendations made to help sell a product.
- Recommendations based on studies published without peer review.
- Recommendations from studies that ignore differences among individuals or groups.

What Nutrients Do We Need?

Nutrient is a general term that refers to any dietary substance that nourishes the body in some way. Sugar, for example, provides energy (calories) to the body. But sugar is not an *essential nutrient*, a very carefully defined term: An essential nutrient is defined as a substance *required* in the diet for health, normal development and reproduction, and its omission from the diet produces adverse effects. This definition is used to include or exclude nutrients that are proposed as essential.

The definition is not perfect, however. Vitamin D, for example, can be made in the body when the skin is exposed to sunshine (ultraviolet light). For many people, vitamin D is thus not required in the diet. But some people do not get adequate sunshine. For them, vitamin D is an essential nutrient. As another example, bacteria that reside in our intestine can make vitamin K for us. The point is that although all vitamins are essential, sometimes they can come from sources other than the diet.

In testing for reality, one must know which are the essential nutrients. How else is one to know that vitamin B-6 and vitamin B-12 are essential nutrients, but "vitamin B-15" (pangamic acid) and "vitamin B-17" (laetrile) are not? (Pangamic acid has been touted, but has no known value, for treating various ills. Laetrile was popularized, but is ineffective, as a cure for cancer.)

"Vitamin B-15" made its debut in ads stating, "NEW STARTLING VITAMIN… Vitamin B-15 in its safest most effective form!" [10] Startling, indeed!—especially since these ads appeared in 1975, and no new vitamin has been discovered since 1948. Simply naming these substances "vitamins B-15 and B-17" didn't make them vitamins, but helped make millions of dollars for their promoters.

The essential nutrients (see Table 1-1) are discussed only briefly here and will be given more detailed attention in upcoming chapters.

Energy-Providing Nutrients— Carbohydrate, Fat, Protein

Carbohydrate, fat, and protein are typically grouped together as the energy-providing (*calorie-containing*) nutrients. (Alcohol—a fermentation product of carbohydrate—is also a rich source of calories.) They are needed to fulfill basic energy needs, but are fairly interchangeable for this purpose. One can use carbohydrate or fat or protein as a source of energy. Fat and protein, however, contain substances that are needed for purposes other than providing energy.

Minerals

Various minerals are needed in the body for a wide variety of purposes. As examples, calcium is needed in bone structure, and iron carries oxygen in red blood cells. The essential minerals are commonly divided into two categories— *major minerals* and *trace minerals*, based on the amounts needed.

Vitamins

Vitamins are categorized as either *water-soluble* or *fat-soluble*. This came about because, in discovering the vitamins, scientists found out there was something in a water extract of food (water-soluble vitamins) that was essential to life. But there was still something missing. Using fat solvents, they extracted the missing nutrients (fat-soluble vitamins) from fat in food.

The hodgepodge of names given to vitamins can be confusing. In 1920, it was thought there were three vitamins—vitamins A, B, and C. It soon became apparent that vitamin B was more than one vitamin, and the alphabetical orderliness of the vitamins fell apart.

Vitamin B turned out to be eight vitamins, and some proposed ones, e.g., "vitamin B-11," did not turn out to be vitamins after all. The naming of vitamins was then in confusion, and vitamins were given alternate names. Vitamin B-12, for example, was also named cobalamin since an atom of cobalt is found in its center. There is some comfort in knowing that the naming of the vitamins did at least begin with a systematic method.

Will the Real Nutrition Expert Please Stand Up?

Anyone can call oneself a nutritionist. After all, a *nutritionist* is simply someone who specializes in nutrition. But the real nutrition experts are those who have a formal education in nutrition or a closely related field and who base their knowledge on information acquired via the scientific method. For example, nutritionists who teach and/or do research at accredited colleges and universities and who serve on blue-ribbon committees that set the Recommended Dietary Allowances (RDA) are all real nutrition experts. Some people call them "conventional" nutritionists.

They did not name themselves conventional nutritionists—any more than plumbers call themselves conventional plumbers. They are called "conventional" or "establishment" as a form of criticism or even ridicule by those who call themselves "natural" or "holistic" nutritionists. These "natural" nutritionists typically do not base their information on scientific reality, and make no bones about it.

Fit for Life's Harvey Diamond says, *"I don't care whether scientific evidence exists or not. I ask people to combine their foods for one week, then tell me how you [sic] feel. One million people are interested in it despite what the scientists think."*[11]

The public is drawn to such "unconventional" authors. Their "glow of health" is literally worth millions of dollars. They garner testimonials from the celebrities that people are so enamored with, and more importantly, they tell the public what they want to hear. Who wants to hear about sensible weight-loss plans where one loses weight gradually by exercising more and eating less? The "same old thing"—how boring! We would much rather hear, *Calories Don't Count! Shed an easy 15 pounds in a week!*

What we want is what Merv Griffin said about *Fit for Life* on the back cover, *"You feel so good... so much energy and absolutely no deprivation. It makes losing weight a pleasure."*[12] Of course, if it were so easy and such a pleasure, everyone should be thin by now. We are reminded once again that what sounds "too good to be true" usually isn't true.

When it's so hard for the public to tell who are the real nutrition experts, who does one go to to get reliable nutrition information? *Registered Dietitians* (R.D.) are one of the most reliable sources. They are credentialed by the American Dietetic Association after completing a curriculum in nutrition and food science from an accredited college, serving an internship, and passing a qualifying exam. They also must take continuing education courses to maintain their credential.

No other academic credential guarantees sound training in nutrition. Even a Ph.D. in nutrition can be from an unaccredited university. Many medical schools offer little or no nutrition education. Study in other branches of the sciences may or may not lay a foundation for sound nutrition information.

What Do You Know?

The best preparation for separating myth from reality is to be armed with a basic knowledge of

Table 1-1: Essential Nutrients.

Energy-Providing Nutrients
Carbohydrate, Fat, Protein
Minerals
Major minerals: Calcium, Phosphorus, Magnesium, Sodium, Potassium, Chloride
Trace minerals: Iron, Zinc, Iodine, Selenium, Copper, Manganese, Fluoride, Chromium, Molybdenum
Vitamins (alternate names in parentheses).
Fat-soluble:
Vitamin A (retinol, retinal, retinoic acid)
Vitamin D (ergocalciferol, cholecalciferol)
Vitamin E (tocopherol, tocotrienol)
Vitamin K (phylloquinone, menaquinones, menadione)
Water-soluble:
Vitamin C (ascorbic acid, ascorbate)
B-vitamins:
Thiamin (vitamin B-1)
Riboflavin (vitamin B-2)
Niacin (nicotinic acid, nicotinamide, niacinamide)
Vitamin B-6 (pyridoxine, pyridoxal, pyridoxamine)
Folate (folic acid, folacin)
Vitamin B-12 (cobalamin)
Biotin
Pantothenic acid

physiology, nutrition, and food composition. Then, you can test what you are told against what you know to be true. As the jargon of the unscientific becomes more sophisticated, and the marketing of dietary products becomes more clever, one needs a solid base of information to sort out the factual from the phony.

Suppose a physician says that cells from the brain often break loose into the bloodstream and attach to receptors in the stomach and heart. The doctor has the right academic credentials. He is debonair, warm, and eloquent. A famous talk-show host calls him brilliant. He goes on to say that this is the reason that we have "gut feelings" and we "feel from the heart."

Mental illness, he says, develops when a vitamin imbalance leads to an abnormal growth of these translocated brain cells, and the brain can no longer overpower them. As a result, the mind feels divided and scattered and progresses to mental illness. The cure is simply a matter of taking the correct balance of vitamins (a month's supply for only $49.95) to return these errant brain cells to their normally benign state. Feeling rather scatter-brained at times, we might be tempted to spend the $49.95—unless we know a bit about physiology and nutrition.

We are constantly bombarded by nutrition information and dietary advice, from all types of sources—the Internet, diet and health books, sports and fitness magazines, government committees, advertisements for dietary supplements, food labels, quacks, nutrition experts. Often, the information is tied in with products to sell. It is easy to become bewildered.

Knowing something of the physical realities of nutrition—the chemistry of foods, the chemistry of the body, and the interactions of the two—can give us some stability amid a flood of scientific and not-so-scientific information. Ultimately, the aim is to be able to answer the simple question, *What should I eat?*

Summary

As ancient peoples sought the link between nutrition and life, food was endowed with magical powers to heal or to make ill. Ancient physicians provided theories of how nutrition was related to health, but it was centuries before these theories could be tested by science. Even then, it took more than a century of work by thousands of scientists to acquire more than the most superficial information about the composition of foods and how that composition affects our body.

Today, we know nutrients—carbohydrate, fat, protein, vitamins, minerals, and water—to be the ingredients of life's chemistry. We have learned that health depends on balancing these nutrients with life's need for their chemical ingredients.

Despite scientific knowledge to the contrary, myths about nutrition persist. We are continually bombarded by nutrition information, some of it scientific, some not-so-scientific, some outright bogus. Some ways to separate nutrition myth from reality are:

• Learn enough about nutrition so that you can evaluate the nutrition claims that come your way. This is not only the best way to separate nutrition myth from reality; sometimes it is the only way. Good credentials are no guarantee of reliable information, and false nutritional claims can be made to sound very "scientific." To confuse things even more, true scientific facts are often intermingled with half-truths and false-hoods.

• Some claims for food can be evaluated simply by looking up the food's nutrient content in food composition tables, e.g., the claim that food cooked from fresh is higher in vitamins than food cooked from frozen can be evaluated this way.

• Be familiar with the essential nutrients. Then, if someone makes claims for a vitamin you never heard of, you will be rightly suspicious. "Vitamin B-15" is an example of such a "non-vitamin."

• Ask if the information is based on scientific fact—knowledge based on information acquired via the scientific method. Erroneous nutrition information does not survive scientific scrutiny and is often based on testimonials.

• Try to determine if the person giving the advice is one who bases information on scientific fact. Registered Dietitians (R.D.) are one of the most reliable sources of dietary advice.

Part 1

Energy and the Human Machine

Chapter 2

Food Power—Use and Storage

Is there any good in calories? It doesn't sound like it. We so often tend to refer to them negatively, as "excess calories," "unwanted calories," "unhealthy calories," etc. That seems strange though, when we are told that calories are a measure of energy. Energy is what we all want more of, isn't it?

The truth is that energy and its sources are very important in understanding how food nurtures and provides fuel for the complex human body. So if calories are another word for energy, they can't be all bad. But why do they so often seem to be too plentiful?

Of course some people don't have a problem with "excess calories." Do they have more will power? Or do they really get that much more exercise? And how do we know how much is too much food?

When we learn the facts of human energy use, we find that some of our fondest beliefs don't hold up. More importantly, we are starting down the road of learning how our bodies function, and the roles that food plays in sustaining health.

When we think of food and our reasons for eating, pleasure is often the first to come to mind. Many of us simply love to eat. Any reason will do. As Dodgers' manager Tommy Lasorda has put it, "When we lose, I eat. When we win, I eat. I also eat when we're rained out."

But the body chemistry sees food differently. The first reason for eating is to provide the fuel to meet our constant need for energy.

In this chapter, we look at various aspects of energy and energy balance: on one side, the energy demands of our body; on the other side, meeting those demands. We examine how energy is defined in scientific terms, and how our energy expenditure and the calories in food are measured. Finally, we see how we efficiently store excess energy as body fat, and how heredity can affect how much we store.

The Bodily Energy Crisis

When we want to drive somewhere, we put fuel into a car and go. When we want to vacuum the rug, we take out the vacuum cleaner, plug it in, and turn it on. When we are finished with these machines, we simply turn them off, knowing that we can start them up again whenever we need them.

But once the human machine has been turned off for more than a few minutes, it doesn't turn on again. To stop it is to destroy it. It's turned on at the moment of conception, and from that moment it must run continuously until the moment of death. This means that we require an uninterrupted supply of fuel. If we run out of fuel, we die.

The demand for fuel fluctuates, but it never falls below a fundamental "idling" rate (basal metabolic rate) that keeps our body functioning at its most basic level. Energy is needed continuously for such basic functions as pumping blood throughout our body and breathing.

Less obviously, a lot of fuel is needed to maintain the brain. Contrary to popular belief, the brain functions at much the same level whether we're studying intensely or sleeping. When we're resting, the brain uses more than 20% of the body's total energy use. Even during sleep, the brain is

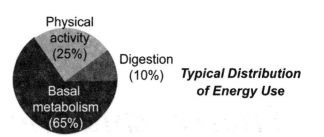

Typical Distribution of Energy Use

busy—messages are going continually from the brain to every limb and organ, and other messages return. If this weren't happening, we wouldn't turn over when our arm cramps; we wouldn't wake upon hearing a baby's cry or smelling smoke; and we wouldn't pull up the covers when a cold gust of wind blows in through the window.

Still more subtly, our body is a cooperative colony of trillions of cells, each of which needs energy to perform specialized functions. The cells need fuel to produce the more than 100,000 biochemicals, as well as to generate the heat we need to stay warm.

These are our basal, involuntary, and unstoppable energy demands. We also require energy for our voluntary activities, which are just as necessary for our survival. We couldn't even begin to find food or care for ourselves without them. We also expend energy in digesting and assimilating food—this energy need is about 10% of caloric intake.

Basal metabolic rate (BMR): the rate at which energy (calories) is used for involuntary bodily functions.

So our total energy needs are basically a combination of the demands of basal metabolism, of voluntary action, and of digesting and assimilating food. Together they constitute an unremitting energy drain. No matter how much we restrict our activity, our energy need is still quite large. Unless we're extremely active, chances are that basal metabolism accounts for about two-thirds of the energy we use.

An energy supply must be constantly on hand, readily available. If we had to get the fuel immediately for each use, we'd be in constant danger. A missed meal or snack could mean death.

In our affluent society, we rarely are aware of true hunger, and we tend to look upon the ease with which we become fat as a curse. In fact, the ease with which we fill our fuel-storage system is an essential mechanism for human survival.

Fat Cells—Friend or Foe?

For our prehistoric ancestors, food was a sometime thing. It depended on the luck of the hunt and the success of the forage. It depended on the seasons. In summer and fall, the land was lush with ripening berries and nuts; flocks of birds were everywhere; and the game grew fat on abundant forage. But in winter, the trees and shrubs were bare; the flocks had migrated; and the ground was frozen too hard to dig for roots. As the eating became sporadic, what fueled the body machine through the hard days? To find the answer, we must examine the fat that lies beneath the skin (subcutaneous fat).

To the naked eye, this fat appears to be a yellowish, inert mass. But under the microscope, we see a crowd of adipose cells ("fat cells"). Each of these cells is like a collapsible thin-walled tank that grows larger as it fills with fat, and smaller as it's emptied.

> Some people call lumpy-looking fat under the skin "cellulite." In fact, it's just ordinary fat. The strands of connective tissue that hold the fat in place can cause dimpling in the skin. The lumpiness can go away when the fat layer is thinned by ordinary weight loss. We can't pound or massage it away, as ads and popular articles would have you believe.

The body takes any excess fuel, beyond that needed to meet current energy demands, and converts it to fat, which is then stored in the fat cells (see Fig. 2-1). Fat is used for this reserve because, as we will see, it's the most compact body fuel.

So when the hungry days came for the caveman, his body could simply draw upon the fat cells for fuel. The release of fuel might have been (and still can be) triggered by many things—too many hours without eating, or a high fever, or by a sudden need for energy to pursue game or escape from an enemy. It's easy to see the urgent practicality of such a fuel-reserve system. One could hardly stop for a snack while being chased by a saber-toothed tiger.

The blanket of plump fat cells under the skin serves in other ways, too. It's an excellent insula-

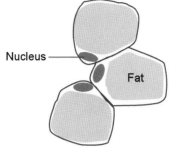

Figure 2-1: Fat Cells. The cross-section of a fat (adipose) cell is aptly described as a signet ring.

Nucleus

Fat

tor against heat and cold, particularly important when one remembers that the body functions well only within narrow limits of internal temperature (usually 98°-99°F). The fat is also a good buffer against injury, a shock absorber against blows, a shield to keep a cut from reaching internal organs. When we fatten, a fair amount of fat forms around these organs, providing additional protection.

The alternating cycles of feast and famine, of leisure and violent activity probably set up a nice energy balance for prehistoric man. Fat cells continually filled and emptied, and in the end there was probably little obesity.

But now, the food supplies of our modern society have affected our delicate fat-storage balance—with supermarkets, vending machines, fast-food outlets, and convenience stores nearby; cans of soft-drinks and beer stockpiled in the refrigerator; packages of frozen dinners and ice cream tucked in the freezer; and packages of instant ramen, microwave popcorn, and ready-to-eat cereal safe in the cupboard. Like our primitive ancestors, we feast when food is abundant and store even the smallest excess of fuel as fat—but unlike the time of the caveman, for most of us now the food is always there.

Ironically, to empty some of this unwanted storage from our fat cells, the primitive plan is still the only one that really works. We must either reproduce the historic days of caloric deprivation, or the vigorous, physical exercise—or a combination of the two.

Even when we are slim, our energy reserves are large. Our bodies range from the 5% fat of the very thin man to the 30% fat of the moderately obese woman.

To get some idea of how much stored energy this fat represents, consider a young woman of

Figure 2-2: Energy Balance—Fat vs. Thin.
Weight maintenance, without gain or loss, balances energy intake (food) and energy expenditure (basically, basal metabolism plus physical activity).

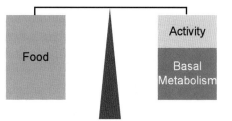

normal weight, at 5'5" and 125 pounds. About 25 of those pounds are in fat. This much fat is enough to meet her energy needs for about 45 days.

This suggests one reason why it's hard to make rapid headway against excess fat. For it takes a significant energy shortage, over a substantial period of time, to draw down large excess reserves.

Suppose the young woman had an additional 60 pounds of fat and weighed 185 pounds. In societies ravaged periodically by famine, the excess weight would serve her well. And our 185-pound woman is really only at the margin of a height-weight definition of obesity (see Chap. 3).

Although obesity in primitive societies may have been unusual, there's good reason to think that an obese woman might have been considered beautiful. In the Sahara where famine is a threat, some brides-to-be were forced to drink several quarts of camel's milk daily until they became obese—and more sexually attractive in their culture. During a famine, a large store of body fat would be expected to carry them successfully through pregnancy and breastfeeding.

Food and Body Fat as Fuel

When we understand how much of an energy deficit is needed to make real headway against even moderate fatness, we can see that the most common promises of so many weight-loss schemes are unrealistic. Fat can't be lost quickly without starvation, illness, or extraordinary physical activity. Dramatic weight loss is usually dramatic water loss. But we don't want to believe it. We all would like something for nothing—weight loss without effort.

How can we test the reality of the rosy vision that fat can be lost quickly without hunger or ex-

traordinary effort? We can test them against the basic formula for determining fat gain or loss:

Energy Intake (food) - Energy Expenditure = Fat gain or loss

There are no other factors. Fat is fat, not "cellulite." Each morsel of food contains a specific amount of energy to fuel the body.

The focus is on calories, rather than on the foods themselves. The body seeks only to meet its energy needs. In this respect, it's similar to a rechargeable battery. It doesn't matter to the battery whether the electrical energy used to recharge it comes from the burning of oil, coal, or even wood. In turn, the ability of the battery to provide energy for work is simply a question of how many energy units—in the case of a battery, watts—it can take in and hold. For us it simply ends up as a matter of calories.

Measuring the Energy of Food and Work

The energy unit in the human body is the calorie. This word calorie takes us into a bit of confusion. The word itself comes from the worlds of physics and chemistry, as a measure of heat—the amount of heat needed to raise the temperature of one gram of water by one degree centigrade (1°C). But this amount of heat is quite small, and the energy in food is quite high.

A gram of water is only about one-fifth of a teaspoonful. The food energy in a single almond can add 1°C to two gallons of water. An ounce of hamburger could do the same to 20 gallons.

The physicist's calorie turns out to be an inconveniently small measure for nutrition science. So nutritionists use a kilocalorie (kcal) or Calorie (with capital C), 1,000 of the small calories of physics, as a measure.

What gets confusing is that in reality, the public, the press, the government, the law, and food labels all now ignore the capital C and use calorie with a small c to mean kilocalorie. In effect, they ignore the tiny unit of measurement used by the physicists. So does this book.

The Energy in Food

How do we find out how much energy a food can supply to the body? We start by measuring how much heat is produced when we burn a sample of that food.

The body uses food energy differently. It doesn't burn its fuel as a log burns in the fireplace—combining rapidly with oxygen at a high temperature. Nevertheless, by actually burning a food sample in the laboratory and measuring the heat produced, we can find out how much energy a food potentially can give us.

That energy potential is essentially the same no matter how we put it to use. Burning food as we would a log would be an inefficient way to derive its energy. If the body operated this way, the fuel would be used up very fast, without much regard for how much energy was really needed at that moment or whether energy was needed for heat or for work. It would also be quite uncomfortable for our innards.

The body does use its fuel (food) through a kind of chemical "burning," and it does combine with oxygen in the process. But fuel burning in the body is an intricate matter, a kind of extremely slow burning which goes through many steps and is exquisitely controlled.

The point is that the amount of energy elicited from a given fuel is much the same whether the fuel is used rapidly or slowly. Whether gasoline is sipped by a Prius, gulped by a Hummer, or exploded in a Molotov cocktail, the energy potential of the gasoline is the same. In a similar manner, the caloric potential of a food is much the same whether it's burned in a flash in the fireplace or burned slowly in the body.

To learn how many calories a specific amount of food will yield, a sample of the food is burned in an instrument called a bomb calorimeter (see Fig. 2-3). The food sample is placed in the chamber, together with oxygen. The container is sealed, and the oxygen is ignited electrically and burns the food in a flash (*like a bomb*). The heat of the burning food heats the surrounding water, and the rise in the water's temperature is a measure of calories of energy released.

Caloric vs. Non-Caloric: When it's said that an apple has 80 calories, this isn't exactly correct. It would be more accurate to say that an apple can provide the body with about 80 calories. If the caloric content of an apple were measured in a bomb

Figure 2-3: Bomb Calorimeter.

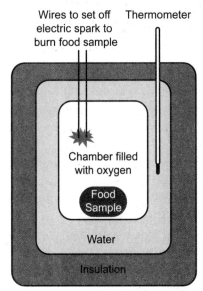

Wires to set off electric spark to burn food sample

Thermometer

Chamber filled with oxygen

Food Sample

Water

Insulation

calorimeter, it would be found to have more than the 80 calories that the body can use.

All of the calories in a food can't be used if the food isn't completely digestible or isn't completely "combusted" to carbon dioxide and water in the body. An apple contains fiber, for example, which has calories as measured in a bomb calorimeter. But since we can't digest this fiber, it doesn't provide us with energy (it's "non-caloric")—just as a chewing a pencil doesn't provide us with any calories.

Another example is saccharin, the non-caloric sweetener. It has energy value as measured in a bomb calorimeter and is readily absorbed by the body, but our body can't break down saccharin and release any of its energy. Thus, saccharin does not provide us with any calories and is excreted in the urine.

When it's said that fiber and saccharin don't have any calories, what's meant is that their energy value is of no use to us. The caloric values we're familiar with are actually physiological fuel values of food (calories that are available to the body). These values have been determined in numerous human studies.

Energy Used By the Body

In much the same way we measure food energy in a bomb calorimeter, we can measure how much energy the body uses. This method is known as

Table 2-1: Calories/Minute for a 140-lb Person.

Calories/minute above that used when resting*	
1 cal	Sitting while reading, knitting, talking, etc.
2 cal	Writing, driving, lab work, playing cards
3 cal	Walking 2 miles per hour (mph), washing dishes, cooking, carpentry
4 cal	Walking 3 mph, washing the car, house-cleaning, playing ping pong
5 cal	Swimming leisurely, plastering a wall, dancing a waltz
6 cal	Downhill skiing, playing tennis, climbing stairs, bicycling 6 mph
7 cal	Sawing logs with a handsaw, mowing the lawn with a hand-mower
8 cal	Pitching bales of hay, playing football, digging a pit
9 cal	Cross-country skiing, playing basketball, dancing the polka
10 cal	Running 6 mph, strenuous swimming, snowshoeing in soft snow
11 cal	Jumping rope (125 times/minute), playing racquetball
12 cal	Running 7 mph

*At rest, a 140-lb man (10% body fat) uses about 1.1 cal/min., and a 140-lb woman (20% body fat) uses about 1.0 cal/min. Asleep, we use about 10% fewer calories than when resting.

direct calorimetry (*heat measured directly*), and the apparatus used is analogous to the bomb calorimeter. It's costly and cumbersome, because it entails enclosing a person in a chamber (a small room). The heat (calories) generated by the person's metabolic and physical activity is reflected in the increased temperature of the water that surrounds the chamber. Of course, the measurements take much longer since the body doesn't burn (oxidize) its fuel in a flash.

It goes without saying that this method isn't very practical if we want to know how much energy the body expends cutting stalks in a cornfield or playing tennis. So for such measurements, another technique is used—indirect calorimetry.

With this method, a person wears a gas-mask-like device, a respirometer (*respiration measurer*), to measure the amount of oxygen consumed while, say, playing tennis. Because the amount of oxygen needed to combine with fuel and generate a certain number of calories is known, the calo-ries expended can be determined indirectly by measuring the amount of oxygen consumed.

Measurements obtained by the two methods—measuring heat production (direct calorimetry) and measuring oxygen consumption (indirect calorimetry)—agree within a fraction of 1%.

By such means of measuring food energy and bodily energy use, science has developed two sets of basic data. One consists of tables of the caloric values of foods, the other of the number of calories used during various activities—from sitting to washing dishes to jumping rope (see Table 2-1). These two bodies of information provide keys to testing the reality of ideas about energy production and energy use by humans—and hence, about weight control.

Energy—A Confusing Use of the Word

We use the word energy rather loosely. For instance, we say that we feel full of energy when we wake up in the morning feeling good, anxious to "hit the books" or go to work. In science, however, energy is a very specific term. Energy is defined as the capacity to do work. From a scientific standpoint, we're really full of energy when we have that extra layer of fat stored under our skin.

Adding to the confusion, the word energy is used even more liberally by those selling dietary supplements or diet plans. As the best-selling book, Fit For Life says:

Because you will be eating to free up energy you will have more energy than you ever had before. Consistently optimizing your energy is a critical part of FIT FOR LIFE.[1]

This made sense to those who made this book a best-seller, but it's nonsense to the scientist.

Much of the confusion over the word energy results from its everyday use to mean both energy in the scientific (physical) sense and vigor. Vigor is, of course, a very real thing, a reflection both of one's physical and one's emotional status, and might be described as a feeling of readiness to do work.

The psychological aspects of this feeling can be crucial. The ancient warrior who has just eaten the raw meat of a lion and the runner gulping a handful of dietary supplements may both feel physically ready to triumph, for much the same psychological reasons. They may or may not be physically fit. Someone in the best physical and nutritional condition may, on the other hand, have no vigor at all after a romance turns sour.

The physical side of vigor is equally important, and lack of vigor can certainly have a nutritional basis. A person who consumes plenty of calories and has ample energy reserves of fuel may, if that person hasn't been consuming enough of some nutrients, suffer from a condition like anemia, which hampers the use of energy by delivering less-than-normal amounts of oxygen to the tissues. He or she will lack vigor.

Because the body's use of fuel is so basic to nutrition, and because all concepts of weight control are so absolutely dependent on how we use and store fuel, it's worthwhile to look deeper into how food provides energy, and how the body puts that energy to work.

ATP—The Secret of Our Energy

The same natural laws are followed whether it's food that's furnishing power to a person or gasoline furnishing power to a car. In both cases, the fuel is combined with oxygen to yield energy, carbon dioxide, and water.

In the engine of a car, the gasoline is mixed with oxygen from the air. An electric spark ignites the mixture, and the gasoline burns in a mini-explosion. Each mini-explosion propels the car forward a bit. The mini-explosions are set at proper intervals (the timing of the engine) so that the car drives smoothly.

Like a car, the body also needs energy for work. But instead of mini-explosions, the body releases energy from its fuel in an exquisitely controlled process. This process is a part of metabolism, which will be discussed in more detail in Chapter 11. When energy is released in metabolism, some of the energy is released as heat, but a good part of the energy is captured in a high-energy substance (ATP—Adenosine TriPhosphate) for use in bodily processes that require energy.

When the body needs energy to, say, run a marathon, the muscles respond by generating energy (ATP) to fuel the muscle contractions of running.

The high-energy ATP is made as needed from the breakdown of the body's fuel. The runner doesn't gather ATP ahead of time as the starting gun is anticipated. Just a bit is already there; the ATP fueling the continuous muscle contractions is made then and there as it's needed.

Muscle naturally contains creatine phosphate, which helps replenish ATP. Creatine supplements can help in "explosive"-type activities like weight-lifting and sprinting.[2]

A lot of ATP is needed for a long-distance run. Fortunately, even the leanest athlete has a more than ample store of fat to fuel a marathon. As the runners start their motion, nerves signal the muscles to contract, and there's action. ATP provides the energy for that action, and the ATP used is rapidly regenerated for the continuing action.

The energy in ATP is released by the breaking of a special "high-energy" bond within the molecular structure of ATP. The process is similar to releasing an arrow from a bow (see Fig. 2-4). The high-energy bond within ATP is like a drawn bow. And once you break the bond and let fly, you need to reload.

With a regular bow, of course, the string can be drawn over and over again. All you have to do is get another arrow and use some energy to pull. So it is with ATP. The energy released from fuel is used to regenerate ATP. In effect, it fits another arrow to the bow and draws back the string. The body doesn't need a lot of bows; it can put arrows to those bows very quickly.

Suppose we want to scratch an ear. A signal goes from the brain to the nerves and is flashed to the muscle cells in the hand. At once, the energy in ATP is released. As thousands of cells in the hand are similarly energized with the production of ATP, the finger bends back and forth to scratch the ear.

Fuel Efficiency

When the body "burns" its fuel to generate ATP, more than half of the energy is "lost" as heat—like the heat produced by an automobile engine (which is why it needs a cooling system). The heat generated in the body this way can be useful (e.g., to maintain normal body tempera-

Figure 2-4: High-Energy ATP.
A. ATP is shown as the arrow of a drawn bow, "bonded" to the bow with a store of energy behind it. **B**. When needed, energy is released as the arrow flies off.

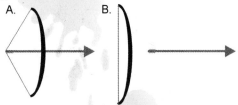

ture), but it also can make us uncomfortably warm when we exercise .

In an endurance event, ATP is used and regenerated at a rapid rate, and the large amount of heat produced as a by-product is in a way wasteful. The athlete would rather that more ATP be produced for power than "wasted" as heat. Also, rapid heat production can hurt performance if the heat can't be dissipated fast enough.

The slender lean body of a typical marathon runner is ideal for getting rid of heat. A slender shape provides relatively more surface area from which heat can escape, and the minimal amount of fat stored under the skin (along with minimal clothing) facilitates the loss of body heat.

In contrast, the heat generated by vigorous and sustained exercise can easily become more than an obese person's body can tolerate. There's less surface area relative to body weight, and the thick layer of fat provides a greater layer of insulation that hinders heat loss.

Why Do We Become Overfat?

The public has a wide variety of ideas about how to cure obesity, but it appears to share one basic idea about its cause—gluttony. Anthropologist Margaret Mead said: "As the obese often describe themselves (echoing the beliefs and attitudes of those around them), they are people who can't resist indulging their gluttonous greed."[3]

The idea is worth testing. Many of us are already eating somewhat less than we'd like, and avoiding a number of foods in the belief—often mistaken—that they "make us fat." This, of course, is especially true for those of us who are already a little fatter than we'd like to be. Thus, it can seem that maintaining our weight—let alone

reducing it—means resigning ourselves to a life of eating without joy.

Such a depressing point of view can discourage people from even attempting to deal with what's a very real problem. Just facing a need for weight control can evoke deep feelings of shame and guilt, in addition to the prospect of unending self-sacrifice.

But how true is the idea that gluttony is the central cause of obesity? When the nutrition scientist applies the facts of energy to the question, it's found that gluttony isn't a requisite for overweight. Only small differences in our intake and use of energy can make great differences in fat storage. From this analysis, we can learn much about how to manage our fatness.

An Analysis of Fat Storage

Often our attention is focused on a few sporadic episodes of extravagant over-eating—which can lead to guilt, despair, and a feeling of helplessness. Let's imagine a very limited sort of glutton, a man who—in addition to the food energy he needed each day—ate an extra ounce of choice porterhouse steak. Very roughly, this amounts to about 125 calories a day.

Using our energy data, we divide these calories into the 3,500 which approximate a pound of body fat and find that every 28 days, this man would gain a pound, assuming all else (e.g., his physical activities) remain the same. In a year, he'd gain 13 pounds.

If we start him on this pattern at age 20 when he weighs 180 pounds, by the time he's 40 he will have gained some 260 pounds and will weigh 440 pounds. You have only to think of how many people you know who weigh 440 pounds, and you will see how few people are gluttonous even to the extent of an extra ounce of steak a day.

The typical overweight American is perhaps 10-20% overweight. Thus, in reality, our 180-pound young man might weigh between 200-220 pounds at age 40—and think of himself as fat. If we put our equations into reverse, we can find how much extra daily food he would have eaten on the average: He would have gained one or two pounds a year during 20 years. That averages out

Table 2-2: *Small changes in diet can lead to big changes in weight IF we don't eat more of other foods to compensate!*

Current Diet	Change To	Calories Saved	How Often	Loss/Year
1 cup whole milk (150 cal)	1 cup 1% fat milk (105 cal)	45 cal	2x/day	9 lbs.
20 potato chips (210 cal)	20 pretzel sticks (40 cal)	170 cal	2x/week	5 lbs.
12-oz. can cola (150 cal)	12-oz. can diet cola (2 cal)	148 cal	3x/week	7 lbs
1 cup granola (515 cal)	1 cup 40% bran flakes (160 cal)	355 cal	3x/week	16 lbs.

to an excess of less than 10-20 calories a day. For a smaller person, say a 128-pound woman who gets a little pudgy, the excess would be even less.

To measure the caloric value of one's diet to an accuracy of 10-20 calories a day is virtually impossible even in the laboratory.

Of course, in practical terms our food intake varies from day to day. Chances are that any excesses are sporadic. We sometimes overeat extravagantly and sometimes, even, undereat. But we remember the excesses and tend to overlook the small daily habits that are usually the real culprits. Occasional episodes of gluttony are relatively unimportant in terms of our overall caloric balance.

We might want to try to keep track of our "overeating" by counting every calorie we eat. But most of us don't have the time or patience. Remember, also, that the neat food tables of caloric values are averages. The same food will vary in calories and composition according to the variety grown, the soil, the climate, fertilization, the amount of sun, and many other factors. For example, changes in climate cause changes in the sugar content of grapes, which is one of the reasons why wines differ in different vintage years.

Careful as we may be, how accurately can most of us guess the exact size of a mound of mashed potatoes on our plate? How about the weight of a steak within an ounce? And remember what a difference an ounce of steak can make.

There are also individual differences in how our bodies use food and energy. After all, even two cars of the same make and model can use fuel at different rates. Not only are we a good deal

more subtle and complex than automobiles, but each of us is a unique model from different manufacturers.

Not all of the differences are yet fully understood. But there's far more knowledge than most people suspect about how fat we are, how we got that way, how lean we should be, and what we can do to change ourselves. For while few of us are gluttons, many of us are losing some of our potential for health to our own fat-storage cells.

The Genetic Factor

Fatness has a strong hereditary component. To measure the importance of this effect, consider your odds of becoming fat. If neither of your parents is obese, your risk of obesity may be less than 10%. With one obese parent, the risk of fatness rises to about 40%. If both parents are obese, your chance of becoming so is about 80%.[4]

At one time, this familial pattern was largely attributed to the eating habits of obese parents, which supposedly determined the food choices of their children. To an extent, this probably has some reality. A child who's taught to savor fatty foods may favor them in adulthood. Meat, for example, simply may not taste right without gravy. Potatoes may not seem good without lots of butter.

Today, the eating habits taught by parents are thought to have more of an impact in terms of the ways in which food is used. For example, the habit of eating everything on one's plate—like it or not, want it or not—can be more destructive of energy balance than what's on the plate. Then there's the effect of accustoming a child to use food as a way of dealing with stresses. ("There, there, have a cookie and you'll feel better.")

Learned personality patterns can also lead to using foods to deal with stress. This may cause a person to engage in episodes of overeating as stress increases.

Aside from such factors, studies have shown some clear genetic bases for obesity. For example, identical twins brought up separately, in different environments with different adult models, have shown a remarkable tendency toward similar fatness or thinness.[5]

In one study, 12 pairs of identical twin brothers monitored in a dormitory with restricted physical activity were fed an excess of 1000 calories per day for 4 months. The 12 sets of twins differed a lot in how much weight, body fat, and lean mass they put on, but each set of twins (the two brothers) responded similarly.[6] What causes this similarity?

Differences in Body Type

One genetic factor is our inherited body type. The shape, and to some extent the composition of our bodies can be as predetermined as the color of our hair, the family nose, or the family chin. Body shapes are generally assigned to one of three categories (see Fig. 2-5); but most of us are a blend of all three, with a preponderance toward one or two of them.

Ectomorphs are slight of frame—reed-like when seen in profile. They typically have long thin hands and feet, narrow and tapering fingers, a tendency to develop wiry or stringy muscle, and a low fat-storage capacity.

Endomorphs appear almost as an opposite—softly rounded in style, often with narrow and sloping shoulders, and a torso which bulks toward the abdomen and hips, suggesting a sort of pear shape. The hands and feet are likely to be pudgy and short and, like the fingers, rather flame-shaped. Their muscles tend to be soft and not well defined, and there's a lot more fat-storage capacity.

Mesomorphs are sometimes described as between the other two types, but this isn't really accurate. They are the football types—broad shoulders, deep chests, with heavy bones and sturdy legs. Their hands are likely to be squarish, with blunt-shaped fingers, and they have bunched, well-formed muscles. Their fat-storage is greater than the ectomorph, but less (and more evenly distributed) than that of the endomorph.

While pure body types are unusual, there's a tendency to speak of people according to predominant type or types, such as "endomorphic" or as "a meso-endomorph." It's probably obvious that there's a relationship between inherited body type and capacity for fat-storage.

Figure 2-5: Body Types.

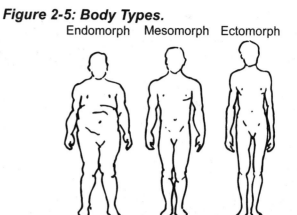

Endomorph   Mesomorph   Ectomorph

Body Shape and Composition

The composition and shape of our body affects our energy needs and the tendency to become overfat. For example, the energy needed to keep our body functioning at its most basic level (basal metabolism) is between 10 and 20% higher for men than for women. One reason is that men have more muscle and less fat than women do, by about 10-20%. Some of this may be due to muscle development, but some is definitely a sexual characteristic.

Lean tissue uses more energy than fat tissue. So leaner people of either sex have a higher basal requirement. Suppose we have two men who weigh about 150 pounds. One is thin, and the other is a bit plump. At rest, the thin man burns about 1.26 calories per minute, and the plump man 1.16 calories.

The difference, a tenth of a calorie per minute, doesn't sound like much. But if both men eat the same amount of food, the plump man treats that tenth-of-a-calorie difference as an excess and stores it. That's 6 calories per hour, or 144 extra calories a day, which theoretically could add a pound every 24 days.

Normal % body fat is about 10% for young men and about 20% for young women.

Thus, an inheritance of muscularity can mean an ability to accommodate greater caloric intake without getting fat. But heredity goes further. For the shape of the body helps to determine the total body surface. A long, thin person will have much more body surface than a short, plump person of the same weight. Since the greater the body surface, the greater the heat loss, a tall, thin body shape means a higher basal metabolism. It can also influence how many calories of energy are used up during activity.

We can see a vicious circle emerging. The thin and lean have more muscle relative to fat, have more body surface, and burn more calories at an idling speed than a stockier or fatter person of the same weight. In this way, nature tends to exaggerate the problems of the heavy and perpetuate them. There can be some reality to the complaint of the stocky man married to the slight woman who says, "She eats like a horse and doesn't gain an ounce; I starve myself and get fat." More often, because of the inherently greater fatness of women, the complaint is the reverse, with females burning less energy for each pound of body weight.

Trial By Calorie

Our tremendous concern about how fat we are supports a multibillion dollar diet industry. Ironically, the industry prospers in large part because most weight-loss schemes are doomed to fail. In other words, the success of this industry depends on the consistent failure of its products. Let's look at some simple tests of reality that we can apply to the alluring promises of so many weight-loss schemes.

A key number in weight control is 3,500. This is about the number of calories in a pound of body fat. Thus, a person must take in at least 3,500 extra calories to make a pound of fat. And a person must expend about 3,500 extra calories to use up a pound of body fat.

In terms of food, 3,500 calories represents about 50 slices of bread or some 135 Hershey chocolate kisses. One would have to eat this much extra to gain about a pound of fat. Therefore, unless drastic and probably unhealthy measures are taken, fat gain or loss isn't going to be very great within a short period of time. Claims of fast weight-loss are suspect, as is the common fear (or hope) that a

person has gained (or lost) several pounds of fat over a weekend.

Common sense tells us that unless we step up our energy output with more exercise, we can't take 3,500 calories out of our daily diet unless we are eating at least this much food to begin with. Consider again the woman of 5'5" who has 25 pounds of excess weight and weighs 150 pounds. Can dieting alone make her lose a pound a day?

In a normal day, she probably eats food providing about 2,300 calories, which without much exercise, her body uses. So even with complete fasting, she can't lose a pound of fat (3,500 calories) in a day unless she adds significantly to her normal activities. If she ate nothing, creating a resting deficit of 2,300 calories, the remaining 1,200 calorie deficit necessary to meet her goal of 3,500 calories would require exercise equivalent to running about 10 miles a day.

People are often drawn to the various plans, schemes, and nostrums that tout unrealistic notions of easy weight-loss. Such sudden changes in weight are usually due to a gain or loss of body water. Weight that's lost so easily isn't fat, and is also easily regained. The dieter is alternately drier and juicier. What's in fact left are lighter wallets and a heavy sense of failure.

Losing excess fat within a relatively short period of time is hard. No wonder we'd rather not believe that the size of our fat stores is simply a matter of consuming more energy than we expend. To help us face this simple truth, we might begin by reminding ourselves that the ease with which we become fat isn't a curse upon the human race or a highly visible punishment for gluttony or inactivity. It's instead an essential evolutionary mechanism for human survival.

Summary

The body has a constant need for energy: a baseline amount to maintain our involuntary bodily functions (basal metabolism), plus the energy used for physical activity. We meet these energy needs by eating and by using fat stores when not eating.

The energy potential of foods and the energy expenditure of our bodies are measured in calo-

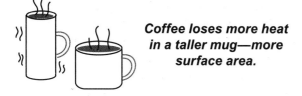

Coffee loses more heat in a taller mug—more surface area.

ries. The number of calories in food is determined by measuring the amount of heat produced when the food is burned. The body's caloric expenditure is measured directly by measuring the amount of heat we produce, or indirectly by measuring the amount of oxygen we use.

When the body "burns" energy, part of the energy is captured as ATP; the remainder is lost as heat. This ATP is then used to provide energy for such needs as protein synthesis, muscle contraction, and brain activity. We feel warm when we exercise because of the increased heat production that accompanies the increased production of ATP for the muscle contractions.

When we consume more calories than we need, we store the excess as fat. Even at a normal weight, we have considerable fat stores. This is the body's insurance against running out of fuel.

Although obesity may bring forth images of gluttony, excess body fat is typically the result of just small and steady excesses of calories. Small differences in either our caloric intake or our caloric needs can mean the difference between being lean or fat.

Genetics, including its influence on body shape and composition, plays a key role in our capacity for and tendency towards fatness. A long, thin body shape and more lean body mass both increase basal energy needs.

Fat tissue contains about 3,500 calories per pound. Thus, fat is gained or lost only gradually, since a person must take in or expend about 3,500 extra calories to gain or lose a pound of body fat. It's much easier to gain fat than to lose it. The tendency to overeat when food is abundant has ancient roots as a key to survival in lean times. In contrast, losing weight doesn't come naturally to those of us in an affluent society—we don't face famine regularly, and survival doesn't require strenuous activity.

Guest Lecturer: *Albert Stunkard, MD*

Theories of the Causes of Obesity

[In a 1986 lecture[7], Dr. Stunkard, a pioneer in obesity research, reflected on his research of the preceding 30+ years—before today's era of identifying specific genes. This is an excerpt from that lecture.]

Our understanding of the causes of obesity has progressed since the days when obesity was considered "the presenting symptom of a basic personality disorder" and "a particular way of handling one's poor relationship with oneself." Current approaches are far more modest. They start from a finding so simple that it was largely overlooked in the days of overarching theory. Despite its simplicity and uncontroversial nature, this finding has been intensively scrutinized until it was firmly established: obesity runs in families. Thirty years ago, this finding would have hardly seemed worth mentioning. Today it is a starting point for research.

Why does obesity run in families? Is it due to genetic influences or to environmental influences?

Environmental Influences

Until recently, most of the evidence favored environmental influences. This early evidence was uncovered in an unexpected way, in one of the surprises that makes research such a delight. We had started out to assess the extent of mental illness of obese people in the Midtown Manhattan Study, "Mental Health in the Metropolis." Then we got sidetracked by a factor we had not considered—socioeconomic status.

Social class showed a striking relationship to obesity. Obesity was six times more common among lower class women than among upper class women. Furthermore, the Midtown data enabled us to go beyond simple correlations and infer causation.

The Midtown Study had assessed not only the social class of the respondents themselves, but also their social class of origin—the social class of their fathers when they were eight years old. Social class of origin strongly predicted obesity. A person's social class of origin was almost as strongly related to obesity as was his or her own social class. The social class into which you are born, particularly if you are a woman, strongly detemines whether or not you will be obese.

Among men, the relationship is less clear: sometimes, as among women, the lower the socioeconomic status, the greater the prevalence of obesity; sometimes it is the reverse. Among children (of both sexes) usually no relationship is found. Only as they grow into adulthood do the distinctive relationships develop.

Whatever the nature of the social forces that determine obesity or thinness, they have a pervasive influence. Even pet animals seem susceptible. A report in the English veterinary literature revealed that 44% of the dogs of people "of obese physique" were obese as compared with 25% of the dogs of those of normal weight!

Genetic Influence

Evidence of a genetic influence on human obesity is of very recent origin. It was obtained by the use of the classic method of assessing genetic influences on humans, twin studies. The rationale of twin studies is simple: identical twins share both a common environment and common genes. Fraternal (nonidentical) twins share a common environment but only half their genes.

The differences in correlations in weight between pairs of identical twins and between pairs of fraternal twins were calculated. Since the environments of twins of either type are presumably similar, any difference between the correlations of the different kinds of twin should be due to genetic influences. The data showed a strong genetic influence extending across the entire spectrum from thin to fat.

Conclusions from the Twin Studies

The research thus shows that both genes and environment play roles in determining human obesity. Genetic influences may largely determine whether or not an individual becomes obese. Given this genetic vulnerability, it is environmental influences that determine how obese the person becomes.

These twin studies have three limitations, however. First, they may overestimate the influence of heredity. Second, they are confined to men. Third, because they are confined to men who could pass a physical examination for entry into the armed forces, they effectively excluded those with childhood-onset obesity.

Adoption Studies

These limitations made it desirable to supplement the twin studies with other methods, and we have done that with two adoption studies. The rationale of adoption studies is straightforward. Adoptees are compared with both their biologic and their adoptive parents for obesity. A relationship between biologic parents and adoptees bespeaks a genetic influence; a relationship between adoptive parents and adoptees indicates an environmental influence.

The first of our adoption studies used the Danish Adoption Register, which had been employed successfully in previous studies on schizophrenia and on alcoholism. We obtained height and weight data for 3,590 adoptees who were living in Copenhagen at the time of the study, and whose average age was 42 years.

We next ascertained the heights and weights of both the biologic and adoptive parents, and compared them with those of the adoptees. This comparison of the relationship between biologic parents and adoptees indicated a genetic influence.

Not surprisingly, this finding confirmed the results of the twin study. What was a surprise was the absence of any apparent effect of the early family environment. The weight class of the adoptees was not related to the weight classifications of their adoptive parents. Whatever the influence their adoptive parents may have had when the adoptees were children, there were no traces of it when they reached middle age. The dire consequences of faulty childhood eating habits, so often blamed for the developments of obesity, have been, to say the least, exaggerated.

Both twin and adoption studies thus show that heredity influences human obesity.

The Role of Genetics

What role then does genetics play in human obesity? Is human obesity determined at conception, like hair color and eye color, and can people do nothing to alter their fate? As far as obesity is concerned, are genes destiny?

The answer is "No!" Obesity is not determined at conception. What is inherited is a vulnerability, which requires a suitable environment in order to be manifested.

Our current understanding of the genetic vulnerability to obesity provides no basis for personal despair or therapeutic surrender. Countless formerly obese people have shown how courage and effort can overcome even the most unpromising heritage. With increased understanding of genetic influences on human obesity, we shall be able to identify people at increased risk and help them to cope in a more informed manner. Understanding their greater vulnerability to obesity can be a prelude to better control.

The Environmental Challenge

The environmental circumstances that contribute to obesity in the United States today are probably extensive. Americans consume a diet high in calories and expend few calories in physical activity. Our diet is high enough in fat to produce obesity in thin rats, and our labor-saving devices are so efficient that we become fat on a diet that now has 1,000 fewer calories than it did at the turn of the century.

The issue in human obesity is not one of heredity or environment, or heredity versus environment, but of heredity and environment, or genetic vulnerability and environmental challenge. This issue affects all of psychiatry, indeed all of medicine. It may well set the agenda for medical research for the foreseeable future.

The Set Point Theory

Another theory whereby genetic and environmental influences both may exert their effect is the set point theory of obesity. Arguments for this theory begin with the observation that the body weight of animals is regulated. Not only does their body weight remain at a relatively constant level when circumstances remain constant, but it is also defended at that level when circumstances change; it responds to environmental challenges.

The remarkable ability of animals to regulate body weight is exemplified by animals that migrate and hibernate. They not only regulate body weight at a constant level under ordinary circumstances, but also perform extraordinary feats of anticipatory regulation. Before its 600 mile flight across the Caribbean Sea, the ruby-throated hummingbird overeats to produce fat stores of precisely the amount necessary for this long flight. Too much fat and it could not get off the ground; too little and it would fall into the sea short of its goal. Similarly, the golden-mantled ground squirrel overeats to produce the exact amount of energy stores it needs for its months of hibernation.

For many years, evidence of the regulation of body weight was confined to animals of normal weight. Then a number of investigations revealed that the body weight of obese animals. is also regulated. One way of explaining their obesity is that their body weight is being regulated at an elevated level by an elevation of their set point.

Studies of hoarding behavior support the existence of regulation. When food intake is restricted and rats lose a certain percentage of their body weight, they begin to hoard food. The weight at which hoarding begins can be interpreted as a body-weight set point, and rats will hoard enormous amounts of food as their weight falls below this level. Hoarding behavior occurs in obese rats as well as in normal-weight rats when their body weight falls below a certain critical level.

Evidence for the existence of a body weight set point in humans is limited to two studies of men of normal weight. In the landmark Minnesota starvation study, volunteers lost 25% of their body weight, whereas in the Vermont prison study, men gained 50 or more pounds. In each study, when subjects were allowed to control their own food intake, their body weight rapidly returned to normal.

Normal weight people can apparently regulate their body weight. We have no information about the regulation of body weight of obese humans, and the constraints upon experimentation with human subjects make it unlikely that further experiments of this type will be carried out. As a result, much of what we learn about the regulation of body weight in humans must be extrapolated from research with animals.

Albert Stunkard, MD is a Professor of Psychiatry at the University of Pennsylvania School of Medicine. He has published more than 400 articles, and was the first to describe binge eating. Recent publications include his studies of the night-eating syndrome.[8]

Chapter 3

Putting the Laws of Energy to Work

What if you want to lose weight? And, you're looking for a weight-loss program that really works.

It's probably not the first time—in fact it probably seems like the zillionth time—but there's still a mixture of hope and readiness to believe. What's new and different about the parade of weight-loss diets on the best-seller lists?

Is there hope? Will it make any difference if you know something about what has worked and what hasn't worked?

Put it this way: If you know only that everything you've ever tried has failed, you're set up to be doubly vulnerable—you won't know the responsible from the phony, and you'll have made your odds against success even greater with your expectation of failure.

If you're well informed, at least you will have some subtle but important tools. You will know that there is no magic of chemistry or faith healing that will do your work for you. And you will have realistic expectations—a critical ingredient of any long-term weight-control program.

Attempting to lose weight might be classified as a national obsession, when one considers the time and effort we put into dieting and the amount of money spent on diet foods and diet plans. Many of us diet solely for cosmetic reasons, but obesity has an important bearing on health—it increases risk of such diseases as diabetes, stroke, and heart disease.

There's thus a substantial health benefit from losing excess fat. Unfortunately, despite all the advances made in other areas of science and medicine, there has been relatively little success in preventing or curing obesity.

In this chapter, we look at the more practical aspects of energy balance and how we can tip that balance towards weight loss. How do we assess our own fatness and our individual caloric requirement? What are some reasons for overeating? And finally, what are the components of a good weight-reduction plan?

How Many Calories Do We Need?

As we've seen, the energy need for most people is mainly governed by their *basal metabolic rate* (BMR). We also saw in the last chapter how genetics and gender affect basal energy needs, through differences in body type, shape, and composition.

A number of other factors affect our use of energy. For example, the older we get, the less fuel we need. Much of this is due to changes in body composition and chemistry, but a decline in physical activity can also play a big part.

Exposure to extremes of climate also has an effect. If the body is exposed to either high or low temperatures, it must spend energy to compensate for them, for the body must stay at a fairly even temperature to survive. One has only to remember how bad one feels with a fever—an extra couple of degrees of body temperature. The body becomes seriously threatened when its internal temperature is changed by more than a few degrees.

In cold environments, the body must spend more energy to generate heat, often by shivering— a way to use vigorous muscle activity to generate warmth. If the weather is hot, the cooling processes

take energy, in pumping more blood to the skin surface, so that heat can escape. Even sweating takes energy.

And there are endless subtleties. Energy needs are conserved by wearing several layers of clothing in cold weather because this reduces loss of body heat. But then, energy needs are increased by the added weight of the clothing and the drag that the clothing exerts upon movement. Then again, energy needs are reduced when bulky clothing—or hot weather—restricts our physical activity.

Thus, energy needs depend on a complex interrelationship of many variables, such as physical activity, body size and composition, age, and climate. In general, while it's common to speak of energy balance as a rather tidy and precise matter, it's neither tidy nor precise.

What this means is that even scientists can't predict energy use, storage, etc., as accurately as they'd like. But this doesn't mean that we can't predict and plan energy use in approximate ways which have great practical value.

Making a Personalized Energy Budget

There are many ways to analyze energy output, and all of them lead ultimately to only general approximations. Nevertheless, it's possible to personalize this information to some extent.

Calculating Your Basal Energy Needs

There are many methods for finding an approximate basal metabolic rate (BMR), some of which are quite complex. One can begin by measuring body size and using BMR tables which show averages. But however carefully these averages are determined, they encompass a rather broad range, with variations of 20% and more. This is a huge variation when we consider the fact that small variations in energy balance can make a dramatic difference in long-term weight gain or loss.

Without a basal metabolism test, you might still get a fairly good idea of your daily energy need for basal metabolism from a simple rule of thumb:

• For women: Add a zero to your weight in pounds. Add to the result, your weight in pounds.

• For men: Add a zero to your weight in pounds. Add to the result, twice your weight in pounds.

By this rule, a 128-pound woman adds a zero, making 1,280 calories, and then adds her weight (128), for a total of 1,408 calories a day.

Correcting for Age: The rule-of-thumb calculation makes no allowance for age, and BMRs change with age. The changes are a reflection of an increase of fatness, a decline in muscle, and changes in various hormones.

To correct your BMR for age, simply reduce it by 2% for each decade above age 20. Therefore, a man of 30 with a basal need of 2,000 calories would subtract 40 calories (.02 x 2,000 = 40) from his basal need.

Basal metabolic rates of children are a special matter, especially those of infants, and the energy-calculating methods shown here don't work for them. Among other things, their body proportions are different from adults, and the factor of growth enters in. The small, growing body uses an impressive part of its fuel as building material. This is one reason why children can take in so many more calories for their weight than adults can.

Correcting for Body Shape and Composition: Going back to the rule-of-thumb calculation of basal need, there's a simple way to make this reflect our individual body shape and our fat-lean composition. It goes like this:

• If you're thinner than average, *add* 5% to what you'd otherwise calculate to be your total basal need. You need more calories for your weight.

• If you're pudgier than average, so that you might describe yourself as "plump," then you are probably some 5% higher in fatness. So *subtract* 5% from your basal calorie need.

• If you'd have to describe yourself as "fat," or about 10% higher in fatness than the average, then you should subtract 10% from your basal calorie need. (Note that % of greater fatness is not the same as % above desired weight.)

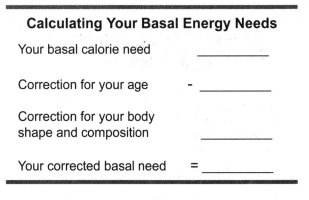

Calculating Your Basal Energy Needs

Your basal calorie need	_____
Correction for your age	- _____
Correction for your body shape and composition	_____
Your corrected basal need	= _____

Adding Calories for Physical Activity

To our basal calorie need, we need to add calories for physical activity. In the last chapter we were given some idea of the calories needed for various activities. But even if we could measure to the minute how we spend our days, it's very hard to use activity tables to estimate the number of calories we need for physical activity on a day-to-day basis. Also, we tend to overestimate how active we are.

Keep in mind that when an activity is strenuous, it's hard to sustain that activity for long —we have to stop to "catch our breath." One might spend an hour "working out," but most of that time may be spent resting between lifts and strolling from one piece of exercise equipment to the next. Weight-lifting, for example, is very hard work, but a lot of time is spent resting between lifts.

In reality, the calories we need in a day is the amount of calories we take in when we are neither losing nor gaining weight. Of course, what this amount is, is hard to figure. Practically speaking, all we can do is use another rule-of-thumb to estimate the calories expended per day above basal needs, based on our general level of activity:

• **Sedentary** (mostly activities like reading, typing): Add 50% to basal calorie needs by multiplying your corrected basal need by 0.5.

• **Lightly active** (mostly activities like laboratory work, cooking): Add 60% to basal calorie needs by multiplying your corrected basal need by 0.6.

• **Moderately active** (mostly activities like carpentry, housework): Add 70% to basal calorie needs by multiplying your corrected basal need by 0.7.

Calculating Your Energy Need for Physical Activity

Your corrected basal need   _____

Multiplied by activity
factor (0.5-1.0)   x _____

Calories for physical
activity   = _____

- **Very active** (mostly activities like unskilled labor, running, dancing): Add 80% to basal calorie needs by multiplying your corrected basal need by 0.8.
- **Strenuously active** (like professional athletes during training): Add 90+% to basal calorie needs by multiplying your corrected basal need by 0.9-1.0.

For a sedentary person with a basal calorie need of 1,400 calories, the calories for physical activity would be 700 (0.50 x 1400 = 700), for a total of 2100 calories. An additional 10% (210) is added for the digestion and assimilation of food, making a total calorie need of about 2,310 (1,400 + 700 + 210) calories per day.

Your Total Energy Needs

Corrected basal need   _____

Physical activity need   + _____

Total (basal + activity)   = _____

10% of Total*   + _____

Total Energy Need   = _____

*Calories used to digest and assimilate food
 (about 10% of caloric intake).

How Much Should You Weigh?

The question should really be, *How fat should you be?,* because weight and fatness aren't the same. True, weight is one indicator of the amount of fat we store. But it can be a deceptive indicator. Consider the illusion wrought by water loss

in some reducing diets. Remember, too, the wide variation in body shape and composition. Bone and muscle weigh more than fat. A stocky, burly person can weigh half again as much as the thin ectomorph of the same height.

Does this mean that the burly person is overweight? Does it mean that the thin person is underweight? In one perspective, the answer to both questions is yes. For if we measure these people against the charts of height and weight, one is above and the other below "normal weight." But relative body weight isn't a reliable index of fatness except in the extreme. Someone who is 5 feet tall and weighs 300 pounds is indeed likely to be fat.

As early as World War II, interest in standards for physical fitness led to studies that compared overweight to fatness. Football players, for example, averaged well above U.S. Army height-weight standards. But they proved to have low body fat. They were overweight, but not overfat.

But in practice, height and weight are easily measured whereas body fat isn't. Body Mass Index (BMI) is commonly used to assess body weight. Its main advantage is that it puts height and weight into a single number. BMI is your weight in kilograms divided by the square of your height in meters (kg/m^2). A short-cut method is to multiply your weight in pounds by 703 and divide that number by the square of your height in inches:

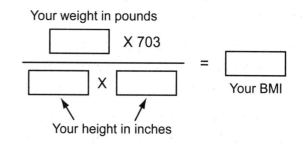

BMI Categories for Adults

		Risk of Disease
Underweight	<18.5	
Normal weight	18.5-24.9	
Overweight	25.0-29.9	Increased
Obese (class 1)	30.0-34.9	High
Obese (class 2)	35.0-39.9	Very High
Extreme obese (class 3)	40.0+	Extremely High

Table 3-1: Height, weight for BMI = 18.5-24.9

Ht	Wt	Ht	Wt	Ht	Wt
4'10"	89-119	5'5"	111-150	6'0"	136-184
4'11"	92-123	5'6"	115-154	6'1"	140-189
5'0"	95-128	5'7"	118-159	6'2"	144-194
5'1"	98-132	5'8"	122-164	6'3"	148-199
5'2"	101-136	5'9"	125-169	6'4"	152-205
5'3"	104-141	5'10"	129-174	6'5"	156-210
5'4"	108-145	5'11"	133-179	6'6"	160-215

Your BMI presumes (correctly in most cases) that excess weight is mostly excess fat, but it doesn't indicate how the weight is distributed (e.g., a big belly). Having a lot of excess fat around the belly (abdominal fat) increases the risk of disease (e.g., diabetes, high blood pressure, heart disease) even if one's BMI is normal.

For those with a BMI of 35 or less, a waist circumference of more than 35 inches in women, and more than 40 inches in men raises the risk of disease to the next category, e.g., a man with a BMI of 24 and a waist of 42 inches has an "increased" risk of disease.[1]

How Fatness is Measured

Measures of weight, height, and waist circumference give a fair estimate of fatness, but more accurate measures are needed by research scientists. Others, such as athletes, also may want to have a more exact measure of body fat. The most inexpensive and easiest measure—especially in studies involving large numbers of people—is the *"pinch test."*

Most of our fat stores can be found under our skin. The underlying fat adheres to the skin when it's pinched, so measures of the width of "pinches" reflect the amount of body fat. Special calipers are used, and the measurements are made by trained personnel.

Typically, a person's skinfold is measured at several sites, since people vary in where they deposit their fat stores. Three sites commonly measured are: the triceps (underside of the arm, midway between shoulder and elbow), the subscapu-

lar (below the shoulder blade), and the subcostal (just below the lowest rib).

Other measures of body fatness include measuring body density by *underwater weighing* (fatter bodies weigh less under water because fat "floats" in water whereas muscle and bone do not), and *bioelectric impedance analysis* (BIA), in which an electrode is attached to an arm and a leg and a mild electric current is passed between the electrodes (lean tissue transmits the current whereas fat tissue impedes it).

Realities of Losing Fat

In theory, tipping the balance of energy, so that the body loses some of its fat reserves, could hardly be simpler. You have only to achieve some mix of more energy expenditure and less caloric intake whereby more calories are used than taken in.

The laws of energy conservation tell us that energy is never really lost. It has to go somewhere, be used somehow, and add up to a neat balance at the end. This basic principle is often overlooked in judging popular weight-loss schemes. If ideas about weight control can't account for an energy balance, they can't be based on reality. You can't have it both ways: you can't "eat all you want," avoid "tiresome exercise," and expect to lose weight.

Most of us seem to settle in at a certain body weight. This weight is popularly referred to as a *"set-point."* This phenomenon is thought to be part of the reason why it's so easy to regain the weight we so painstakingly lose on a reducing diet. The intricacies of how this setpoint works are just beginning to be understood.

Leptin, for example, plays a role as a hormone made by our fat cells in proportion to how much body fat we have stored—it sends a signal to stop eating when our "fat tank" has been replenished. There's substantial evidence that increased exercise can lower the "set-point" in someone who is overweight. In any event, there are many good reasons for being physically active—fat or not.

Looking for More Work

If you're reluctant to eat less, you'll have to exercise more to lose weight. How much more depends on various factors, and it's important to keep several points in mind when estimating the calories used in different types of activities:

- **The energy used in weight-bearing exercises is quite variable.** Not only does the caloric output depend on how far you move, but also on how much you weigh (i.e., how much weight is moved). Someone weighing 120 pounds uses about 70 calories walking a mile in 20 minutes, whereas someone weighing 200 pounds uses about 105 calories walking that same mile. (Good reason to carry an infant in a baby carrier—or books in a backpack—if you're looking to use more calories.)

  This also means that as you lose weight, you will use fewer calories for the same walk (unless the infant you are carrying gains what you lose, or you add a counterbalancing number of books to your backpack).

  The amount of energy used in walking is affected by other factors as well, including the walking surface (e.g., sand or pavement, uphill, downhill, or flat), distribution of weight on the walker's body, the walker's physical fitness.

- **In non-weight-bearing exercise, other physical factors can make a difference in energy output.** In swimming, for example, a more buoyant person expends less energy staying on top of the water.

- **People vary quite a lot in how much energy they expend in a given activity.** Tennis isn't always tennis. Suppose you are much better than your opponent. You return shots while standing at the net, and your opponent runs a lot. But the next day you are outclassed. Now it's your turn to run. You hit harder, stretch further, and pant. The third day you play doubles, and one of the partners is a lawyer who frequently stops to dispute line-calls and asks the score after each point.

Figure 3-1: Activity time to burn about 200 calories.

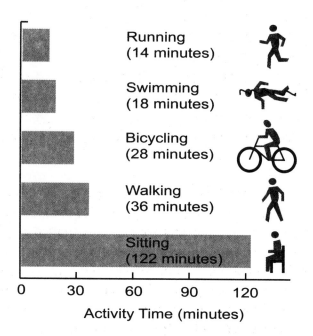

Even in a lecture hall, some people sit at the edge of their seats and fidget. Others are slumped in their seats, barely awake.

Most of us are quick to imagine how we can increase our output of energy. We imagine ourselves deliberately parking a mile away from work, or taking up biking or swimming. But for many of us, such an active imagination doesn't translate into an active body. This leaves us receptive to claims of painless shortcuts. It's important to remember that there are no magic exercises, just as there are no magic foods.

Increasing the output of energy is a fairly obvious matter (see Fig. 3-1). Once an appropriate activity is chosen—one which uses a good bit of energy and which usually involves moving the whole body over a long distance (e.g., a long walk, or a simulated long walk on a treadmill)—the problem is chiefly one of persistence.

Increasing physical activity is helpful in other ways. What we want to lose is fat, but muscle mass is also lost with dieting. Exercise helps maintain muscle mass, and also is a counterbalance to the drop in basal metabolism triggered by a low-calorie diet. Furthermore, if the exercise leads to more muscle mass, basal calorie needs will increase.

Appetite

Increased physical activity can make a crucial difference in the success of reducing regimens, but unless one controls caloric intake, the effort to spend more energy may not accomplish much. One surprising fact that may help is that a moderate increase in activity (increased calorie use) by those who are sedentary doesn't necessarily result in a proportionate in increase appetite.[2,3] (The not-so-good news is that increased physical activity beyond a moderate point generally signals graded increases in appetite.)

Appetite is a rather mysterious phenomenon, intimately involving physical and emotional factors. And a key reason why appetite remains such a mystery, defying many experimental efforts at analysis, is that these two factors are subtly and intricately interlocked.

Appetite was once thought to be controlled mainly by the mechanical effects of food digestion—as seen by such old phrases as "on a full stomach." It was believed that the contractions of an empty stomach were among the main cues for eating. It was noted, for instance, that fats, which leave the stomach more slowly, seem to have greater value for long-term satisfaction

But this theory had to contend with the fact that the stomach usually is emptied within two to four hours of eating (depending on the composition of the meal), without any clear correlation with the arrival of hunger pangs. More sophisticated studies show the process to be a far more complicated one. Food in the stomach doesn't necessarily stop the wish to eat, and an empty stomach doesn't necessarily start it.

The appetite-control mechanism is in the hypothalamus part of the brain, the seat of some of the most basic reactions for survival. It has to do with the control of body temperature, with certain sexual phenomena, and with the primitive "fight-or-flight" reflexes.

The brain mechanism appears to have two parts, one to turn on appetite and the other to turn it off—much like the way a thermostat regulates room temperature. Both of these switches seem to respond to changing blood levels of glucose, the

simple sugar which is a major fuel used to meet the body's energy needs.

There are other bodily mechanisms for assessing how much fuel is coming in, and it's thought that the brain mechanism responds to a number of body reactions and controls that have a joint net effect of leading us to eat or to stop eating. The stomach, for example, makes more of the appetite-stimulating hormone ghrelin before a meal, and makes less of it after the meal.

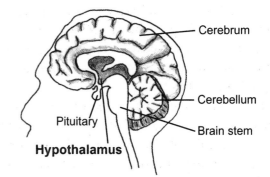

Unfortunately, the fact that big reserves of stored fat are available for energy—and perhaps are even being put to work—doesn't necessarily shut off the drive to eat. Appetite control seems to concern itself mainly with whether or not enough fuel is coming in to take care of current energy needs. The fat person feels just as hungry as the very thin person when lunch time passes without food. And for similar reasons, the person who is trying to lose weight may feel unsatisfied if less fuel is consumed than the body is burning.

On the other hand, contrary to popular belief, experimental evidence makes it rather clear that fatter people don't have an unusually active appetite or find taste extremely stimulating. But it does appear that overweight people are more prone to eat in response to external cues for eating (e.g., a candy dish on the coffee table, or the clock showing it's lunch time).

There's also a difference among people of different body types. The thin ectomorph seems to have a sharper cut-off of appetite than does the bulkier endomorph or mesomorph, who appears to be more inclined to accept some additional food after feeling satisfied ("I couldn't eat another bite—but did you say chocolate?"). The mesomorph may well say to an ectomorph, "You only have a bite of cheesecake left on your plate. Why didn't you finish it?" In fact, the mesomorph may even be tempted to eat that last morsel "so it won't go to waste."

A strong emotional influence runs throughout all these themes, which blurs logic all the more.

Appetite and the Emotions

We've seen that few people who are fat are truly gluttonous—rather they're more likely to be the victims of small steady excesses of intake over need, with perhaps occasional episodes of extreme excess. It's easy to see how even minor emotionally-oriented distortions of the appetite might lead to obesity.

The wish to eat has a powerful emotional aspect. Feelings of all kinds, from joy to pain, can override the physical signals of a need or lack of need for fuel. Feasting is an ancient way to celebrate. Conversely, in the emotional disturbance known as *anorexia nervosa*, young women may suddenly stop eating—until life itself is seriously threatened—with no feelings of hunger.

The psychological effects on appetite are well known to have a strong *placebo effect* for many. Almost any system of dieting, or any kind of pill, will magically wipe away hunger for a number of people, if that's what they're told it will do.

In this case, the placebo effect is a decrease in appetite due to expectation alone. A placebo (from the Latin for "I please") is an innocuous substance or procedure administered to create the illusion of medication or treatment, either to pacify or for test purposes.

This powerful link between appetite and emotion begins in the first hours of life—as we have our first taste of both love and food in our mothers' arms. This maternal nurturing is a key to survival. Love and food are interwoven; the need for both becomes a part of our very will to survive; and food becomes a potent symbol of this whole basic emotional system.

The giving of food quickly begins to symbolize the giving of love, but also begins to embody the sense of healing, and the relief of stress and pain. To the contrary, the withholding of food becomes a sign of love denied, of rejection, hostility, and

an important kind of punishment. Almost every culture greets its guests with food or drink.

As the child develops, a reverse image of these emotions appears: to be loved, one must accept the gift of nurture. How would you feel if you invited guests to dinner, and they sat without eating, saying they just weren't hungry? In many cultures, rejecting an offer of food or drink is an insult.

So, in addition to being a way to soothe and please ourselves, eating also becomes a way to please others. For many parents, the good child is the one who cleans the plate. ("Eat your dinner. I spent hours cooking just for you.")

This subtle kind of reward-and-punishment game can be used in other ways: "If you don't eat your vegetables, you can't have dessert." "Be good at the dentist and we'll go out for ice cream afterwards." A child can thus be taught to view foods as palliatives for the pains and stresses of living.

One of the most widely accepted theories about the emotional development of humans is the internalization of our parents and their ideas. In a sense, growing up is partly the business of becoming our parents. We learn symbolically to slap our own hands if we want to reach for something that doesn't belong to us. We abuse ourselves if we've been wrong and feel guilt. We learn to soothe our own pains, and we learn to reward ourselves for behavior that we think is good.

If our parents have used food for these purposes, then the parents who live in our minds will also use food. Similarly, our early training often leads us to see any deprivation of food as emotional evidence that we are being denied love, or perhaps even being punished for some sin.

Some psychologists have theorized that such feelings on the part of the dieter can lead to repeated episodes of painful crash dieting. It's as if there's a need to punish ourselves for crimes of gluttony.

"Appetite-Killing" Diets

Many reducing diets are advertised with the promise that, though they are low in calories, they are fully satisfying. There can be a thread of truth to such claims, but it's generally exaggerated.

For example, because fat tends to stay longer in the stomach, it can be more satisfying. This does have some reality. But there's the further reality that fat has far more calories than protein or carbohydrate.

Many of the very narrow "crash" diets, such as liquid diets or other monotonous diets, seem to act as limits on calorie intake to some extent simply because they quickly become boring and unappetizing, and people aren't tempted to overeat (or stay on them for very long). An "overdose" of almost anything seems to be a sure way to arrive at some caloric reduction. A diet of all the bread and grapefruit you can eat—but nothing else—can work. And one can expect that a diet of nothing but chocolate ice cream and steak would soon become effective too.

Changes of metabolic function have also been claimed for some crash diets, again with a thread of truth. *Ketosis,* a state which derives from a lack of carbohydrate for fuel (as in an extremely low-carbohydrate diet or starvation), does, for example, produce mild nausea, which, of course, kills the appetite. But purposely altering the body's chemistry in such ways is generally considered to be unwise, especially if the abnormal state is continued for very long.

A "Good" Weight-Loss Diet

What makes a good reducing diet? The simplest answer, of course, is a diet with fewer calories than are used by the body. But when we understand how much time it takes for a realistic caloric deficit to have a real impact on stored fat, we can readily see that a good reducing diet must also be adequate nutritionally.

There's little that the physician—or the self-treating dieter—can do to speed the process of fat loss, despite the breathless stories in hundreds of magazines about magical potions, foods, and diets. Although there are an endless variety of distractions offered in these regimens, all of them generally have a low intake of calories as an essential component.

Are 1,000 calories or less a day okay? We've already seen that in terms of pure survival, one can go a long time without eating and still have

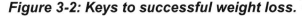

Figure 3-2: Keys to successful weight loss.

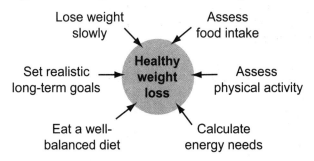

energy reserves to draw upon. And most of us would stop dieting when we became emaciated.

But energy isn't all there is to nutrition. Instructions for most crash diets include the warning to see your doctor first (although few people do) and to "take a vitamin pill."

Yet only some of the needed nutrients are found in vitamin-mineral supplements. We also need the "structural materials"—too "big" to fit into a pill—for the building and repair of tissue. Extremely obese people who are treated with complete fasting, burn not only fat but muscle tissue as well. In a sense, the body consumes its own meat to get needed protein.

The widespread use of so-called *"protein-sparing" diet*—-the most popular of which was marketed as Optifast—was given a lot of publicity. Originally developed by physicians for medically-endangered obese patients, it was designed to be used only with such patients, and under close supervision according to strict medical protocols. Caloric intake was severely restricted, and special supplements provided vitamins, minerals, and protein (to help spare body protein—"protein sparing").

Where used as intended, these liquid diets were useful in achieving rapid weight loss with relative safety. But the rapid weight-loss aspect was so attractive that its use spread. The medical control aspect loosened, and these diets became widespread, under various commercially promoted titles using various supplements and a wide variety of supervisory standards.

As protocols and products have varied, so have long-term results. Health risks come with inadequate supervision and control, and long-term weight-loss was minimal, despite the well-publicized examples of dramatic weight loss.

Figure 3-3: Yo-yo dieting. Repeated episodes of crash dieting—often called weight cycling or "yo-yo dieting"—might be detrimental to health, independent of obesity.

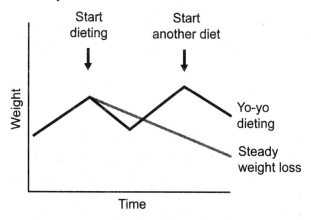

The power of such programs is also its weakness: Participants living for months on liquid supplements don't face up to their regular exercise and eating habits or perceptions about food—elements which are essential for true weight control by the chronically overweight.

So pills and potions aren't the answer. Eventually, the dieter must eat real food. Most dietitians agree that a nutritious diet usually requires at least 1,200 calories a day, and more for people who are larger than average. At this calorie level, much care in food selection is needed to insure sufficient intake of the needed nutrients. So a more generous calorie allotment is better.

At 1,700 calories a day, the expected weight loss for many people would be about a pound a week, depending on one's energy needs. This may seem like a very small amount, but the aim is to lose body fat rather than lean tissue—and fat doesn't come off easily. Unlike lean tissue, it's concentrated in calories and doesn't hold water. It also helps to remember that more gradual weight loss is often easier to maintain—and that the accumulation of excess body fat was gradual, as well.

There are about 3,500 calories in a pound of body fat. This means that one must "go into debt" this many calories to lose a pound of body fat. Losing a pound of body fat a week means a caloric deficit of 3,500 calories a week, or 500 calories a day (3,500 calories/7 days).

For a person who requires 2,200 calories a day, a deficit of 500 calories a day means a diet of 1,700 calories. This simple arithmetic makes it clear why losing one pound a week is reasonable if the aim is to lose fat. Losing weight much faster, one can assume that lean tissue and water are being lost—and any loss of water and lean tissue is very soon restored after the return to a normal diet.

In designing weight-reduction diets, two key principles are usually followed. The first is to limit the intake of *"calorie-dense" foods*—foods which have a lot of calories packed into a small amount of food. Foods rich in fats and oils and sugars are typical.

> As we shall see in later chapters, a good reducing diet is fundamentally the same as a general, healthy diet—both focus on a diet rich in grains, vegetables, and fruits.

Foods with low caloric concentrations should be favored—foods with high content of water and fiber, such as grains, vegetables, and fruits. Their high bulk, relative to their calories, makes them good reducing foods.

A second principle is that of choosing *nutrient-dense foods*—foods that have a lot of nutrients for the calories (e.g., carrots). The simplest way to understand the principle is to think of calories as money. We want to use our limited "budget" of calories to buy as much good nutritive value as we can (see Table 3-3).

This concept explains why sugar is usually restricted in reducing diets. In effect, it "dilutes" foods nutritionally. If we compare canned peaches packed in heavy sugar syrup (75 calories/half-peach with liquid) with those packed in fruit juice (45 calories/half-peach with liquid), we see that portions equivalent in calories will have very different nutritive value. With heavy syrup, we get less peach for the calories. Thus, for reducing purposes, we would choose the more *nutrient-dense* peaches packed in juice.

Reduced-Calorie Foods

There's a variety of commercial food products one can substitute for commonly consumed foods at a lower caloric value. The product may be a tiny packet of an artificial sweetener, such as Equal. It

Table 3-2: Popular Weight-Loss Diets

Type:	**Moderate and general**, e.g., Weight Watcher's, American Heart Association Diet
Key features:	Moderate calorie restriction, - encourages behavior modification and exercise.
Evaluation:	Slow weight loss; more likely to maintain loss over long-term
Type:	**Very low carbohydrate**, e.g., Atkins, South Beach Diet
Key features:	Less than 100 grams carbohydrate/day, restricted food choices
Evaluation:	Ketosis, nausea, water loss, faster weight-loss, hard to maintain loss
Type:	**Very low fat**, e.g., Dean Ornish Diet
Key features:	Mostly vegetarian, high fiber
Evaluation:	Very restricted food choices, hard to stay on diet
Type:	**Liquid formula**, e.g., Slimfast
Key features:	Formulated products for dieting, low-calorie, nutrient-loaded
Evaluation:	Boring, hard to maintain, low fiber
Type:	**Pre-packaged meal plan**, e.g., Nutri-System, Jenny Craig
Key features:	Centers around pre-packaged meals sold as part of plan; behavior modification, exercise encouraged
Evaluation:	Expensive; hard to maintain weight loss once off plan
Type:	**Novelty diets** (e.g., Grapefruit Diet)
Key features:	Emphasis on "magical" foods, nutrients, or food combinations
Evaluation:	Tend to be nutritionally poor

may be a soft drink sweetened with NutraSweet instead of sugar. Or it may be "light" sour cream, low-fat cheese, or non-fat milk.

Even if switching from high- to low-calorie versions of food doesn't lead to an overall reduction in calorie intake, nutrient intake is usually better.

But the body's controls over caloric intake are quire good. If we short-change ourselves on calories at one meal, or with one food, we tend to make up for it with another. So what can we do?

We eat by volume, so if we have fewer calories in a larger volume, we feel more satisfied and are less likely to overeat. Dr. Barbara Rolls has done extensive research in this area.[4-6] She has shown that people given lower calorie versions of a food (e.g., a large bowl of soup instead of small casserole of the same ingredients and calories) eat fewer calories, and that eating such foods (fewer calories per volume) are associated with sustained reductions in calorie intake.

What Works and the Low-Carb Myth

Diets work in the short-term, simply because we eat less. Keeping those pounds off is another matter. Most fail in the long-run because we go back to eating the way we did before. When we start a diet, we're motivated and focused, and lose weight. Even the most creative diet plans aren't all that creative because they use tried-and-true ways to get us to eat less.

- **Smaller portions**: Another no-brainer. We eat more when there's more there. Why not the bigger cup of soda if it's only 10 cents more? "Better" yet, free refills. We eat more from a big bag of chips than from a smaller bag. Bagels, muffins, portions of movie popcorn—have ballooned in size.

- **Doesn't taste as good**: Low-fat, low-carb, low-calorie stuff simply doesn't taste as good as "real" ice cream, cookies, cheese, chips, candy, and beverages. It's a no-brainer that when food doesn't taste as good, we eat less.

- **Costs more**: Sugar, refined grains, and oil/fat in various combinations give us the most calories for our dollar. A diet of snack food and fast food costs less and is more convenient than a diet of whole grains, vegetables, fruit, fish, and lean meat. Low-carb dieters aren't charged less for leaving the bun (and its calories) off the hamburger. Low-carb foods like steak and lobster are expensive. If a food costs more, we buy—and eat—less of it.

- **Keep track**: We're sure to eat fewer chips or cookies if we must write down how many we eat. Most of us can't eat whatever and whenever we want without putting on weight. When we keep track—whether it's calories, times we eat, carbs, or portion sizes—we eat less.

Table 3-3: Calories in Lunch from High vs. Lower Calorie Foods.

Lunch:　　　1 tuna sandwich
　　　　　　　　1 cup milk
　　　　　　　　2 canned peach halves

755 Calorie Version
Tuna sandwich:
　　　2 slices bread (140 cal)
　　　2 oz. tuna packed in oil (110 cal)
　　　1 small dill pickle, chopped (5 cal)
　　　2 Tbs. mayonnaise (200 cal)
1 cup whole milk (150 cal)
2 peach halves canned in heavy syrup (150 cal)

515 Calorie Version
Tuna sandwich:
　　　2 slices bread (140 cal)
　　　2 oz. tuna packed in water (75 cal)
　　　1 small dill pickle, chopped (5 cal)
　　　2 Tbs. low-fat mayonnaise (100 cal)
1 cup 1%-fat milk (105 cal)
2 peach halves canned in juice (90 cal)

•**More—or less—convenient:** A very convenient plan, such as a liquid meal in a can or a low-cal frozen meal, works. So does a not-so-convenient plan, such as having to make our own food using special recipes. This plan could even let us eat potato chips whenever we want—we just have to make them ourselves, starting with a raw potato. When you go to your kitchen for an evening snack, what do you find? Cookies, chips, ice cream, frozen pizza, and more? Or is there only fruit, popcorn, carrot sticks, frozen non-fat yogurt, bread, and the like?

Lowdown on Low-Carb

What about the low-carb diets? Yes, we love the shrimp, steaks, and bacon, and we may go wild on them at first, but low-carb pasta, bread, and sweets don't taste as good and cost more. The reality is that we can't have the pastries or bagels next to the office coffee pot, nor any fries with our bunless hamburger. Most or all of what's in the vending machine is off limits. Dining at a restaurant, we can't touch the bread basket, unless we want to eat the butter without the bread. The entrée comes with rice or potatoes or pasta, but

we can't eat that, nor any of the tempting desserts on the menu. We don't need much math to figure out that this adds up to eating fewer calories.

It's ironic that we use low-carb diets to lose weight, because low-carb is a metabolic signal for starvation. It sets in motion a way to prolong life in the continual famines that have beset human history. The usual reason why people aren't getting any carbohydrate is that there's no food—they are starving.

Our brains need and use glucose relentlessly. When we starve, our body stores of carbohydrate (glycogen) are quickly converted to glucose and depleted. Fat can't be made into glucose, forcing us to break down body protein to provide the amino acids that can be converted to glucose. We break down the least essential proteins first, and then move up the hierarchy until we reach the final stage of having to break down the essential protein structures in organs like the heart to provide the brain with glucose.

Our bodies buy time by slowing the process of tearing down body proteins. The low-carb signal triggers the body to increase the production of an alternate fuel for the brain—ketones.

Ketones are normally made in only small amounts from body fat. Muscles and such can burn fat itself for fuel. The brain can't. Even skinny people have a lot of calories stored as fat, so it makes sense for the body to make those calories available to the brain when we're starving to death. The brain keeps using glucose made from amino acids but, now that more ketones are available, it uses much less.

Those of us on low-carb weight-loss diets certainly aren't starving to death. What we like about the abundant ketones is that it can cause us to lose our appetite (sometimes to the point of nausea). In addition, some of the ketones overflow into our urine, pulling water along with it. This reduces, by pounds, the amount of water our body retains, buoying our spirits on the bathroom scale. Some ketones are also lost in our breath. (The ketone lost is acetone, the key ingredient in fingernail-polish remover, giving our breath a fruity odor.) The ketones lost in urine and breath do have some caloric value, but a relatively trivial amount.

Bottom Line

What's the bottom line on weight-loss diets? It's what we're tired of hearing: we need to eat fewer calories than we use. A better way to say it is that we need to use more calories than we eat. Being more physically active has, of course, many health benefits besides using calories.

We get a lot of health benefits simply by losing excess weight (lower blood pressure, better blood-cholesterol levels, less risk of diabetes and heart disease and some cancers, more endurance, less strain on our joints—the list goes on). This, in fact, makes it hard to compare the relative risks and benefits of various diets.

In the short term, anyway, the many beneficial effects of the weight loss itself can override any effects of the specific dietary components (low carb, low fat, etc.). When studies compare diets where the short-term weight loss is greater in one of them, better blood-cholesterol levels, for example, could very well be from the greater weight loss rather than the diet itself.

Whatever method we use to eat fewer calories, we want one that's healthful and that we can stick with for the rest of our lives. The best plan is a permanent change to a healthy diet and lifestyle.

Psychological Aids to Weight Control

Because emotions can affect how much we eat, influencing the emotions can be an important factor in weight reduction. The theory is good, but it's as hard to carry out as the nutritionist's simple injunction to "eat less and exercise more."

We've noted that the use of food to deal with emotional stress is instilled very early, and early psychological imprintings run deep. This helps to explain why traditional psychotherapy may or may not be successful in motivating patients to control their eating. If deeply rooted "oral" personality patterns can be dealt with—powerful tendencies to depend on nurturing situations and relationships as ways of dealing with pain or fear—the patient doesn't need to rely so much on eating or drinking to manage stress.

Psychiatrists have observed that some patients have mixed feelings about their weight, and mixed perceptions of themselves. Some patients who lose large amounts of weight become seriously depressed and anxious. Often they continue to think of themselves as fat people.

Attempts to make such basic changes in psychological orientation and function are both costly and time-consuming. Therefore, there have been many efforts to find more practical short-term routes to deal with obesity.

Using Group Support

One route uses the psychological pressures of the group—in club-like meetings of the overweight. Principles of dieting and nutrition may be taught to these groups, sometimes rather thoroughly, sometimes in a limited way. Such programs vary widely in quality. But for all of them, the approval-disapproval power of a group of peers and the sharing of common problems is an important part of the method. Having to pay to participate is also an added incentive to lose weight.

But all too often, as soon as the participants are out of the group, they founder. The situation can be much like children who behave very differently when their parents aren't watching.

Behavior Modification

Another route tends to be labeled loosely with the popular term "behavior modification." The term itself is, of course, a very broad one. In a sense, anything we teach people about nutrition is intended to change behavior for the better.

Behavior modification usually refers to a special kind of training, using various techniques to alter eating habits. Originally it began with the theories attributed to the social scientist B.F. Skinner, in which desirable behavior is rewarded and undesirable behavior is punished. As it developed, it dealt with issues like food cues, individual patterns of eating, and rewards and reinforcements for not overeating.

One focus of behavior modification is to increase awareness of food and the act of eating—to make it a more conscious act. Subjects might be taught to count bites of food, with the aim of reducing the number of bites taken each day, so that eating isn't a kind of blind, unthinking behavior.

A basic feature of such programs is record-keeping: Where, and under what circumstances did each eating episode take place? Participants learn to track the places they eat, and to avoid places like the couch in front of the television, that foster automatic, unconscious eating. Again, the aim is to teach a greater awareness of one's eating habits.

After several years of trial and error, the fact remains that in terms of long-term success, some weight-loss programs that use behavior modification techniques have achieved better results than have more traditional methods. Increasingly, specific behavior modification techniques have been incorporated in weight management programs, along with more traditional counseling on diet and exercise.

Obesity can be likened to a lifelong problem—a vulnerability that can be controlled, but for which there's no "cure." People who would lose weight in a nutritionally and medically sound way, must accept the truth that they have to eat fewer calories and/or be more physically active. They must understand the insurmountable facts of energy balance. They must be able to compare nutritive values as well as calorie counts. And they must make permanent changes in their dietary and/or exercise habits.

In the long run, shortcuts are likely to be only self-deceptions.

Anorexia and Bulimia

People with anorexia nervosa (often simply called *anorexia)* and bulimia take extreme measures to control their weight (see Personal Story at end of Chap. 18). Their eating disorders have their basis in a pathological fear of being fat. In this sense, they are emotional disorders. *Anorexia* means *without desire,* and refers to a lack of appetite for food. *Nervosa* refers to its being a "nervous" (emotional) condition. *Bulimia* literally means *to eat like an ox.*

In contrast to anorexics (people with anorexia),

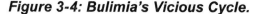

Figure 3-4: Bulimia's Vicious Cycle.

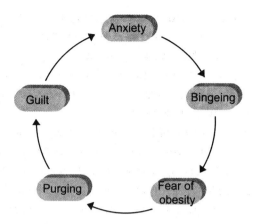

bulimics go on eating binges, consuming huge amounts of food at one sitting. Anorexia and bulimia have their own distinctive characteristics (see Table 3-4), but some people exhibit some of the symptoms of both. Sometimes the disorders are referred to together: *bulimarexia* or *bulimia nervosa.* Both disorders are most common among young upper-middle-class white women (but occur in men and other social and ethnic groups as well). Strong social pressures in this group to be slim are undoubtedly contributing factors, but the exact causes of these disorders aren't known.

Anorexics falsely see themselves as fat, even when they're emaciated to the point of near starvation. Typically, they refuse to eat much, and they exercise compulsively—a sure recipe for weight loss. As a result, they typically are 20 to 40% underweight. Many anorexics have to be hospitalized and fed intravenously to keep them from starving themselves to death.

In contrast, bulimics tend to be of normal weight. They maintain their weight by following their bingeing episodes (gorging themselves with thousands of calories worth of food—usually "junk food"—at one sitting) with induced vomiting, and often laxatives and diuretics as well (see Fig. 3-4). The bingeing and purging is almost always done in secret, and frequently goes undiagnosed.

The dentist is often the first to diagnose bulimia, because of the otherwise unexplained appearance of demineralized enamel. The repeated vomiting brings stomach acid into contact with the enamel of the teeth, causing it to dissolve.

Table 3-4: Anorexia Nervosa and Bulimia. *Having some of these characteristics doesn't diagnose the disease but should cause a person to reflect on their eating habits and related concerns.*

Anorexia Nervosa	Bulimia
• False body perception—thinking "I'm too fat," even when emaciated; relentless pursuit of thinness	• Secretive binge eating; never overeating in front of others
• Rigid dieting causing dramatic weight loss	• Eating when depressed
• Rituals involving food, excessive exercise, and other aspects of life	• Bingeing followed by fasting, laxative abuse, self-induced vomiting, or excessive exercise
• Maintenance of rigid control in lifestyle; security found in control and order	• Shame, embarrassment, deceit, and depression; low self-esteem and guilt (especially after a binge)
• Feeling of panic after a small weight gain; intense fear of gaining weight	• Fluctuating weight resulting from alternate bingeing and fasting
• Feelings of purity, power, and superiority through maintenance of strict discipline and self-denial	• Loss of control; fear of not being able to stop eating
• Preoccupation with food, its preparation, and observing another person eating	• Perfectionism, "people pleaser;" food as comfort/escape in carefully controlled and regulated life
• Helplessness in the presence of food	• Erosion of teeth, swollen glands
• Lack of menses after the normal age of puberty	

The medical problem of most concern is the regular large losses of electrolytes, such as chloride through the vomit (stomach acid is hydrochloric acid), and potassium from the use of certain diuretics. This can disrupt the beating of the heart which can, of course, be fatal.

The "gag me with a spoon" line in the song Valley Girls refers to the self-induced vomiting of bulimia. Actress Jane Fonda and singer Elton John had bulimia; it caused singer Karen Carpenter's death.

Clearly, anorexia and bulimia can have dire consequences and should be diagnosed and treated as early as possible. Treatment should be a team effort, including family members and health professionals such as physicians, psychologists, and dietitians.

Summary

Our total energy need is the number of calories we take in when we aren't gaining or losing weight. Since this number is elusive, we estimate our basal caloric need based on our body weight, gender, age, shape, and fatness. We add to this an estimated number of calories for physical activity, based on how active we are.

Obesity is defined in terms of Body Mass Index (BMI), calculated from height and weight. Obesity raises the risk of several diseases, as does excess abdominal fat (waist bigger than 35 inches in women, and 42 inches in men).

Fatness clearly has a genetic component, but environmental influences also are a determining factor. Obese people are particularly responsive to outside signals that remind one of food or eating (e.g., finding it hard to walk by a bakery without stopping to get a tidbit). An important part of weight control can be to minimize exposure to those cues.

To lose fat, we have to eat less or burn more calories to tip the energy balance towards that goal. This, of course, isn't so simple. There are deep-seated emotional reasons for eating, and the powerful pull of appetite makes it hard to tip the energy balance. For example, when we exercise more, we are usually hungrier. An important exception to this rule seems to be that the appetite of those who are sedentary and overweight doesn't seem to fully compensate for a moderate increase in physical activity.

Other advantages of increased physical activity for weight control include increased lean body mass, which increases basic calorie needs, and possibly a lower "set-point" weight. Also, added exercise may be a way of dealing with stresses that might otherwise lead to over-eating. Increased physical activity can make a crucial difference in one's ability to achieve significant and long-term weight loss.

Weight loss of about 1 lb/week is reasonable, considering the fact that the aim is to lose excess body fat, which requires a caloric deficit of about 3,500 calories per week. The best reducing plan is one that includes at least moderate physical activity, a diet that is nutritionally adequate, and behavior modification techniques to change eating and exercise habits so that long-term weight control is possible.

Anorexia Nervosa and Bulimia are eating disorders that take weight control to such extremes that health—and even life itself—can be in danger. Anorexics typically exercise compulsively and hardly eat, because they falsely see themselves as fat, even when they are dangerously emaciated. In contrast, bulimics mostly maintain their weight by inducing vomiting after eating huge amounts of food. These disorders should be diagnosed and treated as early as possible.

Part 2

Carbohydrates and the Foundations of Food

Chapter 4

The Trapping of the Sun

The forests of the earth have been the subject of passionate controversy. Nature lovers deplore the deforestation of virgin wilderness. Battles have raged over the logging of "natural habitats" of this or that "endangered species." Scientists have voiced concern over the relationship between forestation practices and global warming. It has even been asserted that trees cause pollution.

Are forests important to us for more than beauty and commerce? Is there indeed a wholeness in nature, between plants (including trees) on the one hand, and animals (including humans) on the other?

We are told that the ultimate source of all life-sustaining energy is the sun. Yet we humans cannot get our energy from just sitting in the sun. We must get it from our food. But how does it get into the food?

The answers to these questions involve an understanding of the wondrous interdependence of animals and plants. Each of us thrives on what the other produces—as if we were made for each other.

Lying on the beach on a summer day, we can feel the warmth of the sun. But we may not be aware of how much more the sun provides for our bodies. When we stroll over to the hot dog stand, do we think about how the energy for the stroll, as well as the calories in the hot dog came originally from the sun? We—and all other forms of earthly life—are intimately and ultimately dependent on the sun.

In this chapter, we look at how the sun gives birth to our food by a process called photosynthesis, and then we look at carbohydrate, the most abundant energy-providing nutrient in the world.

The Basic Equation of Photosynthesis

Joseph Priestley was a somewhat radical English minister and politician, who was eventually forced to emigrate to the United States for political and religious sanctuary. But he's best remembered for his secondary interest, chemistry, which led to the untangling of some of the first mysteries of photosynthesis.

One day in 1780, Priestley lit a candle that stood in a shallow dish of water. Then he inverted a jar over the candle, the water sealing the jar from the outside air.

He was limiting the ability of the candle to keep burning, since a candle burns by oxidation. The carbon in the wax combines with oxygen from the air and the reaction produces heat and light. The inverted jar was sealed, so the candle burned only as long as oxygen remained in the jar. As the oxygen was exhausted, the candle flickered and went out.

Air, of course, is a mixture of several gases, mainly nitrogen. But of these gases, only the oxygen could support the flame. In the burning, the oxygen from the air combined with the carbon of the candle wax to yield carbon dioxide. So what Priestley now had was a dead candle in an atmosphere of carbon dioxide and some other gases—and one thing more.

He had also placed a sprig of mint in the jar, with its stem in the water. The mint could receive light through the glass, and water through its stem.

A few days later, Priestley tested the gas from the inverted jar and found "...that the air would neither extinguish a candle, nor was it at all inconvenient to a mouse which I put into it."

In other words, somehow the living sprig of mint had used light and water and turned carbon dioxide back into oxygen again.

Within three years, French scientist Antoine Lavoisier had grasped the basics of the other side of the equation. Lavoisier found that animal life used up oxygen (just as Priestley's candle did) and gave off carbon dioxide (in which Priestley's mint had grown). In the process, heat was given off, as it was by the candle.

By 1800 it was becoming clear—with parts of the puzzle coming from scientists in many countries—that there was a balance between plants and animals, and that that balance involved the use of energy.

Dutch scientist Jan Ingenhousz had followed Priestley's lead and reported, "I observed that plants not only have the faculty to correct bad air...by growing in it...but that they perform this important office in a complete manner in a few hours; that this wonderful operation is by no means owing to vegetation of the plant, but to the influence of light of the sun upon the plant."

Closing the ring, Swiss scientists showed that both carbon dioxide and water were used up by plants during photosynthesis. And finally, in 1842, German surgeon Julius Mayer drew the correct fundamental conclusion about how it all worked. It was simple. He explained it in one sentence: "The plants take in one form of power, light; and produce another power, chemical difference."

The Chemical Birth of Food

It can be said that all our food begins with plants. For example, when we drink milk or eat beef, we get the energy that the cow stored by eating grass and other vegetable matter. And that vegetable matter got this energy from the sun— by a process called *photosynthesis*, which means "putting together with light."

The light in this case is, of course, the light of the sun ("solar energy"). What this light links together are two chemicals which the earth has

Figure 4-1: Cycling of Energy, CO₂, and O₂
Plant and animal life produce a natural balance: Plants produce oxygen and food using the sun's energy. Animals take in that oxygen and food, and use its energy, while turning it back into carbon dioxide and water.

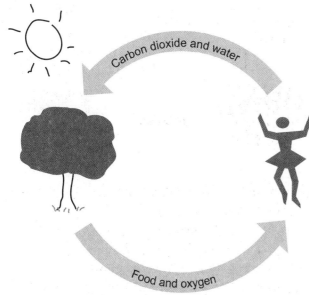

in abundance—carbon dioxide and water. If our body could put these two chemicals together itself, we could create our own energy sources. But it can't. We could sit all day in the sun, taking in both water and carbon dioxide by sipping carbonated beverages, and we'd end up with only a sunburn.

But plants have something we don't have—the phenomenal green chemical, *chlorophyll*. In the presence of chlorophyll, plants can use the sun's energy to combine carbon dioxide and water.

So plants combine the three atoms found in carbon dioxide (CO_2) and the three found in water (H_2O), and use solar energy to reassemble them. They end up with two products: two of the oxygen atoms join together to become oxygen gas. What is left over is a combination of one carbon, two hydrogen, and a single oxygen atom. In effect, the carbon has been combined with water ($C-H_2O$). The carbon has been hydrated—thus *carbohydrate*.

Photosynthesis's juggling act is:

$$H_2O + CO_2 + Energy = C-H_2O + O_2$$

In actuality, this hydrated carbon ($C-H_2O$) is combined with other hydrated carbons into the many forms of a plant's carbohydrate family.

The carbohydrate form that's a major source of energy for us is starch—a carbohydrate that has thousands of these hydrated carbon atoms. We, in fact, get energy from starch by "undoing" starch back into carbon dioxide and water (see Fig. 4-1).

Hydrate: To combine with water.

It could be said that we are solar-powered, since sunlight is the original source of the energy in the food we eat.

In nature, CO_2 in the atmosphere is kept in balance by animal life making CO_2, and plant life using CO_2. This balance can be upset by more CO_2 produced (e.g., more people; burning of gasoline, wood, coal) and less CO_2 removed (e.g., destroying forests). CO_2 is a "greenhouse gas" in that it traps solar heat. An increasing amount of these greenhouse gases causes global warming—the warming of the earth's surface and lower atmosphere—that can be ecologically disastrous.

Sugar Sweet

Sugar is the basic unit of carbohydrates. On the tongue, most sugars are immediately perceived as sweet. Some biologists speculate that sweetness is almost always perceived as pleasant because sweetness is the hallmark of carbohydrate. And a mix of carbohydrate-rich foods—fruits, vegetables, grains—form the core of nutritious diets throughout the world.

It should be noted that not all sweeteners are sugars. NutraSweet (aspartame, Equal) for example, is a laboratory-made sweetener made up of amino acids (the basic component of protein). It is two amino acids (phenylalanine and aspartic acid) linked together, with the caloric value of protein (4 cal/gm). It's a low-calorie sweetener because so little is needed for sweetening—it's about 150 times sweeter than table sugar (see Table 4-1).

Saccharin, Acesulfame-K, and cyclamate are also non-carbohydrate laboratory-made sweeteners. They are non-caloric: Although they are absorbed from the intestine, they can't be metabolized to produce energy, and are excreted in our urine.

Table 4-1: Approximate Relative Sweetness of Some Sweeteners.

10,000	Neotame
800	Sucralose (Spenda)
500	Saccharin
200	Acesulfame-K (Sunette, Sweet One)
180	Aspartame (NutraSweet, Equal)
100	Cyclamate
30	Tryptophan (an amino acid)
1.7	Fructose (sugar)
1.0	Sucrose ("table sugar")
0.7	Glucose (sugar)
0.5	Mannitol, sorbitol, inositol (sugar alcohols)
0.3	Maltose, lactose, galactose (sugars)
0	Starch

Figure 4-2: Single Sugars Glucose, Fructose, Galactose. Each is a different arrangement of 6 carbons, 12 hydrogens, and 6 oxygens. The molecules form rings of either 5 or 6 carbons.

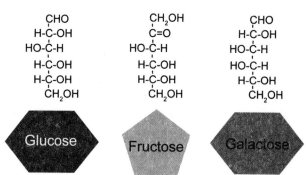

Single Sugars

The simplest sugars are called *single sugars (monosaccharides)*. Those found most commonly in food are *glucose, fructose*, and *galactose*. All three of these sugars have 6 carbons, 12 hydrogens, and 6 oxygens, but differently arranged (see Fig. 4-2).

Glucose (also called dextrose) is the most common single sugar. Glucose is also a component of the double sugars sucrose, lactose, and maltose (Fig. 4-3) and is the repetitive unit in starch, glycogen, and cellulose.

Fructose is about twice as sweet as glucose and is found naturally in such foods as honey and fruit. High-fructose corn syrup is commonly used to sweeten food products. It's much less expensive than sugar extracted from natural sources like sugar cane, and much sweeter than glucose or sucrose, so less is needed to sweeten a product. This markedly lowers a food company's cost of a product when high-fructose corn syrup is the main ingredient—as in most non-diet soft drinks.

High-fructose corn syrup is half glucose and half fructose (see Fig. 4-7), as is sucrose (table sugar) and honey, so there isn't any metabolic basis for it being "worse" than honey or regular sugar. Its main "problem" as a sweetener is that it's so inexpensive. Would we buy that Big Gulp® 32-oz (1 quart) or Double Big Gulp® 64-oz (half-

gallon) "cup" of a soft drink if it weren't so cheap and if it didn't taste so good?

Galactose is found mainly as a part of "milk sugar" (lactose, a double sugar) and is not very sweet—about half as sweet as glucose.

While we will not make deep forays into organic chemistry here, let's look a bit at the construction of these sugars—just to see the pattern by which Nature weaves the same few components into very different substances, each with its own special role.

Glucose, fructose, and galactose are all 6-carbon sugars—they're made up of six hydrated carbons. But these simple sugars aren't the smallest ones. There are some with only three carbon atoms and some with five.

Characteristically, the smaller sugars often appear as indispensable parts of some of the most complex chemicals of life. Consider the 5-carbon sugar called ribose. It's from this that the B-vitamin *riboflavin* takes its name. From ribose also come the names of the key chemicals of genetics, RNA and DNA—ribonucleic acid and *deoxyribonucleic* acid.

Ribose, important as it is, doesn't have to be consumed in foods. The body can make it from other carbohydrates. This suggests two principles that are contrary to popular belief:

• It isn't true that carbohydrates serve only the purpose of supplying energy. Although they aren't essential in the diet, carbohydrates also supply some of the important building blocks of life.

Figure 4-3: Double Sugars.

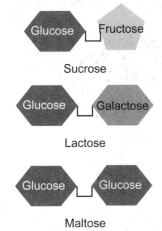

• A substance that's essential in the body—such as ribose (and cholesterol as well)—isn't necessarily essential in the diet. In fact, one might expect that the body, in its wisdom, would make its most essential substances rather than rely on dietary habits to provide a supply of them.

Double Sugars

The *double sugars (disaccharides)* are two single sugars linked together (see Fig. 4-3). Glucose and fructose—two single sugars that are common in the plant world—are very often combined. When one of each joins the other, we get *sucrose* (glucose + fructose)—common table sugar.

Table sugar is sucrose, a double sugar made of glucose and fructose.

It's hard to find a sweet-tasting fruit or vegetable which doesn't contain at least a little sucrose. And often there's more sucrose than either glucose or fructose alone. This is certainly the case of the sweet wild plant called *sugar cane*. Its sap runs rich with sucrose. Refining sugar is simply a matter of separating this sugar from the rest of the plant, which is almost entirely indigestible, as anyone knows who has chewed a stalk. (The same is true for the abundant sucrose in the sugar beet.)

The other most common double sugars found in our food are *lactose* and *maltose*. *Lactose* (glucose + galactose) is the sugar in milk and is the only carbohydrate of animal origin that is consumed in significant quantities. Maltose (glucose + glucose)

is the breakdown product of starch, and is the "malt" in malted milk and in the malted barley used to make beer.

When Sugars Get It Together

As plants trap the energy of the sun by making sugars from carbon dioxide and water, they also use that energy to assemble these sugars into chains. The ability of plants to chain sugars together is great indeed. The chains can be straight or branched, and they can run to thousands of sugars in a single chain.

When many sugars are chained together, the chains are called *polysaccharides* (many sugars) or *complex carbohydrates*. Chained together in this fashion, they are no longer sweet. Starch and cellulose are complex carbohydrates (see Fig. 4-4).

Digestible vs. Indigestible

Complex carbohydrates can be digestible or indigestible—depending on whether or not the digestive tract has the *enzymes* needed to digest them. The sugars that make up the chain can be linked together differently, and we can digest a particular complex carbohydrate only if we have the proper enzymes to break those particular links. Starch and glycogen are digestible. The dietary fiber cellulose is indigestible—a complex carbohydrate for which our digestive system has no enzymes.

"Digestible" means we have the enzymes to break the sugar-links. "Indigestible" means we do not.

Both starch (digestible) and cellulose (indigestible) are chains of glucose, but the glucoses are linked together differently (see Fig. 4-4). We only have digestive enzymes that break the links in starch, making starch digestible, but cellulose not. Plants contain both digestible and indigestible carbohydrates (see Fig. 4-4 and Table 4-2).

Enzymes

Enzymes are biological *catalysts*—they speed up life's chemical reactions. Without enzymes, the chemical reactions necessary for life would rarely occur. A reaction that would spontaneously

Figure 4-4: Complex Carbohydrates—Digestible and Indigestible.

Digestible:

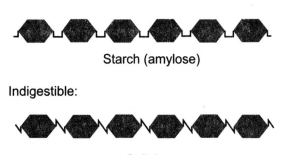

Starch (amylose)

Indigestible:

Cellulose

Figure 4-5: The enzyme sucrase breaks sucrose apart into glucose and fructose.

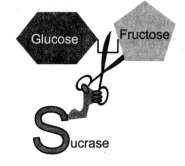

occur once in a thousand years could occur in one second with the help of an enzyme.

Heat, high pressure, and changes in acidity are commonly and conveniently used in laboratories and kitchens to speed chemical reactions. But in living things, severe changes in heat, pressure, and acidity are fatal.

Each enzyme is very selective as to what substance it will act on and what it will do. Our body has thousands of enzymes to catalyze the thousands of chemical reactions that occur in our body. Which enzymes our body can make dictates which chemical reactions take place.

An enzyme is usually named by adding the suffix *-ase* to the root name of its target substance. Lactase acts on lactose, sucrase acts on sucrose, etc. (see Fig. 4-5).

Starch

Starch is found in plants, and is made of hundreds to thousands of glucoses linked together. The glucose units are linked together in one of two patterns—a single straight chain or a highly branched chain—a complex carbohydrate indeed! The straight-chained form is called *amylose;* the highly branched form is called *amylopectin*. Plants contain a mixture of both forms of starch, but the proportions of the forms vary and give the various starches different characteristics. Amylose, for example, is a more effective thickener than amylopectin; thus starches higher in amylose (such as cornstarch) are more effective in thickening gravy.

Sugar is sweet and starch is not. Since starch is made of sugar, why is this? The sweetness of

a substance is determined in large part by how it fits into the receptor of the taste bud. Starch, being a very large molecule, is too large to fit into the receptor, and so—although it's composed entirely of glucose—it doesn't taste sweet. But if you chew a cracker and hold it in your mouth, it develops a sweet taste. This is because a digestive enzyme in our saliva (salivary amylase) has begun to break down the starch, releasing some maltose (a sweet double sugar made of two glucoses) into our saliva.

We can taste the result of sugar being converted to starch. Young corn, for example, is very sweet. But it becomes less sweet as it ages because more of its sugar is being converted to starch. The same is true of many other vegetables such as peas and carrots.

Why is starch formed as a vegetable matures? The answer lies in the demands of reproduction, which usually take precedence in the world of biology. Peas, for example, are really seeds for new plants. Until the new pea plants have been able to grow root systems and leaves—so that they can photosynthesize their own energy from sunlight—the infant plants must draw upon the energy reserves of the seed. In plants, starch is a more compact form of energy than sugar. Thus, as seeds mature they pack in energy as starch for the next generation.

Starch, then, is most concentrated in seeds and roots. These parts of plants are the major sources of calories for people throughout the world. Rice (a seed) is the staple food for nearly half of the world's population.[1] Wheat and corn (also seeds) and cassava and potatoes (roots) are other predominant staple foods.

Figure 4-6: Parts of wheat kernel. Starch is a digestible chain of glucose: amylose (straight chains), amylopectin (branched chains). Cellulose is straight-chained and indigestible.

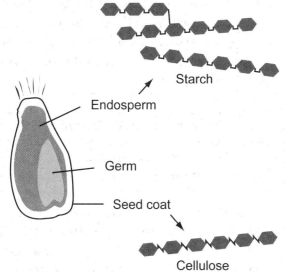

Table 4-2: Carbohydrate Production by Plants

A. Carbon dioxide (CO_2) and water (H_2O) combine to form hydrated carbons ($C-H_2O$) and oxygen (O_2) (see Fig. 4-1).

B. Six hydrated carbons combine to form the most common single sugars: glucose, fructose, and galactose (see Fig. 4-2).

C. These single sugars combine to form the double sugars (see Fig. 4-3):
   sucrose (glucose + fructose)
   lactose (glucose + galactose)
   maltose (glucose + glucose)

D. Hundreds of single sugar glucose units combine to form a digestible chain called starch. It can also be combined into an indigestible chain—the fiber cellulose (see Fig. 4-4).

Fruits tend to have less starch—and their seeds are likely to be the parts we don't eat. (When we do eat the seeds, they are largely indigestible.) The function of the flesh of fruits seems more for attracting animals and insects to dine, so that the seeds will be exposed and distributed over the ground. The edible portion of many fruits (bananas, peaches, etc.) become sweeter with ripening, as their starch turns into sugar. This sweetening makes them more likely to be eaten.

Ingested, undigested seeds become part of the stool—seeds surrounded by "natural fertilizer."

Corn is a major crop in the U.S. and a major part of our food supply. There's whole corn, corn oil, corn meal, cornstarch, corn syrup, high-fructose corn syrup, and corn is also fed to animals we eat. Understanding how carbohydrates are related, we can see how cornstarch (a glucose polymer) can be broken up into individual glucose molecules (dextrose) and liquified (corn syrup), and that converting half of the glucose molecules to fructose gives us high-fructose corn syrup.

Glycogen

Glycogen is the complex carbohydrate found in animal tissue. Like the amylopectin in starch, it's made entirely of glucose units, and is highly branched. Glycogen is sometimes called "animal starch."

Glycogen is an insignificant source of energy in food since there are only trace amounts in the meat we eat. But in the body, glycogen is an important source of glucose, because there's a substantial amount in terms of the whole body, and because this glucose is readily available. Although low in concentration in tissues, the body has a lot of tissue, and, therefore, glycogen represents a sizable store of glucose and potential energy.

The body stores about 300 grams (~11 oz) of glycogen. Carbohydrate has 4 calories per gm, so 300 gm of glycogen can provide 1,200 calories.

Glycogen is stored in two places—liver and muscle. About a third of the glycogen is found in the liver. The liver uses glycogen to store and release glucose, as needed, to keep glucose levels in the blood within a normal range. The other two-thirds of the glycogen is found in muscle, where it's used to fuel muscle activity.

The quick availability of this glucose source is the result of glycogen's highly branched structure. Glucose is released at the ends of the chains. The branching gives many more ends from which glucose can be released. If the glucose chain were a long, single strand, as in amylose, there would be only two ends from which glucose could be released. The highly branched structure of glycogen allows for a very rapid release of glucose when it's needed to raise blood-glucose levels or to fuel muscle activity.

Fiber

Fiber is a general, collective term for the indigestible, but edible, parts of plants. Fiber is not necessarily made of sugars, but most of them are chains of sugar or sugar-like substances. Fiber generally serves as the supportive component of plants. For example, the fiber content of celery, rhubarb, and asparagus is high because they are stems. Vegetables such as cabbage are also fibrous; the thick stems of their leaves form their supportive structure.

With all the current talk about fiber, it should be pointed out that fiber isn't always the coarse stuff that gets caught between your teeth. There are a wide variety of fibers, including some found in soft and even liquid foods.

The original chewing gum was a fiber—a chunk of chicle (the dried sap of the Mexican sapodilla tree)—today's chewing gum is made from synthetic polymers (e.g., polyvinyl acetate).

Based on whether or not they dissolve in water, they are divided into two basic groups: soluble fibers and insoluble fibers. (Soluble fibers tend to make things more viscous rather than coarse and chewy.) But fiber isn't easily categorized. Some kinds of fibers fall into both groups. For example, some hemicellulose fibers are soluble in water whereas others aren't. Also, various fibers are partially fermented by bacteria in the colon, producing varying amounts of short-chain fatty acids that we can absorb and use.

Insoluble Fibers

The insoluble fibers include *cellulose, lignin,* and some *hemicellulose.* Cellulose, in fact, is the most abundant plant product on earth. Plentiful in celery, it's also the main constituent of most wood, and represents virtually all of cotton.

Like the amylose in starch, cellulose is a straight chain of many glucose units linked together (see Fig. 4-4). But in cellulose, as discussed earlier, the glucose units are linked together differently than in amylose, making cellulose indigestible by humans.

Although our digestive enzymes can't break the links between the glucose units in cellulose, many microorganisms can. Ruminants, such as cows, have bacteria residing in their rumen that can break apart the cellulose in grass and hay, enabling the cow to absorb the resulting sugars. In other words, grass is fattening for cows and non-fattening for us.

A *ruminant* is an animal with several chambers in its stomach, one of which is called the *rumen.* After food goes through the rumen, it's regurgitated back into the mouth where it (the cud) is chewed a second time. This is why *ruminating* also means *thinking it over.*

Like starch, cellulose absorbs water. Hemicellulose is also effective in holding water. Since cellulose and hemicellulose pass through the digestive tract undigested, their holding of water adds bulk and softness to stools. Prunes, peanuts, and bran are good sources of cellulose and hemicellulose.

Soluble Fibers

The soluble fibers include *pectin, gums,* and some *hemicellulose.* Pectin is one of the most common soluble fibers, and is made of galactose and other less-familiar sugars. Apples, oranges, and carrots are good sources of pectin. Pectin can form gels and is thus useful in thickening jams and jelly.

Pectin can also bind to bile products in the intestine and promote their excretion in the stool. (Cellulose doesn't have this property.) As will be discussed later, bile-binding substances such as pectin can be helpful in lowering cholesterol in the blood. Since apples are a good source of pectin, perhaps it's the pectin in "an apple a day [that] keeps the doctor away."

Some soluble fibers are common food additives. Because they form gels, they're useful as stabilizers, emulsifiers, and thickeners in food products such as ice cream and salad dressing. *Carrageenan,* for example, is a soluble fiber taken from red seaweed. It's not only added to food, but is also added to lotions and medicines because of its moisture-holding capability and its gel-like consistency.

Table 4-3: Fiber Content of Some Foods

Grains:	
1/2 cup cooked barley	4 gm
1 slice whole-wheat bread	2 gm
1/2 cup cooked brown rice	2 gm
1 corn tortilla	1 gm
1 cup popcorn	1 gm
Breakfast cereals:	
1 cup Grape Nuts or 40% Bran Flakes	7 gm
1 cup Crunchy Bran or Shredded Wheat	5 gm
1 cup Wheaties, Total or Cheerios	3 gm
1/2 cup cooked oatmeal	3 gm
1 cup Alpha Bits, Golden Grahams	1 gm
Legumes (cooked):	
1/2 cup pinto beans	7 gm
1/2 cup garbanzo beans or peanuts	6 gm
1/2 cup kidney beans or navy beans	5 gm
1/2 cup split peas	4 gm
1/2 cup lentils	3 gm
2 Tbs peanut butter	2 gm
Vegetables (cooked):	
1/2 cup corn, green peas, or okra	3 gm
1/2 cup carrots, broccoli, or cabbage	2 gm
1/2 cup mushrooms or onions	2 gm
1 potato	2 gm
1/2 cup green beans, celery, or kale	1 gm
Fruit:	
1/2 cup blackberries or raisins	4 gm
1 avocado or pear	4 gm
1 apple, orange, or kiwi	3 gm
1 banana, peach, or nectarine	2 gm
4 prunes	2 gm
1/2 cup sliced strawberries	2 gm
1/2 cup cantaloupe or honeydew	1 gm
1 lemon, lime or tangerine	1 gm

Algin and *agar* are also gelatinous fibers taken from seaweed and added to foods. (Agar is perhaps more well-known for its use in solidifying the broth—agar plates—used to grow bacteria in the laboratory.) Gums are also soluble fibers taken from various plants and used in food products, and include *gum arabic, locust bean gum,* and *guar gum.*

It should be noted that the fiber in food comes as a mix. Carrots and apples, for example, are rich in pectin, but they also contain some cellulose, hemicellulose, and lignin. Fiber may be quite subtle, so that you're really not aware of it at all. By the time the carrots and celery in your stew have simmered for several hours, you may not suspect that you are eating fiber.

Fibers can be relatively short-chained. For example, beans have fibers containing chains of only three or four sugars. Like other fibers, these can't be digested because we don't have the digestive enzymes to take them apart. But some of the microbes living in our lower intestine do have the enzymes to break apart some of these particular fibers in beans. And they do split up some of those sugars, with a waste product of mainly carbon dioxide and water. The carbon dioxide from this bacterial digesting is a cause of some of the intestinal gas that often results from eating beans.

Remember, too, that our definition of these substances as indigestible is very human-centered. One species' fiber is another's meat and potatoes: The shells of lobsters and grasshoppers are made of a long-chain carbohydrate known as *chitin*, which snails flourish on. And termites dine gloriously on the cellulose of wood. The fiber content of some foods is shown in Table 4-3.

Carbohydrate-The Staple Diet

A high-carbohydrate diet is common for much of the world's population. The typical American diet—high in fat, low in fiber—is the rather odd one.

People have been subsisting mainly on carbohydrates for thousands of years, ever since the development of crops made civilization possible and ended dependence on the hunt. According to anthropologists, the change started between 8000 and 6000 B.C., perhaps earlier.

Some domestication of animals developed about the same time—some kept for milk and others for meat. But a lot of land was needed to supply food for each animal, land which could yield food for many people when planted with grains. The result wasn't surprising. Animals as food became mainly the luxury of the rich.

The general situation hasn't changed very much. Except for the hunting peoples of the earth, the poor must live largely on plant foods. Since the world remains mostly poor, most of the people on our planet are dependent on grain (rice, wheat, corn) and roots (cassava, potatoes) for their calories and protein.

It's true that we find most of our real malnutrition among these people. But this isn't mainly attributable to the fact that the bulk of their food comes from plants. Rather, the main problem is their poverty. For when the world's food supply is short, or when local crops fail, prices rise and drive the poorest from the market. They stand last in line.

Poverty also tends to confine such people to narrow and monotonous diets, with the vast majority of their food coming from just one or two kinds of plants, such as cassava, sorghum, or rice. There's an important lesson here: Much of their malnutrition provides eloquent testimony for the nutrition principle that variety is the best guarantee of good nutrition—and that monotony is the handmaiden of bad nutrition.

At any rate, it's perhaps ironic that the typical American diet can be improved by eating more of the poor man's carbohydrate-rich plant foods—foods which are generally low in saturated fat and calories, rich in fiber, and devoid of cholesterol.

Back to Sugar

Some of the most cherished myths about food and health involve carbohydrates. For example, a common myth is that sugar is poison to our body. While sugar can cause tooth decay (discussed in the next chapter), it's hardly a poison. All carbohydrates are absorbed from the intestine as single sugars.

Let's suppose that we've just taken a bite of Thanksgiving candied sweet potato. Like virtually all foods, it has many components. It has a large number of chemical compounds, some of which play a role in nutrition and some of which do not. But since the chief nutrient substances in the dish are two classes of carbohydrates—starch in the potato, and sugar in both the potato and the candied topping—we can learn some principles by following a bite.

The starch and sugar in the sweet potato are digested to single sugars (monosaccharides) before they're absorbed into the bloodstream (details

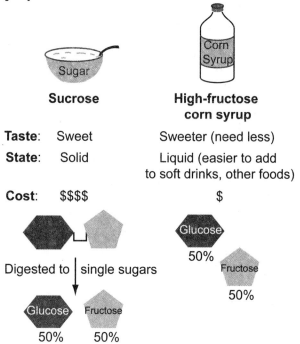

Figure 4-7: Sugar vs. High-Fructose Corn Syrup.

of digestion will be discussed in Chap. 10.) Our sweet potato is now quite unrecognizable. Its usable carbohydrate is thoroughly broken apart into the single sugars, like the blocks of a child's building set. For it's only in very simple forms that nutrients can actually enter the bloodstream to take part in life processes.

We use the example of sweet potatoes. But whether we begin with Fruit Loops, organically-grown turnips, high-fructose corn syrup, or our sweet potato, what passes through our intestinal wall into our bloodstream is mainly glucose and fructose, with perhaps some galactose if milk is poured over the Fruit Loops.

Different foods release their sugars at different speeds, depending on particle size, fiber content, etc. Starch in brown rice, for example is digested slower than starch in white rice. Glycemic Index is a measure of how high a particular food raises your blood sugar. As you'd expect, jelly beans have a much higher Glycemic Index than pinto beans.

Once these sugars enter the bloodstream, their origin matters no more to the cells that will use them than do the origins of oxygen matter to the lung—whether from an ocean breeze, or a scuba tank. Glucose is glucose. Fructose is fructose.

Figure 4-8: Corn is used for many products.

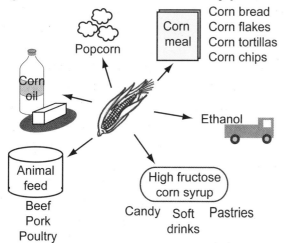

Indeed, the next step is toward even greater simplicity. The blood coming from the intestine goes directly to the liver—and the final simplification of the sugars. Virtually all the single sugars which aren't already glucose are converted by the liver into glucose.

If you've ever wondered why hospitals tend to provide caloric supplementation to patients by using only simple glucose (also called dextrose), the reason should now be clear. Ultimately, glucose is the sole carbohydrate used by most body cells for energy.

Alcohol

Alcohol is a fermentation product of carbohydrate. Yeast converts sugar to alcohol, using enzymes for this conversion. The first enzymes were, in fact, discovered in yeast, and the word *enzyme* comes from the Greek words meaning *in yeast*. Alcohol has an energy value of about 200 calories per ounce (7 calories/gram).

Yeast use sugars—not starch—in fermentation. For this reason, sweet liquids, such as the juice of sweet fruits (including wine grapes) are good starters for making alcohol.

Starch must be first broken down to the sugar maltose or glucose before the yeast can use it. One way to do this is by a process appropriately called malting: Grain is allowed to germinate (sprout) for a few days; this produces enzymes that convert starch (the plant's stored form of energy) to maltose and glucose (providing the fuel for the seedling).

There are other ways of converting starch to sugars for alcohol production. One particularly interesting method was used in Peru in the 16th century:[2] Corn was ground and soaked in a pot of water. People then chewed this soaked corn, thereby breaking it into smaller pieces and mixing it with a digestive enzyme in saliva that breaks the cornstarch into maltose. Rather than swallowing the mixture, it was spit into a pot, where the action of the enzyme continued. Then, the entire mixture was boiled for several hours. This killed microbes from the saliva and concentrated the sugars by evaporating the water. The mixture was then filtered, providing a clear liquid rich in sugars, ready for fermentation.

In wine, grape juice typically provides the sugar that's converted to alcohol; in beer, malted barley commonly provides the sugar. Such wine and beer thus have some of the nutrients that are in grapes and barley.

Wine and beer also have a limited alcohol content because yeast can't grow once the alcohol reaches about 15-20% by volume. Wine is about 12% alcohol, beer about 4%.

In order to make high-alcohol liquors (hard liquor), the alcohol must be distilled (vaporized and condensed). Alcohol vaporizes at a lower temperature than water, so when a mixture of alcohol and water is heated, the alcohol will vaporize first, separating and concentrating it.

Alcohol content of distilled liquors is designated by proof. Doubling the % alcohol in the liquor gives its proof, e.g., liquor designated as 100 proof is 50% alcohol by volume. Brandy (~80 proof) is distilled from wine; whiskey (~90 proof) from beer; and rum (~90 proof) from fermented molasses.

Distilled liquors are not only a concentrated source of calories because of their high alcohol content, but are essentially devoid of nutrients. The small amount of nutrients in the original fermented product is left behind in the distillation process. For some people, more than half their caloric intake comes from alcohol. It isn't surprising that people who drink a lot of alcohol are susceptible to nutrient-deficiency diseases, as well as the toxic effects of alcohol itself.

An increasing amount of our corn crop is being used to produce ethanol to partially replace gasoline (see Fig. 4-8). But this isn't very energy-efficient, because the energy in the alcohol produced isn't much more than the energy in the fossil fuel used to produce it (ratio 1.4). In contrast, Brazil uses sugar cane to produce alcohol, and gets ten times as much alcohol-energy than the fossil-fuel energy it puts in (ratio 10.2).[3] Brazil produces 4.2 billion gallons of alcohol per year, and doesn't need to import oil to meet its energy needs.[3]

The production of biofuels from corn is economically feasible in the U.S. because the production and the corn crop are government-subsidized. The diversion of corn for alcohol production raises the price of many foods, including meat from corn-fed animals, corn tortillas, food sweetened with high-fructose corn syrup, and even our movie popcorn (see Fig. 4-8).

The U.S. Dept. of Energy is backing refineries to make ethanol from cellulose,[4] e.g., from corn cobs and husks, expected to be completed in 2009-2011.[4] The energy-efficiency of making ethanol from cellulose (ratio 10.0) is similar to making ethanol from sugar cane, but the process is much more difficult.[3,4]

Summary

Carbohydrates are created by photosynthesis: The energy of the sun is captured by the green chlorophyll in plants to create hydrated carbons—carbohydrates—from carbon dioxide and water. In fact, plant life and animal life provide a natural balance—plants produce food and oxygen, and animals take in that food and oxygen and turn it back into carbon dioxide and water.

The simplest carbohydrates are called single sugars (monosaccharides). The single sugars most common in food are glucose, fructose, and galactose. When two sugars are linked together, they are called double sugars (disaccharides). The most common ones are sucrose (glucose + fructose), lactose (glucose + galactose), and maltose (glucose + glucose).

When many sugars are linked together, they are called polysaccharides or complex carbohydrates. We can digest only some of them, depending on whether we have the proper digestive enzymes. (Enzymes are biological catalysts that enable life's chemical reactions to take place.) The digestible complex carbohydrates include starch and glycogen. Starch is the storage form of glucose in plants; glycogen is the storage form of glucose in animals.

There are various indigestible complex carbohydrates, which are collectively called fiber. In fact, the definition of fiber is simply the edible but indigestible parts of plants, since fibers aren't necessarily complex carbohydrates. But most fibers, are chains of sugar or sugar-like substances. Fibers include a wide variety of substances, classified according to whether they dissolve in water—soluble fibers and insoluble fibers.

Insoluble fibers include cellulose, lignin, and some hemicellulose. These form the structural components of plants and add bulk and softness to stools. Soluble fibers include pectin, gums, and some hemicellulose. Many of these impart gel-like qualities to food, and can bind to bile products in the intestine. All plants contain an intimate mixture of various fibers which vary in their physical properties, health effects, and how well they are fermented by bacteria in the colon.

Carbohydrate-rich foods—plant foods—are the staple food for most of the world's population. The typical American diet—a high-fat, low-fiber diet—can be improved by including more of these plant foods.

Carbohydrates have a caloric value of 4 calories per gram, and must be broken down to single sugars (monosaccharides) before they are absorbed from the digestive tract. Practically speaking, fiber, indigestible as it is, has no caloric value (though short-chain fatty acids produced from some fibers by bacterial in the colon do). Alcohol, a fermentation product of carbohydrate, has 7 calories per gram.

Chapter 5

Of Carbohydrates And Health

There are a lot of popular perceptions of carbohydrate ("carbs"), many of them not very flattering. One is that whatever it is, it makes you fat, and you'd better stay away from it if you're concerned about weight (which means quite a few of us).

Part of the negative image is certainly tied to the identification with low-carb diets and with "sugar." For many, carbohydrates are synonymous with sugar—and of course many of us have been taught that sugar is bad. Another word with unfortunate associations is "refined," which a lot of carbohydrates seem to be. If a food once had some virtues, it (like some people) clearly lost them when it became refined.

On the other side, the government and the professional health community has been urging us to eat more complex carbohydrates. Are there good carbs and bad carbs? Are they related? How can we tell the difference?

The basic story of carbohydrates is quite simple. It can easily straighten out several popular misconceptions. And it can equip us to judge popular health claims and make important food choices that we know make sense.

Low-carb diets wax and wane in popularity. Are carbs really the cause of obesity, as some popular writers would have us believe? Are sugars to blame for diabetes and hyperactivity? How real are these ideas about carbohydrate and its effects?

We begin our look at the health implications of carbohydrates by looking at the scientific view of blood sugar. We then examine some other aspects of carbohydrates and health, including the relationship between sugar and tooth decay, and the possible role of fiber in reducing the risk of diverticulosis and colon cancer. The chapter ends with a look at the role of carbohydrates in athletic performance.

The Doctor Looks at Blood Sugar

By the time carbohydrates from food reach the bloodstream, they've been broken down by digestion into single sugars, mostly glucose. Other single sugars are readily converted to glucose.

Glucose in the blood (blood glucose) is kept within a normal range by the action of two *hormones* made in the pancreas: *insulin* and *glucagon*. After carbohydrate is ingested, blood glucose rises, and insulin is secreted in response. Insulin promotes the entry of glucose into cells, thereby lowering the level of blood glucose (see Fig. 5-1).

Hormone: A chemical messenger secreted in one location, carried in the bloodstream, and having specific effects elsewhere. e.g., the pancreas secretes the hormone glucagon, which causes the release of glucose from the liver.

When one hasn't eaten for a few hours, blood glucose falls, and the pancreas secretes glucagon in response. Glucagon triggers the release of glucose from liver glycogen (the body's storage form of glucose). This raises blood glucose (see Fig. 5-1).

Insulin and the Causes of Diabetes

The most common blood-glucose-related medical problem is *diabetes mellitus,* characterized by an abnormally high blood-glucose (see Fig. 5-2). Some of this glucose "spills over" into the urine,

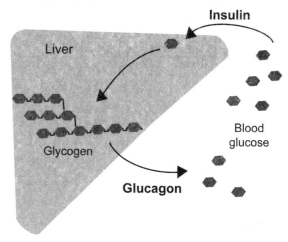

Figure 5-1: Insulin and glucagon use liver glycogen to maintain blood glucose. When blood-glucose falls, glucagon releases glucose from liver glycogen. When blood-glucose rises, insulin promotes glycogen production and storage.

bringing water along with it. As of 2005, about 21 million people in the United States—7% of the population—have diabetes, and about 6 million of them don't know they have it (haven't been diagnosed).[1]

Unlike low blood sugar, which catches your immediate attention by symptoms like weakness and fainting, high blood sugar itself doesn't make you feel bad. Diabetes is diagnosed when your doctor discovers abnormally high blood-glucose in a routine check-up, or because you've gone in because of a sudden increase in urination or thirst—or because you've developed more serious problems. Early diagnosis and treatment of diabets are important.

Diabetes, from the Greek, means *passing through*, referring to the fact that untreated diabetics urinate often. To this is added the term *mellitus*, derived from the word for honey—the urine of the untreated diabetic is sweet with sugar.

Type 1 Diabetes

About 5-10% of diabetics have type 1 diabetes, characterized by an inadequate amount or a total lack of insulin, due to destruction of the pancreatic cells that make insulin. It isn't associated with obesity, and occurs most commonly among children and adults under 30 years of age. It's controlled with insulin injections, diet, and exercise.

Before insulin was available as a drug, insulin-dependent diabetes was quite rapidly fatal. Present evidence suggests that this type of diabetes is primarily an autoimmune disease that can be triggered by certain viruses. In autoimmune diseases, the body mistakenly sees a normal part of the body as foreign and destroys it via its immune system. In this case, the part seen as foreign is the cells in the pancreas that make insulin.

Human insulin can be made by biotechnology. Before, the only insulin available for diabetics came from extracting animal pancreases.

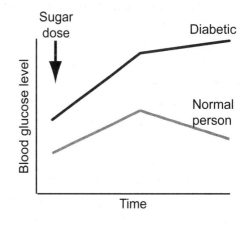

Figure 5-2: Blood glucose levels are abnormally high in untreated diabetics.

Type 2 Diabetes

About 90-95% of diabetics have type 2 diabetes, and most of them are overweight.[2] Not all overweight people develop this disease, however, since a genetic susceptibility is involved. This kind of diabetes is generally characterized by the resistance of cells to insulin action. The cells can't adequately remove glucose from the blood, despite a normal amount of insulin.

The risk of type 2 diabetes increases with age. In the U.S., an alarming 10% of adults over age 20, and 20% of adults over age 60 have diabetes.[1] Type 2 diabetes is typically an adult disease, but as obesity has become more common at younger ages, so has diabetes. It's now seen increasingly in children and adolescents.

Obesity brings out a genetic tendency to diabetes, just as alcohol consumption can bring out a genetic tendency to alcoholism, or a high-salt diet can bring out a genetic tendency to salt-sensitive high blood pressure. An interaction of environment and genetics is a common theme in disease. As obesity has increased, so has diabetes (see Fig. 1-1, 1-2).

Regular exercise, in addition to helping to control weight, increases a cell's responsiveness to insulin. Type 2 diabetes often can be controlled with weight control, exercise, and diet. When overweight, even a small loss of weight is helpful. Various oral medications can be used, and sometimes insulin injections are needed as well.

One of the most severe effects of diabetes (both type 1 and type 2) is damage to blood vessels. Since all tissues are served by blood vessels, the consequences depend most on which vessels are affected and how severely they are affected.

There's wide individual variation in how fast diabetes progresses—some diabetics develop severe symptoms rapidly, whereas others have only mild and non-progressing disease. But overall, adults with diabetes, compared with adults of the same age without diabetes, have twice the death rate, including a 2-4 times higher death rate from heart disease or stroke.[1] Diabetes is the leading cause of kidney failure, and a major cause of blindness, nerve damage, and amputations below the knee.

Whether the cause of diabetes is a lack of insulin or a resistance to the action of insulin, glucose doesn't get into cells as it should, and glucose builds to abnormally high levels in the blood. We see that a high blood-sugar is a result of diabetes, not its cause.

A diet high in carbohydrate doesn't cause diabetes. In fact, the prescribed diet for diabetics is rich in whole grains and vegetables—foods rich in starch and fiber, allowing the glucose to enter the bloodstream more slowly. The diet limits sugars, such as table sugar, corn syrup, honey, raw sugar, and foods high in such sugars. Large amounts of these sugars, rapidly consumed, cause a surge in blood-glucose levels. This can mean trouble for diabetics, with their impaired ability to deal with glucose.

Diabetes Prevention and Treatment

There isn't yet a way to prevent type 1 diabetes (studies are underway). For type 2 diabetes, excess body fat, especially around the belly, increases the risk, so weight control by exercise and diet is important (see Chap. 3). For the overweight, losing weight is hard, and gaining weight is easy, so if one isn't losing weight, the goal should be to not gain more.

Treatment for type 1 and type 2 diabetes focuses on keeping blood-glucose levels in check. Type 1 diabetics do this with insulin injections, diet, and exercise. Some type 2 diabetics can control blood-glucose with only diet and exercise, but many need oral medication, and some also need insulin injections. Weight control in the overweight is also a major focus in the treatment of type 2 diabetes.

Gestational Diabetes

Gestational diabetes occurs in some women during pregnancy; screening is a part of routine prenatal care in the U.S. If blood glucose is controlled by diet, exercise, and sometimes medication, there's no harm to the mother or baby.

The risk factors and treatment are similar to type 2 diabetes. The diabetes usually goes away after pregnancy, but women with gestational diabetes have a 20-50% chance of developing type 2 diabetes within 5 to 10 years.[1]

Are Carbohydrates Dangerous?

Large amounts of sugar cause problems for a diabetic, but what about the rest of us? Can sugar and other carbohydrates in excess be hazardous to one's health? They can, but in the context that all nutrients, even water, can cause problems in large enough amounts.

True, these substances are needed by the body. Therefore, the body has mechanisms for using them, as well as mechanisms for dealing with excesses beyond need. But eventually, there comes a point at which the body's mechanisms for use, and for protection against excess, are overwhelmed.

One of the primary questions when judging food safety is, what is the expected use of the

Figure 5-3: Recommended Diet.

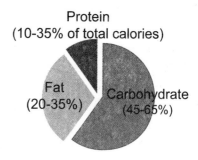

food in relation to the rest of the diet? In the case of carbohydrates, the typical American intake is well within tolerance. Our intake is far less than that of many nations, some of which have diets which are 80% carbohydrate and more.

Another important thing to know about carbohydrates is that if we don't consume any—a difficult trick, for there is some carbohydrate in the vast majority of foods—the body will make some. We can, for example, make glucose from protein.

Does this mean that we don't really need to eat carbohydrate foods? No, it would be unhealthy for us. Grains, vegetables, and fruits—all carbohydrate-rich foods—provide us with an abundant source of vitamins, minerals, and fiber. And compared to protein-rich and fat-rich foods—usually animal foods—they provide us with an inexpensive source of calories.

We need a daily minimum of about 200 calories worth of carbohydrate (50 grams). Otherwise, the body must rely on the conversion of other nutrients to carbohydrates, and there can be an accelerated breakdown of body protein, and dehydration.

But this doesn't mean that such a minimum is desirable. It's recommended that 45-65% of our calories come from carbohydrate (900-1300 calories-worth in a 2,000-calorie diet.) (See Fig. 5-3.)

Is there any recommendation about the kind of carbohydrate? Yes, there is. The overconsumption of overly-refined carbohydrate foods (as well as calorie-dense foods high in fats) reduces our intake of vitamins, minerals, and fiber. That's why nutritionists caution against consuming too much of our diet in the form of refined grains or sugar, and too little in the form of whole grains, vegetables, and fruits.

But this advice can easily be misinterpreted. Let's consider one misinterpretation—the idea that relatively isolated sugars and starches are somehow harmful in themselves, rather than potentially harmful because they may displace other nutrients. This erroneous deduction leads some popular writers to describe isolated sugars and starches as "poisons."

The reality is that a molecule of sucrose remains a molecule of sucrose, no matter what its source. "Refining" refers to what happens to the total food, rather than specific nutrients. So refined carbohydrate foods have substances removed, substances which might or might not have nutritive value. But the sugar or starch itself is likely to be unchanged in the food. In any event, before carbohydrates enter our bloodstream, digestion will have brought them all to the "refined" form of simple sugar.

Honey, maple syrup, corn syrup, white sugar, brown sugar, raw sugar, and white flour are all refined foods, separated—by a tree, a bee, or by a machine—from much that was in their original sources. To our cells, they are no more "toxic" than the same sugars and starch would be in apples, raisins, or wheat.

Reality and Hypoglycemia

What about the idea that we eat too much carbohydrate, and this has resulted in widespread *hypoglycemia* (low blood sugar)? As is often the case in many popular nutrition articles, there's a bit of truth topped with a heap of fiction.

Hypoglycemia is a condition of abnormally low blood glucose. Its symptoms are relieved by dietary sugar. The symptoms range from mild (e.g., dizziness, nervousness, hunger) to severe (e.g., convulsions, coma). The most common cause of severe hypoglycemia is excess insulin taken by a diabetic.

Some people experience mild hypoglycemia as a result of a temporary overproduction of insulin, paradoxically in response to a large amount of dietary carbohydrate. When taken on an empty stomach (e.g., skipping breakfast, and having a soft drink and pastry in mid-morning), the sudden carbohydrate intake causes a surge in blood glucose, in turn stimulating a surge in insulin secretion that can overshoot its mark.

This type of hypoglycemia is appropriately called *reactive hypoglycemia*. The symptoms are fairly mild, occur 2 to 4 hours after eating, and the advice is to ingest smaller "doses" of carbohydrate (e.g., an apple rather than a candy bar for a snack) in more frequent and well-spaced intervals.

Many people decide that they have hypoglycemia when they actually don't. (A true diagnosis must be made by a physician and includes testing blood-sugar levels.) It's a popular diagnosis because the symptoms are quite vague, and a diagnosis of "hypoglycemia" has been effective in promoting an array of worthless products, as well as the pet themes of some misguided health-practitioners and some authors of best-selling diet-and-health books.

Certain popular authors claim that low blood sugar afflicts a major part of our population, and see it as the cause of an endless array of symptoms. It's one more example of an eternally popular and effective general tactic of creating a "non-disease," and then selling its cure. Many who do this are truly sincere—but sincerity isn't the same as scientific evidence.

Some Realities of Sugar

There's one health problem with sugar—as a cause of tooth decay. Otherwise, the main problem is that a sugar-rich diet is often a nutritionally poor one. Typically, a sugar-rich diet is one in which soft drinks and sweets—candy, pastries, ice cream, etc.—displace more nutritious foods. Also, a high-sugar diet is usually high in fat and low in fiber as well.

Sugar and Tooth Decay

Tooth decay is a preventable disease caused by mouth bacteria. The bacteria feast on sugars and excrete an acid waste. Tooth decay results when the acid first demineralizes the enamel and then erodes it, allowing bacteria to infect the tooth (see Fig. 5-4).

Saliva is rich in calcium and phosphorus and can remineralize enamel before it erodes. When we don't provide sugar for the mouth bacteria (between meals, etc.), the saliva returns to its non-

Figure 5-4: Tooth Decay. Cross-section of tooth with decay at two common sites.

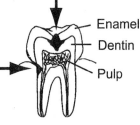

Enamel
Dentin
Pulp

acidic, slightly alkaline state, and can restore some of the minerals—but only at the earliest stages of mineral loss.

This is why constant snacking promotes tooth decay, and why cleaning the teeth promptly after eating helps prevent tooth decay. Sucking on hard candy throughout the day, for example, gives bacteria a steady source of sugar with which to make acid—too much time for mineral loss and not enough time for restoration.

A striking example is "bottle mouth," the rampant tooth decay seen in young children who are put to bed with a bottle of milk (milk has the sugar lactose). Children fall asleep while sucking on the bottle, with a pool of milk in their mouths, and may also suck on the bottle intermittently throughout the night. A bottle of fruit juice or sugared water is, of course, just as bad.

Treating severe tooth decay is not only expensive, but can be traumatic for a very young child

---

Children's teeth are especially susceptible to decay; the enamel of newly-emerged teeth isn't yet completely mineralized ("hardened"). They shouldn't get in the habit of going to sleep with a bottle even if their teeth haven't come in yet— habits are hard to break.

A popular classroom experiment is to dissolve a tooth in a glass of Coca-Cola, to show how sugar "rots the teeth." Children are impressed but, actually, it's the long-term acidity—not the sugar nor any bacteria—that dissolves the tooth in this demonstration. Vinegar (or diet Coke) would do the same thing. In the mouth, the acid made by the bacteria from the sugar is the true villain.

The bacteria don't discriminate between sugars "artificially" added in soft drinks and sugars found "naturally" in raisins. The raisins, in fact, promote tooth decay more than soft drinks. Raisins are sticky and keep their sugars on the teeth longer, prolonging acid production.

Does Sugar Cause Hyperactivity?

Despite claims to the contrary, diet hasn't been found in double-blind studies to cause hyperactivity, criminality, etc. (Nor have double-blind studies found such behavior to be helped by massive doses of vitamins, or dietary manipulations such as eliminating sugar.)

Double-blind studies are essential in investigating such dietary relationships, because evaluations of behavior are subjective and prone to bias. Also, dietary changes may improve behavior without the diet itself being directly responsible.

Double-blind study: A study in which neither the subjects nor the investigators evaluating them know whether a particular subject is in the test group or the control group used for comparison.

Severely restrictive diets drastically change the entire family dynamics. It's thought that this change in itself can reduce a child's hyperactivity— or its perception. More time is be spent shopping for foods; meals are specially planned; and more time is spent preparing them. Children get more positive attention, and they feel better about themselves because they're not held responsible for deviant behavior. Rather, food ingredients are blamed.

Despite the popular belief that sugar causes hyperactivity and adolescent delinquency, controlled studies suggest the reverse—that sugar has a calming effect. This isn't surprising, based on what little we know about "food and mood."

Sugar and Mood

Does what we eat throughout a day affect our mood? As tantalizing as the question is, the scientific tools and basic knowledge needed to explore it fully are only now beginning to emerge. But what little we do know is intriguing.

The brain chemical serotonin has a calming effect; it's made from tryptophan, one of the nine amino acids essential in our diet. Experimental animals fed tryptophan-deficient diets produce less serotonin, and become irritable, hypersensitive to pain, and develop insomnia.

Since tryptophan comes from dietary protein, one might expect that a high-protein diet would raise brain tryptophan and serotonin levels. In fact, the opposite occurs, and this takes a bit of explaining.

Protein has very little tryptophan compared to other amino acids. Since the tryptophan enters the brain in competition with other amino acids in the blood, a high-protein meal brings in more tryptophan, but it brings in even more of the other amino acids. As a result, less tryptophan gets into the brain, and less brain serotonin is produced than without the high-protein meal

---

The brain chemical serotonin is made from the amino acid tryptophan. Some antidepressants, e.g., Prozac, Zoloft, are Selective Serotonin Reuptake Inhibitors (SSRIs) that raise brain serotonin and improve mood.

But a high-carbohydrate meal or snack changes the odds in favor of tryptophan by causing a rise in insulin. (Recall that a high-carbohydrate diet raises blood sugar, which in turn stimulates the secretion of insulin.) Although insulin is best known for reducing blood glucose, insulin also reduces the amounts of certain amino acids in the blood—the amino acids that compete with tryptophan for entry into the brain. Here's the sequence of what's thought to happen:

1. High-carbohydrate meal
2. Increased insulin
3. More tryptophan entering the brain
4. Increased brain serotonin
5. Calming effect

This is theorized to be part of the reason why some people feel sleepy after a high-carbohydrate meal. This calming effect is also theorized to be a reason why people often find comfort ("tranquility") in carbohydrate-rich foods (e.g., candy).

Fiber and Health

Whole grains, vegetables, and fruit, besides being rich in carbohydrate are also rich in fiber. Since fiber, by definition, is the indigestible parts of plants, it's a not a required nutrient, per se. But fiber does add bulk to the diet without adding calories, and in this way can reduce the risk of becoming overweight.

Figure 5-5: Colon with diverticula.

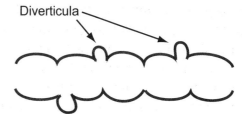

Because fiber is indigestible, it passes down the digestive tract where it may reduce the risk of chronic constipation, hemorrhoids, diverticulosis, and colon cancer. Fiber's possible relationship to diverticulosis and colon cancer will be discussed here; other conditions, e.g., fiber and heart disease, will be discussed in upcoming chapters.

Diverticulosis

Diverticulosis is the outpouching of the wall of the colon, much like a hernia (see Fig. 5-5). It's been estimated that 10% of people in this country over age 40 and more than half of those over age 60 have one or more of these outpouchings, although many don't suffer any ill effects.[3] But pain can result if an outpouching fills with bacteria and feces or becomes ulcerated.

If an ulcer erodes a blood vessel, there can be severe bleeding. If the ulcer erodes completely through the colon wall, there can be severe problems from bacteria leaking out into the normally germ-free abdominal cavity.

With a low-fiber diet, the muscles in the colon have to squeeze hard to pass stool that's too small or too hard. This increases the pressure inside the colon, which eventually may cause outpouchings at weak points in the colon wall. Fiber is thought to help prevent diverticulosis by providing bulk and softness to the stool, which helps the colon move things along with less pressure.

Colon Cancer

Colon cancer is the second leading cause of cancer death in the United States (lung cancer is first). There's thus a tremendous interest in the possibility that diet may affect one's risk of colon cancer.

In looking at colon cancer rates throughout the world, higher rates of colon cancer have been associated with diets low in fiber and high in fat, refined sugar, and animal protein. (All these dietary factors tend to be associated with each other: Diets high in animal protein tend to be high in fat and sugar and low in fiber.) Other studies, such as those comparing vegetarians with non-vegetarians, also show an association between more fiber and less colon cancer.

But these studies show only associations rather than cause-and-effect relationships. Studies with laboratory animals have shown inconsistent results, with some showing protective effects for fiber, some showing no effect, and some even showing an increase in colon cancer.

The probable reason for these variable results is that the diets studied differed in the types and amounts of fiber. Oat bran, for example, isn't the same as wheat bran. Even differences in how fine the various fibers are ground can change the outcome of a study.

As can be seen from the array of high-fiber cereals on the super-market shelves, the possible role of fiber in lowering risk has been well advertised. Although fiber might be helpful in lowering the risk of colon cancer, it could be that other dietary components are bigger factors.

Might the high fat and protein typical of low-fiber diets play a role in colon cancer? Fat and protein both stimulate the secretion of bile in the intestine, and suspected *carcinogens* (cancer-causing substances) include breakdown products of bile. Some kinds of colon bacteria have been shown to change bile acids into carcinogens.

Carcinogen: Any substance that causes cancer.

A study of over 88,000 nurses found that colon cancer occurred $2\frac{1}{2}$ times more often among those who ate beef, pork, or lamb as a main dish every day, compared to those who ate these meats as a main dish less than once a month.[4] Most cuts of beef, pork, and lamb are high in both fat and protein, so this finding supports the hypothesis that a high intake of fat and protein increases the risk of colon cancer.

But the study doesn't prove cause and effect. As discussed in Chapter 1, studies of population groups—in this case a big group of nurses—give clues to causes of disease. Selected aspects of the population (e.g., body weight, diet, exercise habits) are compared statistically to the occurrence of a disease. These studies only show links (people who differ in one way often differ in other ways that may or may not have been considered).

In this nurses study, a daily main dish of meat was linked with an increased occurrence of colon cancer. It doesn't show that meat causes colon cancer. It could be, for example, that those who eat more meat also drink less milk. Dietary calcium may be protective against colon cancer, and milk is the main source of calcium in the American diet.

Fiber-rich foods, by making the stool softer and bulkier, are helpful in preventing constipation, diverticulosis, hemorrhoids, and perhaps colon cancer—good reason to eat more fruit, vegetables, and whole grains.

How might fiber be protective? Fiber might play a role in preventing colon cancer by moving substances faster through the colon. This would shorten the time that the colon is exposed to any carcinogen present. As a general rule, the length of exposure to a carcinogen has a bearing on whether cancer is induced in a cell (e.g., the more a person smokes, the greater the likelihood of developing lung cancer.). But if the time of exposure was the crucial factor, it would be expected that people with a history of constipation would be more likely to get colon cancer. This doesn't appear to be the case.

It's also generally true that the greater the concentration of carcinogens, the greater the risk of cancer (e.g., smoking unfiltered rather than filtered cigarettes raises the risk of lung cancer). By providing bulk, fiber might help prevent colon cancer by diluting carcinogens in the colon.

Clearly, the possible effect of diet on colon cancer isn't simple or straightforward. Based on current evidence, however, it appears that a diet of more fiber-rich foods, fewer fatty foods, and only moderate amounts of protein can help guard against colon cancer. This is consistent with the Dietary Guidelines (discussed in Chapter 18) that we eat more whole grains, vegetables, and fruits, and less animal fat.

Carbohydrates and the Athlete

In terms of energy sources, athletic events can be roughly divided into two groups. Strength-and-power athletes (e.g., weight lifters, gymnasts, sprinters, shot putters) burn glucose to fuel their event, whereas fat is the main fuel for endurance events (e.g., long-distance bicyclists, runners, and swimmers).

Because strength-and-power events are short, normal stores of muscle glycogen provide ample glucose as fuel. So, strength-and-power athletes can perform optimally on a normal diet.

Endurance events require a lot more fuel, and must ultimately depend to a large extent on stored fat. Even the thinnest of athletes has ample body fat to fuel an endurance event. But although fat is the major fuel in endurance events, carbohydrate is also used. In fact, depletion of muscle glycogen causes muscle fatigue and hinders performance. So, despite the fact that fat's the main fuel, the availability of carbohydrates is what limits endurance.

Training enhances an endurance athlete's ability to use fat stores, and thus becomes an important factor in carbohydrate availability. The other main factor is the amount of glycogen stores in the muscles at the beginning of the event.

In preparing for competition, endurance athletes often use a technique called *carbohydrate-loading* to temporarily increase the amount of glycogen in their muscles. About a week before competition, the athlete trains hard, and then tapers off, resting on the day before the event. For 3 days before the event, the athlete eats a high-carbohydrate diet. The earlier, intense exercise depletes the muscles of glycogen. Upon repletion with a high-carbohydrate diet, there's a rebound effect, and glycogen stores are temporarily raised to higher-than-normal levels in time for the event.

Endurance athletes are also helped by drinking carbohydrate-containing drinks during competition if their event exceeds 90 minutes. Consuming drinks containing about 5 to 8% carbohydrate (glucose, sucrose, or glucose polymer) beginning about 30 minutes before fatigue sets in, works best. Most commercial sports drinks contain this amount of carbohydrate (as do most fruit juices diluted with equal amounts of water).

Summary

We require a daily minimum of about 200 calories worth of carbohydrate (50 grams) for normal metabolism. But much more than this is recommended for good health, mainly as a diet rich in whole grains, vegetables, and fruits.

The carbohydrates in our diet are all broken down by digestion into single sugars, mostly glucose, before being absorbed into our bloodstream. The level of glucose in our blood is kept within a normal range by the pancreatic hormones insulin and glucagon: insulin lowers blood glucose, and glucagon raises it.

When blood glucose is abnormally high, the most common cause is diabetes. Normally, insulin allows cells to take in glucose from the blood, thereby lowering blood levels. In diabetes, body cells can't take in glucose normally from the blood because of a lack of insulin (type 1 diabetes) or a resistance to insulin action (type 2 diabetes). In the U.S., about 1 of 10 of adults over age 20, and 1 of 5 of those over age 60 have diabetes. Diabetics have a much higher risk of heart disease, stroke, kidney disease, and nerve damage as compared to those of the same age without diabetes.

Most diabetics in this country have type 2 diabetes. This form of diabetes increases as adults get older, mostly from a combination of obesity and genetic predisposition. Type 2 diabetes has become more common in young adults and children as obesity has become more common.

About 5-10% of diabetics in this country have type 1 diabetes. They require an outside source of insulin because the pancreatic cells that make insulin have been destroyed. This diabetes isn't related to obesity and is typically diagnosed in children and young adults.

Abnormally low blood sugar (hypoglycemia) occurs when there's excess insulin. The most common cause of severe hypoglycemia is excess insulin taken by a diabetic.

Reactive hypoglycemia is a mild form of hypoglycemia that some people experience when they consume a large amount of carbohydrate after hours of not eating. The pancreas temporarily overshoots its secretion of insulin in response to the surge in blood glucose.

Sugar can cause tooth decay by providing food for mouth bacteria. The bacteria make acid, which erodes tooth enamel and allows bacteria to infect the tooth. Otherwise, the main problem with sugar is that sweets tend to displace more healthful foods in the diet.

Sugar doesn't cause hyperactivity in children. In fact, sugar appears to have a calming effect. In animal studies, a high-carbohydrate dose causes a rise in insulin, which in turn, increases the amount of serotonin in the brain. Serotonin is a brain chemical that has a calming effect.

Fiber adds bulk to the diet, bulk and softness to the stool, and plays other roles within the digestive tract. These attributes of fiber are thought to reduce the risk of constipation, diverticulosis, hemorrhoids, and possibly colon cancer.

In endurance events, depletion of muscle glycogen results in muscle fatigue. To delay this depletion during competition, endurance athletes often use a carbohydrate-loading regimen to increase their muscle glycogen at the start of an event. A high-carbohydrate diet follows a depletion of muscle glycogen, resulting in a higher-than-normal deposition of glycogen. Also, carbohydrate-containing drinks are successfully used in competitions lasting more than 90 minutes.

Guest Lecturer: Ellen Coleman, RD, MA, MPH

Glycogen Storage and the Athlete

Muscle glycogen is the preferred fuel for most types of exercise. Replenishing and maintaining muscle glycogen stores during intensive training requires a carbohydrate-rich diet. Depending on the intensity and duration of your activity, you should be consuming 6 to 10 grams of carbohydrate per kilogram of body weight daily. Adequate muscle glycogen stores allow you to exercise harder and longer with less fatigue.

Glycogen depletion can occur gradually over repeated days of heavy training when muscle glycogen breakdown exceeds its replacement. When this happens, your glycogen stores drop lower with each successive day, and your workouts become more difficult and less enjoyable. The deterioration in performance and feeling of sluggishness associated with glycogen depletion is often referred to as "staleness" and blamed on overtraining.

Glycogen depletion is often accompanied by a sudden weight loss of several pounds (due to glycogen and water loss) and you can't maintain your usual training intensity. When you don't consume enough carbohydrate or calories and/or don't take days off to rest, you're a prime candidate. Most Americans consume 5 grams of carbohydrate per kilogram of body weight – about half of their calories.

Carbohydrate Recommendations for Training

You can prevent glycogen depletion by consuming a carbohydrate-rich diet (6 to 10 grams of carbohydrate per kilogram daily) and taking periodic rest days to give your muscles time to rebuild their stores. You should consume 6 grams of carbohydrate per kilogram daily if you're working out hard for an hour each day. Take in 8 grams of carbohydrate per kilogram if you're working out hard two hours each day. A diet providing 10 grams of carbohydrate per kilogram is recommended when you're training hard for three hours or more each day.

A high carbohydrate diet is even more critical for recovery from prolonged, heavy exercise. Cyclists in the grueling Tour de France consume about 12 grams of carbohydrate per kilogram and 6,000 calories each day. By keeping your carbohydrate intake high, you can minimize the chronic fatigue due to muscle glycogen depletion.

The recommendations for carbohydrate are given in grams per kilogram because this is an easy way to determine how much you need. One kilogram equals 2.2 pounds. For example, a 154-pound person (70 kg) who trains strenuously for an hour needs 420 grams of carbohydrate daily.

You can determine the carbohydrate content of different foods by reading food labels.

Carbohydrate Loading

You can improve your performance when you exercise for longer than 90 minutes by maximizing your muscle glycogen stores prior to the event. During endurance exercise that exceeds 90 to 120 minutes, your muscle glycogen stores become progressively lower. When they drop to critically low levels (the point of glycogen depletion), you cannot maintain high-intensity exercise. In practical terms, you've "hit the wall" and must drastically reduce your pace.

Carbohydrate loading can increase your muscle glycogen stores by 50 to 100%. The greater your pre-exercise muscle glycogen content, the greater your endurance potential. You can carbohydrate load using a six-day, a three-day, or one-day regimen.

The graph below gives an overview of the six-day diet and training regimen used for carbohydrate loading. On the sixth day before the event, you exercise hard (about 70% of VO_2max) for 90 minutes. On the fifth and fourth days before the event, decrease your training to 40 minutes. During the first three days, you consume a normal diet providing about 5 grams of carbohydrate per kilogram per day. On the third and second day before the event, you reduce your training to 20 minutes. On the day before the event, you rest. During the last three days, you eat a high carbohydrate diet providing 10 grams of carbohydrate per kilogram per day.

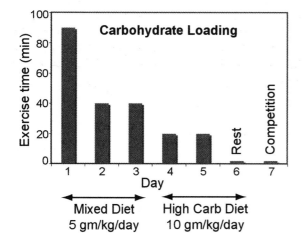

For the three-day regimen, you exercise hard (about 70% of VO_2max) for 90 minutes three days before the event. You rest and eat a high carbohydrate diet (10 grams of carbohydrate per kilogram per day) until the event.

A one-day carbohydrate loading regimen has been proposed to minimize disruptions to your training and competition preparation. On the morning of the day before the event, skip breakfast and warm up for five minutes. Next, exercise at the highest intensity that you can maintain for 2 and ½ minutes followed by a 30 second all-out sprint. For the next 24 hours, rest and consume 10 grams of carbohydrate per kilogram. Start taking in carbohydrate within 20 minutes of completing the exercise.

You must be endurance trained or carbohydrate loading won't work. Also, the exercise to lower glycogen stores must be the same as your competitive event because glycogen stores are specific to the muscle groups used. For example, a runner needs to decrease glycogen by running rather than cycling.

It's essential that you decrease your training the three days prior to competition. Too much exercise during this period will use too much of your stored glycogen and defeat the purpose of the whole process. The final three days, when you taper and eat a high-carbohydrate diet, is the real loading phase of the regimen. If you have difficulty consuming enough carbohydrate from food, you can use a high-carbohydrate supplement.

For each gram of glycogen stored, additional water is stored. Some people note a feeling of stiffness and heaviness associated with the increased glycogen storage. Once you start exercising, however, these sensations will work out.

Carbohydrate loading will help only for continuous endurance exercise lasting more than 90 minutes. Greater than usual muscle glycogen stores won't enable you to exercise harder during shorter duration exercise. In fact, the stiffness and heaviness due to increased glycogen stores can hurt your performance during shorter competitions such as 10 kilometer runs.

Carbohydrate loading enables you to maintain high intensity exercise longer, but will not affect your pace for the first hour of exercise. You won't be able to go out faster, but you will be able to maintain your pace longer.

Sample Carbohydrate Loading Menu 1
About 3,000 calories; 518 grams of carbohydrate

Breakfast	1 cup orange juice
	1 cup oatmeal, with
	1 banana
	1 cup low-fat milk
	2 slices wheat bread, with
	1 tsp. margarine
Lunch	2 slices rye bread
	3 oz. turkey
	1 oz. mozzarella cheese, with lettuce, tomato, mustard
	1 tsp. mayonnaise
	1 cup apple juice
	1 orange
	1 cup lemon sherbet
Snack	8 graham crackers
	1 cup low-fat milk
	1 apple
Dinner	2 cups spaghetti
	$2/3$ cup tomato sauce, with mushrooms
	2 Tbs. Parmesan cheese
	4 slices French bread
	2 tsp. margarine
	$1/2$ cup broccoli
	$1/2$ cup ice cream, with
	$3/4$ cup strawberries
Snack	6 cups popcorn, air popped

Sample Glycogen Loading Menu 2
About 4000 calories; 607 grams of carbohydrate

Breakfast	2 cups corn flakes
	1 cup non fat milk
	2 cups orange juice
	3 sliced cracked wheat bread
	3 tsp. jelly
Snack	2 large bananas
Lunch	6 slices cracked wheat bread
	3 oz. turkey
	3 oz. low fat American cheese
	2 cups apple juice
Snack	2 almond granola bars
Dinner	3 cups spaghetti with non meat sauce
	2 medium rolls
	2 Tbs. margarine
	1 cup green beans
	1 cup non fat milk
	2 large oranges
Snack	2 large apples

References
Bergstrom J, et al. Diet, muscle glycogen, and physical performance. Acta Physiol Scand 71: 140, 1967.

Fairchild TJ, Fletcher S, Steele P, et al. Rapid carbohydrate loading after a short bout of near maximal-intensity exercise. Med Sci Sport Exerc 34:980-986, 2002.

Karlsson J, et al. Diet, muscle glycogen, and endurance performance. J Appl Physiol 31:203, 1971.

Sherman WM, et al. The effect of exercise and diet manipulation on muscle glycogen and its subsequent use during performance. Int J Sports Med 2: 114, 1981.

Ellen Coleman is an exercise physiologist, registered dietitian (RD), and certified specialist in sports dietetics (CSSD) in Riverside, California. She has completed the Ironman Triathlon in Hawaii twice and numerous marathons and 200 mile bicycle races. She has consulted with the Los Angeles Lakers basketball team and Angels baseball team, and is the author of the popular book, *Eating for Endurance*.

Part 3

Proteins–The Masters of Life

Chapter 6

The Protein Confusion

We come now to "the good guys"—protein. If we've been wary of carbohydrates (not to mention sugar), we have only a good feeling about protein. It increases strength, athletic excellence, health, vitality, doesn't it?

And we've heard about amino acids, and we may understand that they are a part of protein. So it makes sense when amino acid supplements are promoted, and we know we will feel like a million when we've spent somewhat less to stock up.

We know there's protein in the juicy steak they used to give football players on game day to make them fierce. But red meat isn't as big a part of our diet these days, and there is still an interest in vegetarian diets. Can we get enough protein from plant foods? If so, how so?

Adequate protein is indeed essential, but at least in affluent societies, it's relatively easy to get all we need, and can use. Again, a bit of information can save us needless concern—and expense.

In most people's minds, the "protein foods" are mainly meats, milk, cheeses, and eggs. Indeed, many think of these foods as synonymous with protein.

The preference for these animal foods seems as old as mankind. The preference has been expensive—most of the world's population hasn't been able to afford them. Even today, the overwhelming majority of the world's vegetarians aren't vegetarians by choice.

This chapter begins by looking at animal foods from a cultural and historical perspective. We then look at protein itself from a scientific perspective—looking at its physical properties, structure, composition, and functions. The chapter ends by discussing plant and animal sources of dietary protein.

Protein and the Rich Man's Diet

In ancient Egypt, bread was the currency of labor. Workers on the pyramid of Cheops were paid three loaves of bread a day and some beer. Yet animal husbandry was well known. Even then, there was grain-feeding of cattle and force-feeding of birds to make plump roasts.

But animal foods were for the rich. The diet of the Greek and Roman peasants was mainly grains, sometimes flavored with honey or wine. People who could afford to eat what they wanted disdained the cheap food of the common folk.

When Alexander the Great swept from Macedonia through all of Greece, an account of one of his dinners tells of starting with chicken, duck, goose, ringdove, hare, pigeon, turtledove, partridge, and young goat. There follows a great pig, stuffed with thrush, warbler, duck, eggs in pea puree, oysters, and scallops. Finally came the main dish of skewered boars.

The cereal foods weren't entirely banned from the tables of the Greek wealthy. But the manner of their use symbolized the aristocrat's feeling about such nourishment. The breads were baked and served—to be used as napkins, to wipe the grease of the meat from the fingers.

The double standard of meat consumption continued through the centuries. The 1840s in England were known as the "hungry forties."

Depression was rife. Wages, for those lucky enough to have jobs, were historically low. In both Ireland and England, the potato—recognized from the 1600s as one of the world's richest yielders of calories per farm acre—was the dietary staple. Supplementary calories seem to have been supplied mainly by gin or beer.

It was in this worst of times that a plant disease—the potato blight—decimated the potato fields. This major food source gone, many people died of starvation, and millions emigrated to the United States.

The New Right to Meat

The land in the Old World was held by a privileged few. Even the hunting forests were the private preserves of the nobility. One of the inducements which led emigrants to the New World was the availability of land.

In America, there was a chance to get land, for little or nothing, and this could guarantee that a family would eat. And there was game. Colonists may have endured much, but they could eat meat.[1] In many areas, farms each had a smokehouse for preserving the game. Especially in the South, pigs flourished on the smallest farms, and barrels of salted pork provided the food staple for many households.

It was only a matter of time before cities grew, forests were pushed back, and game was killed too freely. In areas colonized first, the poor once again were driven toward carbohydrate foods—beans in Boston and corn grits in the South, along with molasses and sorghum to fill the belly. The westward expansion began as a push toward food security, toward open land for farms and forests to supply meat.

Weren't animals raised on the small farms in the first colonies? Yes, but as luxuries. For while grass would feed them in the warm months, the winters required stored animal fodder. It was a luxury to feed grain to a cow and to till land for animal food (see Fig. 6-1).

Not until the 1870s did the great western herds begin to have an impact on the national food supply. Even then it took a lot of money to buy meat in eastern cities. While beef was cheap at the source,

Figure 6-1: Pounds of grain fed to get one pound of meat, poultry or eggs

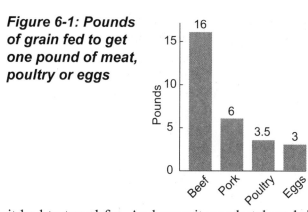

it had to travel far. And once it was butchered, it couldn't be kept fresh for long.

As late as the Depression of the 1930s, the American poor were used to a high-carbohydrate diet. In those dark years, the poor were even hard-pressed to get their carbohydrates, and much of the middle class joined them in the "bread lines." "A chicken in every pot" became a political fantasy.

Then World War II came, just as the Depression was lifting. There was money now, but there was also meat rationing. It wasn't surprising that, with the end of the war, Americans rushed to the butcher shop, hungry for meat, and with a firm belief that meat was needed for protein—and good health.

From about 1950 to the early 1970s, consumption of beef, poultry, and cheese rose dramatically in this country, while demand for beans and grains waned. Encouraged by the popularity of low-carbohydrate, reducing diets (yes, the same diets in different guises that come and go with regularity) and by their suspicions about sugar and starch, Americans viewed meat as the dietary assurance of health. What else was eaten seemed to matter little, as long as meat was on the plate.

Then in the early 1970s, food prices rose dramatically, especially the price of meat. Poorer people felt that they'd been deprived of a right—the right to meat—and complained that their health was threatened by the lack of protein.

It was certainly true that the poorest Americans, those on welfare and at the bottom of the income ladder, had been pushed away from the table of steaks and roasts. But setting aside the social and political questions, what are the nutritional realities of this change? What are the protein needs for health?

In the face of the social protest, some scientists suggested that a limitation on the availability of meat might actually be an advantage. Why was this said? To understand the answer, we must know something more of the science of proteins, of the foods in which they are found, and of the amounts needed for health.

Early Clues to the Protein Mystery

Shortly before Lavoisier made his revolutionary discoveries about the chemical character of life and food, a French scientist named Macquer made some of the first progress toward a scientific understanding about protein.

Protein isn't physically obvious; seldom do we see it in pure form. We don't really see it when we look at meat or cheese. This is in contrast to the other energy-providing nutrients: we see carbohydrate in quite pure form as table sugar or honey, or even the sap of trees. We are familiar with fat as we trim it from the leaner parts of meat, as we toss a salad with oil, or as we french-fry a potato.

We do see pure protein in the white of an egg. Macquer was struck by some of the now well-known characteristics of egg white. Heat it, and the viscous liquid coagulates to a slippery solid. Agitate it, and it assumes yet another form, as when we whip it for the meringue on a lemon pie. Macquer suspected that this coagulation-prone substance in food might be the single fundamental nutrient substance sought since the time of Hippocrates. So he examined other life substances.

The protein in a hen's egg is divided between the white and the yolk. But all of the fat (including cholesterol) is in the yolk. The white is all protein.

Some very essential materials shared this characteristic coagulation of the egg white—blood and semen for example. Perhaps, Macquer thought, this was the stuff which had been sought for so many centuries. "The gelatinous matter of animals," he wrote finally, "is the true animal substance. It constitutes almost entirely the bodies of animals; it is that which nourishes, repairs, and reproduces them." It was thought that this gelatinous matter was the fundamental life chemical.

Table 6-1 The 20 Kinds of Amino Acids Needed to Make Protein

Essential in the Diet (the body can't make these 9)		
Histidine	Lysine	Threonine
Isoleucine	Methionine	Tryptophan
Leucine	Phenylalanine	Valine
Not Essential in the Diet (the body can make these 11)		
Alanine	Cysteine	Proline
Arginine	Glutamate*	Serine
Asparagine	Glutamine	Tyrosine
Aspartate*	Glycine	

*Aspartate and glutamate are also called aspartic acid and glutamic acid.

So it was named *protein,* from the Greek meaning *elemental or primary.*

Early scientists also found that all these protein-containing substances could be treated to give off ammonia. This wasn't true of carbohydrates or fats, both of which have carbon, hydrogen, and oxygen as their basic structure. The ammonia showed that the basic structure of protein had something more—*nitrogen,* for ammonia is made of three atoms of hydrogen and one of nitrogen.

The chemical notation for ammonia is NH_3.

Nitrogen is hardly an uncommon element. It is, in fact, the largest constituent of the air we breathe—there is more than three times as much nitrogen as there is oxygen in air. But while we can use the oxygen in our body chemistry, we can make little use of the nitrogen we inhale. So our bodily nitrogen must come from food.

The Need for Amino Acids

By 1900, researchers knew that proteins were actually made up of much smaller and more fundamental molecules—the *amino acids.* Soon afterwards, scientists found that life didn't depend on protein *per se,* but on the amino acids of which it was composed. Indeed, we could get along very nicely without a single protein in our diet—if we consumed the amino acids that the proteins hold.

It's actually quite possible to do so. Pure amino acids are readily available for purchase. But this plan would be quite expensive, and a jarful of amino acids is hardly appetizing fare.

The day may come when we move closer to eating this way. Algae, the one-celled animals which make green slime in ponds, are much more efficient than ordinary food crops in trapping solar energy and producing amino acids. So far, we're happily stuck with the likes of the juicy roast of the Thanksgiving turkey, mashed potatoes, and pumpkin pie.

What a Few Amino Acids Can Do

Twenty different amino acids are needed to make protein (see Table 6-1 and Fig. 6-2)—11 of these we can make; the other 9 must come from our diet. The awesome fact about this handful of chemicals is that they can be juggled into the whole variety of plant and animal life on earth.

Consider how they're used by our own bodies. Virtually all of life's enzymes are made from them, as are enormous varieties of hormones and *antibodies.* More than this, they are the principal materials that make up our cells—cells of bone and brain, blood vessel, muscle, nerve, skin, intestine, gland, and lung. Our cells make an estimated 100,000 different proteins from these same 20 amino acids, not only to produce the chemicals of life processes, but also to repair and reproduce themselves.

Antibody: A protein that the body makes in response to a foreign substance, creating a defense and immunity against it (e.g., measles antibody made in response to a measles infection or vaccination).

Now reflect that we are only one species, and that these same amino acids are used still differently by other life forms—from mosquitoes to daffodils, from whales to sparrows, from fur and claw to leaf and bark. How is this possible?

The Chemistry of Life's Variety

The potential number of variations of which the handful of amino acids are capable is mathematically huge. (Note that our whole language is

Figure 6-2: Different amino acids join to make a protein.

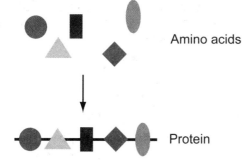

built from just 26 letters, and that these same few units spell out many tongues.)

The rearrangements of these few symbols into such huge systems suggest how just 20 kinds of amino acids can be chained together to make a whole library of proteins. Since the chains of amino acids are so much longer than our words, the possibilities for variation in proteins are enormously greater. For the proteins of life chemistry are usually at least 100 amino acids long, and they commonly range from 500 to 1,000.

Like our language, the proteins can be affected by the slightest change in sequence. Change the sequence of letters in words and you can change the meaning drastically—like going from *baste* to *beats* to *beast*. Thus, the same units serve radically different functions when they're differently ordered. And similar differences occur when you substitute one unit for another, as in *six* and *sex*.

Amino acid changes can have at least as much impact. Consider *hemoglobin,* the protein which carries oxygen in blood. It's a chain of 146 amino acids. Change only the sixth amino acid (valine instead of glutamate) in the chain, and you have the defective hemoglobin that causes sickle cell anemia. Such tiny changes can, in many cases, spell the difference between sickness and health, between life and death.

Sickle cell anemia: An inherited disease caused by defective hemoglobin in red blood cells. Found mainly among those of African heritage.

The *sequence* of amino acids in a protein is known as its *primary structure*. But changes of the *geometric arrangement* of that chain can also alter the characteristics of the protein, multiplying possible variations almost to infinity.

As a very crude comparison, picture the amino acid chain of a protein as a thread. If we drop that thread, perhaps with a twirling motion, it can fall in a variety of patterns as it turns and twists and crosses over on itself.

The geometry of protein molecules is far more sophisticated. Remember our analogy of proteins as words, with the amino acids as letters. Suppose that these extremely long words could be written not only in straight lines but, without actually changing the sequence of the letters, in shapes, each of which had a different meaning, like this:

```
      R        O     T
      P              E  I  N
```

Or perhaps, using the name of the amino-acid phenylalanine:

```
      P
      H  E
         N   YL
              A
      N  A   L
      I
      N  E
```

Recalling that these protein words are often 500 letters long, imagine the potential variety of shapes. But the variety doesn't stop here. So far, we have considered the variety of two-dimensional geographic arrangement, using only the vertical and horizontal dimensions of this flat page. Imagine that, having written out our immensely long word in this wandering pattern, we could further change the meaning by crumpling the paper into a ball. Indeed, protein "words" are written in three dimensions (see Fig. 6-3).

Protein Shapes and Their Meaning in Life

How important is the shape of a protein? It's extremely important because a protein's shape is a key to its action. The hormone insulin (a protein) is an example. There are a few differences in amino acid sequence between human insulin and the insulin of other animals. Yet some animal insulin can work in the human body, because—despite the differences of sequence—the shape and cross-linkages are much the same as those of human insulin.

We've seen that a protein can change its characteristics when heated, agitated, or exposed to certain chemicals, as in the case of egg white. Such alterations are the result of changes in the shape—the three-dimensional structure—of the protein.

These changes in protein's shape are known as *denaturing* (Fig. 6-4). Another example is the co-agulation and color change of the blood and other "juices" on the surface of a broiling steak—also the result of the changing shape of protein.

The fact that denaturing a protein is a matter of changing its shape rather than changing its amino acid content has nutritional significance—denaturing protein by cooking doesn't ordinarily lower its nutritional value.

Cooking, in fact, usually increases the protein value of food—especially plant foods—by making the food more digestible. The nutritional value of rice is markedly improved by cooking, since uncooked rice is quite indigestible. Increasing the digestibility of plants is especially important for people in developing countries, since plants are their major source of both the calories and the protein that are often deficient in their diet.

Denaturing inactivates proteins, including enzymes. And a dim understanding of this has led many well-meaning "health-food" advocates to insist on raw foods, and to worry needlessly about some processing techniques. Enzymes in milk are denatured by pasteurizing, so some people insist on "raw" (unpasteurized) milk. For the same reason, some people demand wheat which has been stone-ground on the theory that more modern milling methods produce somewhat more heat and inactivate the enzymes of the grain.

But while they're correct about the denaturing of enzymes, they fail to understand that the body has no use for a food's enzymes—except as a bit of dietary protein. For a food's enzymes are treated by the body like all other food proteins—they're broken down into amino acids by digestion and have no special value except as contributors of very small amounts of amino acids.One popular myth dear to weight-loss hucksters is that grapefruit enzymes can work some special magic to break

Figure 6-3: *Chain of Amino Acids Forms a 3-Dimensional Protein.* The 3-dimensional shape of a protein is exact. The amino acid chain folds automatically and precisely, based on the sequence of the amino acids in the chain.

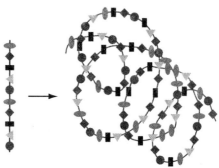

down body fat. Untrue. Grapefruit enzymes are certainly useful—but only for grapefruit.

Cooks—and food companies—denature enzymes for good reason. By blanching *(heating quickly and briefly)* vegetables before freezing them, their enzymes are denatured and thus inactivated, retarding the deterioration of the vegetables. Typically, vegetables are blanched by a short immersion into boiling water—long enough to denature the enzymes, but brief enough to minimize other changes that might adversely affect the flavor, texture, and nutrient content of the vegetables.

Corn loses its sweetness as it ages because its sugar is turning into starch. By blanching the corn, the enzyme needed for this chemical reaction is inactivated, and the sweetness of corn is preserved. Anyone who has tried to add fresh pineapple to a gelatin concoction such as Jell-O knows that it doesn't gel as it should. This mishap is avoided when canned pineapple is used because, in processing, the pineapple was heated, denaturing the enzyme in fresh pineapple that breaks down gelatin.

Proteins can also be denatured—and appear "cooked"—by acidifying their surrounding fluid. In the Latin American dish *ceviche*, raw seafood is marinated in seasoned lime juice and then served. The seafood appears to be cooked because the acid in the lime juice has denatured the protein of the seafood. We also see this acid effect in the curdling of milk proteins when the milk "goes sour," or when we marinate beef in vinegar to make *sauerbraten*.

There can be problems in "cooking" food this way (marinating in lime juice) instead of using heat. In 1991, Peru had a deadly cholera epidemic when contaminated sewage tainted the seafood. Ceviche is a "fast food" popularly sold at food stands along the Peruvian coast. The mild acidity of lime juice doesn't kill cholera organisms; thoroughly cooking the fish does.

Proteins in the body can be denatured by changes in acidity as well. The enzymes in blood and tissue fluids function optimally only when the acidity of these fluids is within its normally narrow range. This sensitivity is to be expected, since a change in acidity alters the shape of the enzymes and, thereby, alters their function.

> Lactic acid is produced in muscles when oxygen and muscle glycogen become scarce during muscle activity, as in endurance events. This will be discussed in Chapter 11.

When athletes feel sudden fatigue ("hit the wall") in endurance events, one explanation is that the lactic acid that has accumulated in their muscles has made the fluids in those muscles more acid—thereby, impairing their function.

The Proteins in Our Food

Evaluating food sources of protein involves looking at the quantity (amount) of protein in the food as well as its quality—how well the *amino acid composition* of the protein meets our needs. Animal foods are generally higher in both quantity and quality of protein than plant foods (see Fig. 6-5).

A 3-oz. portion of chicken meat has 27 grams of protein, whereas a cup of refried beans (weighing over 3 times as much—10 oz.) has 18 grams of protein. And of at least equal importance, the amino acid composition of chicken protein is of higher quality—it's more in line with what we need.

What Makes a High-Quality Protein?

Since the need for protein is actually a need for amino acids, differences in protein quality are based on the ability of foods to supply amino acids in something like the proportions of the body's

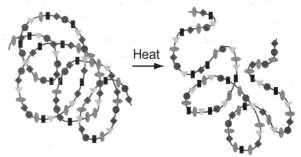

Figure 6-4: Denaturing a Protein. Such conditions as heat can change a protein's 3-dimensional structure—denature it. A protein's function depends on its shape, so denaturing a protein inactivates it.

needs. The key to that quality is how well it supplies one group of 9 amino acids, those which are called *essential amino acids* (see Table 6-1).

Essential Amino Acids

At first glance, this may seem puzzling. For the body must have all 20 amino acids to do its job of making protein. Why then, are some amino acids "essential" while others are not?

The answer is quite simple. It's that 11 of the 20 amino acids can be made by the body (as long as the body has enough nitrogen, the characterizing element of proteins). These amino acids are available to the cells as long as a sufficient amount of protein is consumed, no matter what its origin and amino acid composition. They are thus called non-essential amino acids because they aren't required in the diet.

The nine that can't be made by the body are called essential amino acids because they are required in the diet. If we don't eat foods with enough of these nine amino acids, the body can't make the proteins it needs. We require adequate intakes of these amino acids, just as we require adequate intakes of specific vitamins and minerals.

The quality of a dietary protein refers to its proportions of essential amino acids, relative to our own needs. As might be expected, animal proteins are the highest in quality, since the amino acid composition of these proteins more closely reflect that of our own proteins. The proteins found in our muscles, blood, and organs certainly resemble proteins from a chicken or cow more than proteins from beans or corn.

Plant proteins vary in quality, with soybean protein near the top, and wheat and corn proteins near the bottom. Plant proteins can, however, be combined to improve their quality. Virtually all proteins have some amount of all 20 amino acids. The critical question is whether the total diet has a sufficient amount of each of the essential amino acids.

Egg protein is the gold standard by which other proteins are measured. Its high quality isn't surprising—it represents the compact package of nutrients needed to produce a bird.

The essential amino acid in shortest supply (relative to need) is called the *limiting amino acid*, because it limits protein production. Since all 20 amino acids are needed to make protein, the amount of protein that can be made is limited if there isn't enough of just one amino acid.

The Vegetarian Diet and Proteins

In a vegetarian diet, a low level of an essential amino acid in a plant protein can be compensated for by appropriate combinations of different plant proteins—*complementing the proteins*. The classic example is that of grains (e.g., wheat, corn, rice, oats, barley) combined with legumes (e.g., soy, lima, garbanzo, pinto, kidney beans—and peanuts, which are really legumes, not nuts).

By eating grains (low in the amino acid lysine—the limiting amino acid in grain) with legumes (low in methionine—the limiting amino acid in legumes), the two protein sources help make up for one another's amino acid shortages (see Fig. 6-6).

So grains and legumes are spoken of as being complementary in terms of protein. That is, each protein source helps compensate for the amino acid shortage of the other.

Oftentimes, quantity can make up for quality. If a single plant food that's a fairly rich source of protein is eaten in sufficient amount, there may be enough of even a low-level amino acid. In such a case, complementing plant proteins may not be necessary. For example, even though wheat protein doesn't have much of the essential amino acid

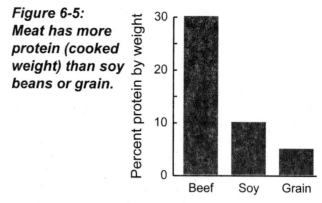

Figure 6-5: Meat has more protein (cooked weight) than soy beans or grain.

lysine, a diet which includes enough wheat can supply enough lysine.

This was demonstrated in an experiment in which subjects were fed a diet which depended for most of its protein on eight slices of bread at each meal. Within a few weeks, it could be shown that the subjects were receiving adequate amino acids, even though wheat is low in lysine.

The problem is that where one food becomes an overwhelmingly large part of the diet, there's always a risk that one or more vital nutrients will not be adequately supplied. A basic tenet of good nutrition is to eat a variety of foods.

In any event, many people throughout the world don't have the luxury of eating the large amounts of plant protein needed to meet their amino acid needs. In some cases, technology has come to the rescue. A large segment of the population of Tunisia has been given wheat which has been enriched with additional lysine. Also, a serious problem of protein malnutrition among the children of Hong Kong has been alleviated by the addition of methionine to a soy milk.

Many people throughout history have survived well on wholly vegetarian diets—plant proteins were combined "properly" long before the discovery of amino acids (see Table 6-2). Traditional combinations, of grains and legumes are tortillas and beans, tofu (soybean curd) and rice, baked beans and bread, falafel (chickpeas/garbanzo beans in pita bread), and the old American standby—a peanut butter sandwich (see Fig. 6-6).

Legumes and seeds (e.g., sesame, pumpkin, sunflower) also make a good combination, as in the middle-eastern dish hummus, a combination of chickpeas and sesame seeds. In a modern

Figure 6-6: Combining Proteins with Different Limiting Amino Acids. **R**=limiting amino acid (aa) in peanut protein; **T**=limiting aa in wheat protein. Each can spell PROTEIN only once (peanut runs out of **R**; bread runs out of **T**). Together (peanut-butter sandwich), PROTEIN can be spelled 5 times.

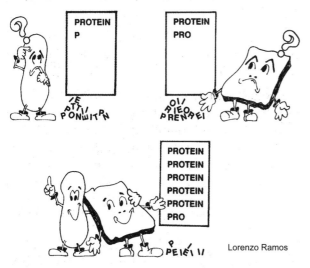

Lorenzo Ramos

Table 6-2: Complementary Plant Proteins

Combine Legumes with:	
kale	beet greens
collard greens	winter squash
mustard greens	sweet potato
swiss chard	yam
Combine Grain or Corn with:	
fresh lima beans	broccoli
peas	asparagus
brussels sprouts	okra
collard greens	snap green beans
spinach	cauliflower
Combine Potatoes with:	
spinach	corn
mustard greens	okra
broccoli	soybeans
collard greens	

twist, Japanese researchers envision the creation of "rice-tofu" by biotechnology—transferring the genes for soybean protein into rice.[2]

How Much Protein in the Food?

In addition to the need for sufficient sources of the essential amino acids, there's a need for an amount of protein in general, to supply—or for the body to make—the non-essential amino acids. In this respect, it's the total amount (quantity) of protein in the food rather than its essential amino acid composition (quality) that must be considered.

As noted earlier, quantity and quality tend to be related, in that foods with the highest quality protein generally have the most protein. Cooked portions of lean beef, chicken, and fish have about 30% protein by weight, soy beans about 10%, and grains about 5% or less (see Fig. 6-5).

Diets that regularly contain animal protein are usually more than adequate in terms of meeting needs for both essential amino acids and total protein. In this country, about two-thirds of the protein in the overall diet comes from animal sources. As might be expected, the amount—and quality)—of protein in the "typical American diet" far exceeds our requirements.

Proteins from Plant and Animal Foods

It follows from what's been said that the amount of protein needed in the diet is higher when the protein comes exclusively or primarily from plants. More is needed because of differences in quality, but also because of differences in digestibility. Animal proteins are about 95% digestible, proteins in refined grains are about 90-95% digestible, and proteins in whole grains, beans, and vegetables are about 80-85% digestible.[3] These small differences in digestibility are significant in diets that provide marginal amounts of protein.

Because of its high quality, animal sources of protein are particularly valuable to growing children. For infants, the need for essential amino acids makes up about 45% of their protein requirement because of an infant's rapid growth (addition of body tissue), whereas the proportion for adults is only about 20% (see Fig. 6-7).

Essential amino acids make up a greater proportion of animal protein than of plant protein, and, therefore, animal proteins are better suited to meet an infant's needs. It's no coincidence that breast milk is an infant's first and best food. A mother's milk is an easily digested, rich combination of nutrients (including essential amino acids) tailor-made for a baby.

Growing children not only need high-quality

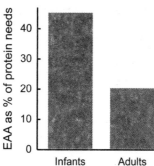

Figure 6-7: Infants need higher quality protein—more of the essential amino acids (EAA).

protein but, as mentioned earlier, need large amounts of protein in proportion to their body weight. They also need more calories in proportion to body weight. Animal sources of protein are not only more concentrated in protein than plant sources, but also provide more fat—a concentrated source of the calories needed by a growing child.

Strict Vegetarian diets (no animal foods) thus aren't generally well-suited for young children. But, as we shall see in the Guest Lecture at the end of this chapter and in the next chapter, vegetarian diets can work well for adults.)

To get a better understanding of our need for dietary protein, we must know something of how the body uses the amino acids once they have been absorbed. This understanding can enable us to choose this most costly part of our food with wisdom, with economy, and with the realistic knowledge of how these foods can support good health.

Summary

Proteins are made up of amino acids that are linked together in a long chain. A basic component of an amino acid, and hence protein, is nitrogen. This is a distinguishing feature of protein; carbohydrates and fat don't have nitrogen as a universal part of their structure.

Proteins are typically more than 100 amino acids long. The order (sequence) in which the amino acids are linked together is known as the protein's primary structure. The structure of a protein is made intricately more complex by the variety of geometric and three-dimensional arrangements that are possible with a long chain of amino acids.

The shape of a protein refers to its three-dimensional structure. Because the shape of a protein is intimately related to its function, even tiny changes in a protein's shape can alter its ability to

do its job. Changing a protein's shape is called *denaturing*. Proteins can be denatured by heat, agitation, and exposures to certain chemicals such as acid.

In both plants and animals, 20 kinds of amino acids are needed to make protein. Nine of these amino acids are called *essential amino acids* because they are required in our diet. The other 11 amino acids are called *non-essential amino acids* because our body can make them. We thus need protein in our diet for two basic reasons—to provide the essential amino acids and to provide enough total protein so that our body can make the non-essential ones.

A food's protein value is assessed by looking at its *quality*—how well the protein's content of essential amino acids matches our body's needs—and the *quantity* of protein in the food. Animal proteins generally rank much higher than plant proteins in both quality and quantity. So when animal proteins make up a substantial part of the diet, it's easy to meet the need both for essential amino acids and for total protein.

For most of the world's population, animal proteins are scarce. But plant proteins can provide adequate amounts of the essential amino acids as well as total protein. When only one kind of plant food is available and there's an ample amount, one can get enough of the essential amino acids and total protein by eating large amounts of that food—so long as protein makes up a sufficient portion of the food. However, any diet based heavily on one food runs the risk of being inadequate in some essential nutrients.

A better way to obtain protein from a diet of only plant foods is to eat certain foods in combination (e.g., grains and legumes), enabling one protein to make up for the essential amino acid shortage of another ("complementing" the proteins). Also, enough of these foods must be eaten to supply sufficient total protein.

When possible, it's generally advised that some animal protein be included in the diet. This is especially true for young children, who need a lot of high-quality protein because of their rapid growth. For many children throughout the world, the kinds and amounts of dietary protein can mean the difference between sickness and health, between life and death.

The Vegan Diet

A vegan (pronounced *vejjan*, as in vegetable, or *veegin*, as in begin) is a person who chooses to eat no animal-derived foods at all. A strict vegan avoids not only red meats, fish, and poultry, but also dairy products and eggs. Some even eschew honey, since it is made by bees, but most vegans consider this unnecessarily orthodox.

Although the term *vegan* is new, the concept has been around for thousands of years. In ancient Greece the ranks of well known vegans included the philosopher and mathematician Pythagoras, a remarkable athlete from Sparta named Charmis, the philosopher arid astronomer Thales, and two great mystics, Apollonius of Tyana and Philo of Alexandria. Each of these men was a prominent figure who attracted many students, and since the custom was for students to live with their teacher and follow his way of life, these examples probably represent not just isolated instances but several ancient vegan communities.

A vegan meal looks simple, austere, and timeless, as if it had been the typical fare of people close to the earth since the dawn of time. But this impression is probably not accurate. Archaeologic findings in Turkey and elsewhere show that certain animals were domesticated as much as nine thousand years ago, and the Leakeys' findings in Africa show that animals have figured in the dietary habits of mankind since the early days of human ancestry. No traditional society that we know of, past or present, has been consistently vegan, except in cases of abject poverty or cataclysmic disruption when no alternative was available.

Vegans in our own society were once rare and adhered generally to an explicit philosophy. In the last two or three decades, though, their number has increased markedly, for reasons that reflect real diversity. There are also many vegetarians who, though not rigid vegans, eat very little in the way of dairy products and eggs. Some people are vegans or near vegans for health reasons: all plant diets tend to be very low in fat and relatively free of chemical residues. Others don't like the way the animals producing these foods are treated on large-scale commercial farms; avoiding animal products eliminates one's own participation in this trade. And many simply find that eggs and milk begin to taste heavy and fatty next to vegetables and grains.

Whatever the reason, just as many omnivores today describe themselves as "almost vegetarians," many vegetarians today are almost vegans. (One of our friends calls himself a "pancake-o-vegan": he faithfully avoids all other sources of milk and eggs, but draws the line at ruling out an occasional buckwheat or buttermilk pancake.) What was a fad is becoming acknowledged as one of many acceptable ways of eating. This trend translates into a real need for up-to-date guidelines on the special nutritional problems of an all-plant diet.

Current Knowledge of Vegan Nutrition

Despite the example of Pythagoras and the rest, it is only today, with a scientific knowledge of nutrition and the available array of special foods and dietary supplements, that it is easy to be a vegan and stay healthy. Uninformed experimentation can be dangerous, because dairy foods are the usual source of certain nutrients that otherwise can only be assured by careful planning.

The main problem areas of a vegan diet are calcium, which is best supplied by milk, and vitamin B 12, which is not supplied by any plant food. In addition, vegans reportedly have high incidence of dental disease and higher than normal risks of iron deficiency anemia. Despite these potential problems, though, a majority of modern-day vegans seem to manage quite well on their austere diet. T.A.B. Sanders goes so far as to suggest that a vegan type diet supplemented by vitamins B-12 and D may be the diet of choice for victims of ischemic heart disease, angina pectoris, and certain hyperlipidemias (conditions of excess fat in the blood). "The few clinical studies made so far in Britain and United States," he adds, "have not been able to identity any real differences in the health of vegans compared with omnivores."

Yet as we have said, care and intelligence are necessary in adopting the vegan eating style. Reports of multiple nutrient deficiencies have surfaced periodically in the literature, especially among children in poorly informed vegan communitics. It is not difficult to avoid such problems, as you can see in the suggestions below.

Vitamin B 12

Since it is not supplied by plant foods but comes ultimately from microorganisms, vitamin B-12 is usually considered the critical nutrient in the vegan diet. B-12 deficiency is a very serious problem, which over time can harm the spinal cord. The problem proceeds unnoticeably and very slowly, but can cause irreversible damage.

Despite this danger, some popular writers today are discounting the vegan's need for vitamin B-12, since deficiency problems have been quite rare in this country. We can't go along with this attitude. The risks involved are so serious, and preventive measures so simple, that it seems foolhardy to disregard them. Please do not court a B-12 deficiency! If you work into your diet the suggestions below, and make them a habit, you can be a vegan without fuss or worry.

One simple way to get your B-12 is by using fortified soy milk. However, commercial soy milk products are often designed not for vegans, but for meat eating children who are allergic to milk, so the amount of B-12 supplied may be too low to he practical. Check the label to see what percent of the recommended dietary allowance (RDA) for B-12 is met by one glassful. If it is as little as 10%, you'll need ten glasses to meet the RDA, and you can suspect that the manufacturer had the allergic omnivore in mind.

Another way to get vitamin B-12 is to eat tempeh or miso every day. Of the two, tempeh is the more reliable source of B-12, but only if it has been specifically fermented with Kiebsiella bacteria along with the usual mold. Other fermented foods, such as natto and even shoyu, may contain B-12, but this should not be counted on.

Some types of nutritional yeast are grown on B-12 enriched media, and these too are reliable sources. Regular nutritional yeast has no B-12 at all, so be sure to check the label.

Finally, you can take a vitamin pill. B-12 supplements generally come in high dosages, so you may need only one a week. The RDA level might also be supplied by daily multiple vitamin pills: again, check the label to see that it lists at least 2 micrograms of B-12.

Calcium

Calcium intake is commonly listed among the vegan's problem nutrients, and our own experience tallies with this. One of our good friends avoided dairy products for fifteen years until he discovered that his bones had deteriorated with severe osteoporosis. As is often the case with this disease, there was no sign of a problem until trivial stress on a bone resulted in a painful fracture. He was under forty years old at the time, very active physically and very well informed about nutrition. While aware that his calcium intake was low compared to the RDA, he had believed that this low intake would be adequate. Now he is using milk and calcium supplements in an attempt to strengthen his compromised bones.

It is not unlikely that this friend has an unusual hormonal problem which causes his body to waste calcium. Most people, evidence suggests, can adjust over time to very low levels of calcium in the diet, by absorbing it with great efficiency. But which of us knows whether he or she is in that fortunate majority? As with B-12, we advise caution: the consequences of error are painful and the remedies simple. We suggest that every vegan monitor calcium intake and make sure that it stays at RDA levels.

Protein and Energy Needs

The medical information available on vegans indicates that they have no trouble getting enough protein. The key, though, is getting enough calories. In our experience, it is possible for a vegan to develop a marginal protein deficiency if he or she simply gets too little food. To be a healthy vegan, in other words, you have to be a big eater. The sheer volume of a vegan's normal meals can give the impression of gluttony. Yet according to the literature, very few vegans are overweight—certainly none we know. It simply takes a lot of food to run a vegan body.

Vegans we know tend to have a sweet tooth. We suspect that this is partly due to a need for calories—plain energy. Some of the medical cautions against too much sugar may not apply here, since the available literature on vegans' blood lipids and ability to handle glucose show that as a group, they are at very low risk for obesity, heart disease, and diabetes. However, as noted earlier, vegans reportedly do have more dental caries than normal. (You can't have everything.)

Actually, the most important threat that sweets pose for vegans may be simply letting sugar, even in fruits, crowd out more nutritious foods. Fortunately, most vegans probably stay clear of junk foods like candy, soft drinks, commercial potato chips, doughnuts, and fast food items, the worst offenders in nutrient crowd-out.

Excerpted with permission from *The New Laurel's Kitchen: A Handbook for Vegetarian Cookery and Nutrition.* Ten Speed Press. Berkeley, California.

Chapter 7

Putting Amino Acids to Work

It's helpful to learn something about protein needs, and about their components—amino acids. But we've seen only part of the picture, until we've learned a bit about the relationship to DNA and the genetic code.

We've been told that protein is an essential nutrient, one that's intimately involved in our basic life processes of growth, repair, and reproduction. But how does this all come about? How do our bodies make the proteins needed for these functions? How is information passed along specifying what's needed?

In fact, the breakthrough discovery of the genetic process has led the way for much of our understanding of how our bodies function at the most elemental levels—how we fight disease, pass on inherited traits and disabilities, and how we conceive and produce our children.

We will find that the story of the formation of proteins leads to an understanding of many basic health concepts, helping us to make wiser choices in what we choose to eat.

Much of life may be thought of as the building up, breaking down, and re-building of proteins. And it's through this ceaseless taking-apart and putting-together that food allows us to grow and reproduce, to act and know and feel.

That miracle is happening at every moment at dazzling speed, not only within us but within all of life—plant and animal. This work of life takes place within cells—life's basic unit.

So we begin by getting a broad view of the cell before focusing in on its genetic material—the blueprints to make protein. Step-by-step we look at how these blueprints are used to assemble amino acids into protein. The bulk of our requirement for dietary protein is for this protein synthesis. Having considered the details of how proteins are made and used, the chapter then shows how this information can help us answer questions of dietary protein and health.

Cells—The Lives Within Our Life

The truth is that each of us is but a society of cells which live and work together to survive and reproduce. Human cells vary enormously in size, but generally they're too small for all but micro-scopic view. Most range in size from half a micron to 20 microns—that is, from about a fifty-thou-sandth of an inch in diameter to something less than one-thousandth of an inch. Nerve cells are our largest, for they serve much like living wires. Many nerve cells are small, but they can be as long as several feet. Some kinds of human cells are shown in Figure 7-1.

To describe the cells as separate lives is no mere poetic license. It's simple fact. With just a few exceptions, each cell, within its own outer membrane, carries its complete hereditary plan and can reproduce itself.

It has its own systems for taking in nutrients. On the average, it produces hundreds of complex chemicals—and some cells make thousands—to break those nutrients down, rearrange its atoms, and replace damaged or aging cell parts. It has its own system of waste disposal and its ways to communicate with other cells. It has its specific work to do in supporting and controlling its fellow cells. It even breaks itself down into harmless chemical bits when death comes.

It's almost too much to believe—that these cells can conduct such lives when, in many cases, a million of them can fit onto the head of a pin. It's hard to comprehend the concept that we have no life aside from these tiny lives, that all of life on earth, from insect to oak tree, is nothing more than colonies of cells.

But it's true. Take away the cells, and we are only puddles of salty, chemical-laden water, with a bit of grease and protein—which the cells have made.

Even for biologists, the concept is a little un-nerving. Yet it explains why some tiny microbes (bacteria are single cells) can strike down man with disease. The invading microbial cells are re-ally at war only with other cells—generally their equals in size and strength. And much of modern medicine is based on the understanding that the war is at this microscopic level. In fact, the vast

Figure 7-1: Some Kinds of Human Cells. (a) Goblet cell. (b) Cartilage cell, (c) Bone cell. (d) Two kinds of blood cells. e) One kind of nerve cell. (f) Cells from the lining of the trachea, or windpipe. (g) Epithelial cells from the lining of the urinary bladder. (h) Cells from the outer layer of the skin. (j) a sperm, male reproductive cell. (k) an ovum, female reproductive cell. (l) a smooth muscle cell from the stomach.

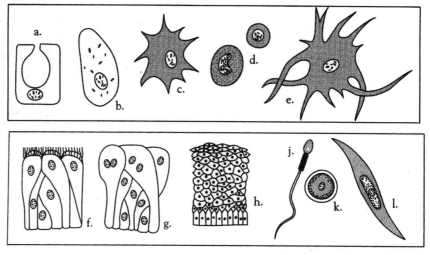

Figure 7-2: Some parts of a "typical" cell.
Mitochondria: where oxygen is used to release energy from food. *Nucleus*: home of DNA, the genetic material. *Ribosomes*: sites of protein synthesis. *Cytoplasm*: fluid that fills the cell.

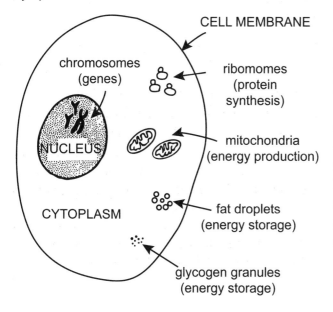

Mitochondria are the power centers of the cell. It's in these tiny bodies that the body's fuel is finally burned to free the energy we need to live. *Ribosomes* are the protein factories of the cell.

Finally, we reach the core of the cell, the *nucleus*. Isolated by its own special membrane, this is the computer, data bank, and administrator of the cell. For it holds the ultimate substance of life—DNA.

DNA is the genetic material passed from generation to generation. To DNA is attributed the differentiation of all life's forms and processes. It determines the difference between a nose and a leaf, between a grape and an asparagus, between a gnat and an elephant. How does DNA provide such a variety of life? How does it control life processes within our own bodies?

DNA—The Secrets in Its Structure

DNA *(deoxyribonucleic acid)* is a chain of chemical units, each made of a *sugar,* a *phosphate* (a combination of phosphorus and oxygen), and a *base* (a nitrogen-bearing chemical which looks like a second cousin to an amino acid):

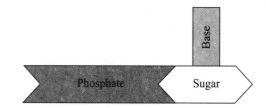

These units join with one another to form a chain, like this:

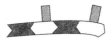

The chain joins side-to-side with another chain. Their bases, which look like "arms" protruding outward, link together like this:

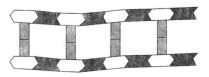

bulk of modern pharmacology—from penicillin to the exotic drugs which combat leukemia, from sulfa to the birth control pill—is aimed at guarding, healing, and controlling, not the whole organ or whole body, but the cell.

Cells differ very widely in some respects. The blood cells which initiate clotting, for example, are extremely small. Other cells, such white blood cells, are especially large and can actually swallow up and digest invading bacteria.

Some cells, such as the muscle cells, can relax and contract. Some cells tend to stack themselves like stones in a wall, as do skin cells. Some have deep indentations, as do the goblet cells in glands. Some rapidly produce chemicals which send electrical impulses along a chain, as nerve cells do.

But all human cells have certain attributes in common. A few key features of a typical cell are shown in Figure 7-2; those which don't concern us here, are omitted.

First, we might notice that the cell has an outer skin, known as its *membrane*. Inside the membrane lies the *cytoplasm* ("cell plasma"), the fluid of the cell. The cytoplasm has a great many small bodies—such as mitochondria and ribosomes—within it. Around these wash nutrients, wastes, and chemicals, circulating freely.

The result is a kind of chemical ladder. The sugar-phosphate parts of the units are now the sides of the ladder. The bases form the rungs. And now the ladder twists into a spiral, thus:

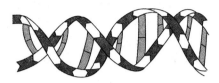

This spiral—the *double helix* called DNA—is the master control of life. Human DNA is estimated to have some 3 billion rungs in its chemical ladder. Within this ladder, lie about 20,000 sets of instructions to make an astonishingly wide array of human proteins.

Where do the instructions lie in DNA? As scientists searched for the answer, it was noted that the bases that make up the rungs of the DNA ladder are varied—that actually there are four kinds of bases. The sequence of these bases seemed random, but the scientists found that the order was the coded plan of life.

So let's focus for a moment on this tiny part of DNA. To give us a simple way of seeing how the code was discovered, let's look at the four kinds of bases as the four suits of playing cards—clubs, diamonds, hearts, and spades:

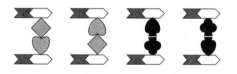

One fact which struck the scientists was that although the bases varied, when they linked up as the "rungs of the ladder," they paired consistently, always in the same pattern. One kind of base will join only with one other kind of base. In terms of our playing-card labeling of the four kinds of bases, clubs link only with spades, and hearts link only with diamonds.

But this wasn't the complete answer—the consistent pattern of the base-matching alone couldn't provide enough variables to code for all 20 amino acids. There had to be more to the code. Scientists were stumped, but not for long.

The breakthrough was the discovery that the code didn't lie in reading one base at a time, but

rather three bases at a time. Each of these groupings of three is called a triplet, and the triplets changed the mathematics drastically, providing 64 possible combinations of the four bases, such as this one:

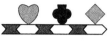

Now the answer to the puzzle rapidly emerged. Sixty-four triplets are more than enough to code for 20 amino acids. By this code—the *genetic code*—the DNA in each cell can use its sequence of bases to call for the amino acids in a specific order and number. Such a chain of amino acids, as we've seen, is a protein.

The sequence of bases in DNA are read 3 at a time; the set of 3 (a triplet) codes for an amino acid.

Using the DNA Blueprints to Make Protein

Thus, a sequence of triplets in DNA is the blueprint for a chain of amino acids—for a protein. The DNA in our cells is much like an extremely long tape—3 billion bases long—on which about 20,000 blueprints for proteins are imprinted. Using these blueprints, the cell gathers the amino acids and arranges them into a wide array of proteins, much as children use a small variety of toy blocks to make a wide variety of structures.

Each blueprint to make a protein is called a gene. Human DNA has about 20,000 genes. These genes are collectively called the human genome.

Let's watch a tiny section of a long thread of our cell's DNA to see how this happens. We see its double strand "unzip" for a short length, letting the two strands separate:

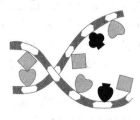

We assume that the body has called for the production of a certain protein. And for clarity, we look at the end of the chain. But actually, the "unzipping" can happen anywhere along the chain, depending on which instructions are needed to make whatever kind of protein is in short supply. The length of the unzipping, of course, is governed by the length of the instructions needed to make that protein.

To keep matters as simple as we can, we will now follow just one side of the unzipped double chain. And we will follow just one *triplet*—the genetic code for a particular amino acid—in the instructions to make this protein.

There are three main stages involved. First, the blueprint for the protein has to be reproduced. Then the reproduction has to be sent out from the nucleus to the cytoplasm of the cell, where the manufacture is conducted. Finally, the needed raw materials (amino acids) have to be brought together and assembled in a chain.

The reproduction of the blueprint begins with certain submicroscopic bits which float freely in the nucleus. These bits are like the chemical units that make up DNA, but differ slightly. One difference is in the sugar which joins with the phosphate and base.

In DNA, that sugar is *deoxyribose* (for *deoxyribonucleic acid*). But in the loose bits floating in the nucleus, the sugar is *ribose,* and thus, the new material is called *RNA* (for *ribo*nucleic acid).

The base of each of the new loose bits is much like the base of one of the four DNA bases, which we illustrated with the four playing card suits (like a single heart, diamond, and so on). And the moment that the DNA spiral unzips, the RNA bits rush in to seize the open places that each matches: a diamond snaps onto the heart of our triplet, a club onto the spade and a heart onto the diamond:

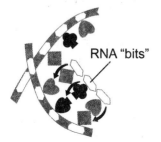

RNA "bits"

As soon as the RNA bits lock onto their opposite numbers in the DNA, they link to one another and begin to make their own chain. When this RNA copy of the protein's blueprint—perhaps fifty triplets long, perhaps a thousand—is completed, the RNA "tape" breaks its bond with the DNA and pulls free.

The first step in protein synthesis is to make a copy of the blueprint for the protein.

The blueprint for a protein has been reproduced, but with a reverse image. If we look back at the drawing of our triplet as it begins to form from RNA bits, we can see that the RNA reproduction is a diamond-club-heart, through the complementary matching of the DNA heart-spade-diamond. One might compare it to the negative of a photograph.

At this point, the newly formed *RNA "tape,"* having freed itself, begins to move. This is the second phase of the process. It leaves the cell's nucleus and moves out into the cytoplasm, where it seeks one of the many tiny protein factories—the *ribosomes.* Because of the function it performs, our wandering RNA is given a more specific name. It's called *messenger RNA.* And it delivers its message through a channel in the ribosome.

The copy of the blueprint to make the protein is called messenger RNA.

The journey looks like this:

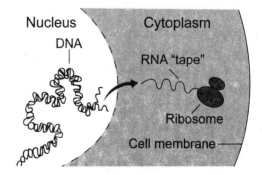

The voyage of messenger RNA. The RNA "tape" breaks free from the DNA spiral, slips through the wall of the nucleus and out into the cytoplasm, where it goes to a ribosome, the site of protein synthesis.

To understand what happens now, it will help if we focus in on our triplet again, as a part of the messenger RNA that feeds into the ribosome.

As we move in closer, we begin to see some odd-looking particles. These particles are called *transfer RNA*. It, too, gets its name from its function, which is to attach to a certain kind of amino acid and bring it to the ribosome. There are at least 20 kinds of transfer RNA—at least one each for the 20 kinds of amino acids needed to make protein.

Each of the 20 amino acids has its own special transfer RNA to carry it to the ribosome.

Each transfer RNA is designed to select and attach itself to a specific amino acid, and also to match up with the triplet code carried by messenger RNA for that same amino acid. At one end, each of these new particles has its own triplet of hearts, clubs, spades, or diamonds in the special combination identifying the particular amino acid. At the other end, the new particles have a curious shape, which looks something like a piece from a jigsaw puzzle. It's a highly specific shape—it's made so that only the particular kind of amino acid coded for will just fit it.

Such a particle might be represented like this:

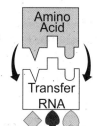

Each amino acid attaches to and is carried by the transfer RNA that carries its triplet code. The shapes of the amino acids are kept simple in the drawings, but they are actually ornate, three-dimensional structures that differ in size, shape, and chemistry.

As each triplet on the tape of messenger RNA enters the channel of the ribosome, it calls for a matching transfer RNA triplet. In the matching process, the "reverse image" sequence of the messenger RNA triplet is paired through a second reversing process with a transfer RNA triplet with the same sequence as the corresponding triplet on the original DNA. Going back to our example, its

diamond club heart triplet attracts one bit of transfer RNA with the complementary heart-spade-diamond sequence.

If we think back to the start of all this, to the triplet we saw on the DNA spiral, it, too, was heart-spade-diamond—DNA's code for a particular amino acid. That amino acid, and no other, is now attached to the other end of the transfer RNA.

As all the triplets on the messenger RNA tape pass through the ribosome, each triplet does the same job. It attracts the right transfer RNA, which in turn holds the right amino acid—until dozens, or hundreds, of amino acids are lined up in the exact sequence called for originally by the corresponding segment of DNA in the cell nucleus. The process looks like this in a very short section of the tape:

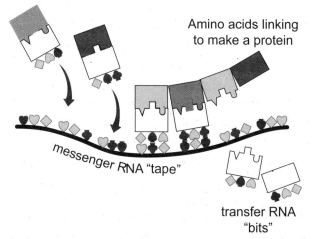

A simplified picture of the ribosome "assembly line" in action. The transfer RNAs arrive with amino acids in tow. These are lined up according to the instructions of the RNA messenger tape. The amino acids are held in proper order until they link with one another. gradually making the entire protein.

Now, as each amino acid falls in line, it joins with the others. And when—according to the blueprint—the chain is complete, the chain breaks free. That chain, of course, is a new protein.

Let us recap briefly. The DNA of a cell has about 20,000 blueprints (instructions) for making human proteins. When a particular protein is to be made, a matching copy of the blueprint to make that protein is made in the form of the tape-like messenger RNA.

The messenger RNA then travels to the ribosome where the protein is assembled. Here, the triplets in the messenger RNA are matched—one by one—by the incoming triplets of transfer RNA. Each matching transfer RNA brings with it the appropriate amino acid. The amino acid is linked into sequence to make one link of the chain we know as protein.

It's as though the messenger RNA had the instructions for assembling a freight train. At the ribosome, which is like a marshaling yard, each type of car needed is summoned up and coupled in line. Once completed, the train is immediately released for its destination. Then new instructions are received, and another train—perhaps a completely different sort—begins to be assembled. A ribosome is capable of putting together any protein which the messenger RNA calls for.

It's by this method that food becomes life. For, protein—as enzymes, and such—is what enables life as we know it.

All of life uses the same genetic code in making proteins. This is why we can use bacteria to make human proteins: Using the techniques of biotechnology, we can snip out a gene in human DNA and insert it into the DNA of bacteria.

Since the body assembles all these proteins from just 20 kinds of amino acids, we can see clearly why our need for dietary protein is so basic. We can also see that the basic need isn't for the proteins themselves, but for the amino acids they contain.

What's truly amazing is that all life forms make their proteins from the same 20 kinds of amino acids, using the same triplet codes for these amino acids, and using the same method of protein synthesis. Each with its own unique DNA as an orchestrator, a tomato seed grows into a tomato by using the same fundamental process and raw materials that a robin's egg uses to become a bird.

Do We Need to Eat DNA?

A doctor recommending a "no aging diet" tells of the importance of DNA and RNA in our lives. He says that the quality of our DNA and RNA goes down as we age, and for good health, "Foods high in DNA and RNA—nucleic acids—are the key."

According to this doctor's thesis, we can counter these aging effects and recapture some of our youth by taking in new DNA from food. Is this a realistic possibility? Luckily not. The DNA and RNA in foods are broken down before being absorbed from the digestive tract. (Our cells make all the DNA and RNA we need—they aren't required in the diet.) But if our cells were able, in fact, to absorb and use the DNA in food—or in certain "rejuvenating" skin lotions—we must consider the consequences.

In the "no aging diet," foods such as sardines, salmon, and the organs of the cow are recommended as "DNA rich." If we were able to use such DNA, we'd begin to make protein according to their blueprints. We'd form the structures and chemicals suitable to fins, horns, and tails. Our rejuvenated selves would be "newer" in the extreme.

Protein and the Questions of Health

Many of us have come to associate a high protein diet with good health. The concept holds some truth and quite a lot of fantasy.

It's true that those nations with diets rich in animal proteins tend to have populations with long lives. Conversely, those nations with low protein diets of mainly plant protein tend to have shorter lives.

Averages in our nation of 300 million can hide millions whose food isn't fully sufficient in protein. The reason can be lack of money, lack of information, or indifference. Also, fad "disease curing" or reducing diets (often consisting of only fruit, or severely limited to only a few plant foods) can be seriously deficient.

But the meaning of this can be deceptive. While lack of protein is a major food problem of developing countries, there are many other factors involved. Animal foods are expensive, and in nations where there's money for animal foods, there's generally money for education, medical care, immunizations, proper sanitation, better housing, and all of the other things which help give people long, healthy lives.

The simple fact is that while protein and amino acids are a basic necessity of life and health, they aren't miracle nutrients, as some promoters would have us believe. When we have adequate protein with adequate amounts of essential amino acids, additional amounts have no further biologic value. As long as the cells have all the amino acids they need, more won't be put to work. To pour excess amino acids into the body is no different than delivering to a mason more bricks than the mason needs to build a house.

Do We Get Enough Protein?

How much protein is needed in the diet to meet the body's protein needs? For most of us, the amount needed is that required to replace normal losses (i.e., maintain body proteins). This replacement need is calculated on the basis of normal body weight. Children and pregnant or nursing women need more protein in proportion to their body weight because children and pregnant women are adding body tissue, and nursing women are "exporting" protein in their milk.

The Recommended Dietary Allowance (RDA) for protein is given in Table 7-1. It's based on needs for growth, maintenance of body proteins, and the composite quality of protein in the U.S. diet, e.g., the RDA for a 150-pound adult who's not over-fat and eats a "typical American diet," is 54 grams (150 x 0.36 = 54) per day. (For a rough estimate of adult RDA, divide normal body weight by 3.)

The average protein intake in the U.S. is well above the recommended levels. Most of us not only get what we need, but much more. Moderately excessive protein intakes are thought to be safe, but it's best to keep it within 10-35% of total calories for those over age 18, 10-30% for ages 4-18, and 5-20% for ages 1-3.[1]

A protein intake of 10-35% of calories is 50-175 gm/day for someone who takes in 2000 calories/day. *[10-35% of 2000 calories = 200-700 calories. Protein = 4 cal/gm. 200-700 cal/(4 cal/gm) = 50-175gm.]*

Most rich protein sources, such as meats, are among our most expensive foods, and when we try to add to a protein consumption which is already

Table 7-1: Recommended Dietary Allowance (RDA) for Protein[1]

Age (years)	RDA (gm/lb)*
0.6-1	0.68
1-3	0.50
4-13	0.43
14-18	0.39
19 and older	0.36
Second half of Pregnancy	0.50
Nursing Women	0.59

*Grams protein recommended per pound normal body weight per day. RDA for pregnant women is based on pre-pregnancy weight, and increases only during the 2nd half of pregnancy.

ample, we waste money. This may not be a burden for our wealthier citizens, but it can be a critical nutrition factor for some people in our society.

What Happens to Excess Amino Acids?

When dietary protein provides more amino acids than we need, the surplus isn't stored. Rather, the nitrogen portion of the amino acid is removed, and what remains is a fat or carbohydrate-like structure (depending on the structure of the particular amino acid) that can be converted to body fat or broken down to provide calories.

Excess protein and amino acids aren't stored.

As for the nitrogen portion, it's a liability for the body, since it can convert to ammonia, which is toxic even in fairly low concentrations. To prevent this toxicity, the discarded nitrogen is made into urea, which is disposed of in the urine. When large excesses of protein are consumed, a correspondingly large amount of urea is formed. The kidneys, in turn, must make more urine. Thus, those taking in large excesses of amino acids need more water—and are thirstier—because they urinate more.

The first step in getting rid of excess amino acids is to remove the nitrogen part, and discard it in the urine as urea.

This need to get rid of urea through urination is one reason why high-protein weight-loss diets can be effective in the short run: the body is forced to dump water in a hurry, often resulting in a sudden loss of weight. Of course the loss is in water, not fat. When the water stores are replenished, the weight goes up.

Do We Need to Eat Sunflower Seeds?

Our food choices are so very broad because the building blocks of protein—the 20 amino acids—are the same for all of life. Mouse protein is just as useful to us as beef protein. We break both down to the same amino acids that our cells require.

This calls into question the claims that certain foods have extraordinary properties as protein sources. Many seeds and sprouts, for example, are sold with this sales pitch.

For protein synthesis, the food source of the amino acids doesn't matter. If the amino acid lysine is what the protein blueprint calls for, the transfer RNA will bring lysine and nothing else—without concern for whether that lysine came from hot dogs, canned tuna, sunflower seeds, soy sprouts, or a bottle of "free amino acids," Nor could the lysine from one source be different from any other. If it were, it wouldn't fit the uniform blueprint and couldn't be used to make protein.

Do Athletes Need More Protein?

The Roman gladiators thought so. During their training, and especially on the night before their trial on the Coliseum floor, they were given meat to make them strong.[2]

Today's gladiators still tend to follow a similar regimen, except now they are much more "scientific" and talk of protein and amino acids instead of meat. Like the gladiators before them, they commonly seek extra protein for their athletic endeavors. But many of today's athletes take their "meat" as spoonfuls of "free amino acids."

How realistic is this idea that athletes need more protein? Contrary to popular belief, heavy exercise requires only a little extra protein. Cross country skiers need only a little more protein when they race 40 to 50 miles a day as they do while relaxing—and they typically already eat much more protein than they need.

The Food and Nutrition Board of the Institute of Medicine, the official body that sets the Recommended Dietary Allowances, states, "It is commonly believed that athletes should consume a higher-than-normal protein intake to maintain optimum physical performance. However, since compelling evidence of additional need is lacking, no additional dietary protein is suggested for healthy adults who undertake resistance or endurance exercise."[1]

Protein is digested into amino acids before being absorbed into the bloodstream, so the body can't differentiate between "free amino acids" coming from ordinary food and that coming from an expensive powder in a jar.

Simply eating more protein doesn't make the body build more muscle. Muscle size is determined by ordinary growth, heredity, and hormones, and by exercise. What we eat merely supplies the materials for making muscle.

When we build more muscle, say, through exercise, don't we need extra protein to make it? Yes, we do need a little more, but the RDA is generous, and also the typical American diet already provides an extra amount—the typical diet of an athlete provides even more.

Vegetarian Diets

As said earlier, most of the vegetarians in the world aren't vegetarians by choice. They would eat animal protein if available and affordable. These people are often suffering from the many ills of poverty, and their strictly vegetarian diet is a poor one.

In contrast, most of the vegetarians in this country are vegetarians by choice and/or religion, and their situation is far different from those in developing countries. Moreover, many of the vegetarians in this country are lacto-ovo vegetarians.

A lacto-ovo vegetarian diet can easily be nutritionally adequate, since dairy products (*lacto*) and eggs (*ovo*) are not only rich sources of high quality protein, but provide other important nutrients as well. Milk, for example, is a good source of calcium and the B vitamins riboflavin and vitamin B-12—nutrients which are often low in strictly vegetarian diets. But milk and eggs are low in iron, so they are vulnerable to iron-deficiency anemia, as are strict vegetarians. As will be discussed in Chapter 17, the iron in plant foods isn't as easily absorbed as iron in meat.

Those who choose to become strict vegetarians (vegans) as adults can have nutritionally adequate diets, when they are knowledgeable about nutrition and foods and apply their knowledge to their eating. Including sources of vitamin B-12 (multivitamin tablets, B-12-fortified breakfast cereal, etc.) is particularly important because B-12 isn't found naturally in plant foods.

Infants and young children are at higher risk of developing nutrient deficiencies on strictly vegetarian diets. They need more nutrients, including protein and calories, in proportion to their body weight, and need higher quality protein than adults. They should eat complementing plant proteins in the same meal to improve protein quality (see Chap. 6). In this country, growth retardation is often the first sign seen in children on strictly vegetarian diets.

Protein Energy Malnutrition

Protein deficiency rarely occurs alone. Typically, there's a deficiency of calories and other nutrients as well. Severe protein deficiency is most commonly seen in children living in poverty in developing countries.

As would be expected, a severe protein deficiency affects the synthesis of a wide variety of proteins in the body and has diverse effects. For example, less of a blood protein called albumin is made. As a result, some of the fluid normally held in the blood by albumin flows out of the blood vessels and into the surrounding tissue. This causes the tissue to swell, and a protein deficient child to look "puffy," especially in the face and belly.

The diseases of protein-energy malnutrition are also known as marasmus (marasmos is Greek, meaning wasting away) and Kwashiorkor (a local term in Gold Coast, Africa for displaced child). When a nursing mother is malnourished, she makes less milk, but the milk she does make is fairly normal in composition (i.e., the milk isn't "protein deficient").

Protein-deficient children are often small for their age and are prone to infection (antibodies are proteins). If their hair is normally black, it may contain light bands of orange, from insufficient pigment to darken it (the pigment melanin is made from the amino acid tyrosine). Brain growth may also be retarded, often starting before birth with a malnourished mother.

Clearly, breastfeeding is of tremendous importance in developing countries where malnutrition and poor sanitation are common. Breast milk is often the only regular source of high-quality protein and other essential nutrients available to an infant. Breast milk also provides calories and some protection against infections. The infants often develop protein-energy malnutrition when they are displaced at the breast by a newborn sibling.

The Need for Energy Comes First

Meeting energy needs is a higher priority for the body than meeting protein needs. If a diet is deficient in calories, the body will "burn" amino acids to meet energy needs rather than use the amino acids to make protein. Thus, when energy needs aren't met, protein needs are higher because some of the protein is diverted for energy production. Inadequate amounts of calories and protein often go hand in hand in many developing countries—a protein deficiency is made much worse by a calorie deficit.

A dilemma occurs in setting requirements and making recommendations for protein intake in developing countries. Should the recommended protein intake be based on the actual average intake of calories, which is often inadequate, or should it be set lower, based on an assumption of adequate calories? This is an important question, because recommendations for protein intake are used in forming food policies, and are used by individual countries as well as world health organizations in providing aid.

Food rich in protein (e.g., meat, eggs, milk) is much more expensive than food rich in carbohydrate (e.g., rice, corn). Using protein-rich food to provide necessary calories is an inefficient use of available resources. Therefore, when resources are limited, the need for inexpensive sources of calories is related to the problem of providing adequate protein.

Moderation in Protein Intake The Middle Road to Good Nutrition

Too much protein can be harmful too. The animal foods rich in high-quality protein are often rich in saturated fats and cholesterol, and high in calories. Meats, milk, and eggs are also devoid of fiber. Thus the same foods that can "cure" the hungry in impoverished countries—foods such as hot dogs, fried chicken, pizza, cheeseburgers, and ice cream—are excessive in the American diet.

In contrast, much of the malnutrition in developing countries stems from a diet that contains only plant foods—foods that contain less and lower quality protein, are devoid of cholesterol, and are generally low in fat and calories. The typical American diet can be improved by more of these foods.

The traditional diets of many countries contain moderate amounts of protein. In these diets, animal sources of protein are not the center of the meal as they tend to be in the American diet. Rather, they are often just one of several ingredients in the main course. Examples include Chinese stir-fried broccoli with bits of beef, an Indian dish of lentils and vegetables mixed with small cubes of cheese, and the Middle Eastern dish of couscous—a flavorful mound of crushed grain topped with vegetables mixed with bits of meat.

We can do the same with our American menus by, for example, eating smaller portions of meat and more generous portions of the plant foods that we often consider the "side dishes." A prudent diet is one that contains a variety of foods, that includes only a moderate amount of animal proteins.

Summary

Proteins are made within cells. The blueprints to make proteins are encoded in the structure of DNA, the genetic material that lies in the center—the nucleus—of cells. Human DNA contains about 20,000 blueprints to make proteins. Each blueprint—the directions to make a particular protein—is called a gene.

DNA is a long double-stranded chain of chemical units, each of which contains a substance called a base. There are four kinds of bases found in DNA, and it's the sequence of these bases along the chain of DNA that encodes the directions to make protein.

The bases are "read" in groups of three. This provides 64 possible combinations of the four bases—more than enough to code for the 20 kinds of amino acids needed to make protein.

A particular sequence of three bases (*triplet*) is the genetic code for a particular amino acid. With this genetic code in hand, one can determine the sequence of amino acids in a protein by "reading"—three at a time—the sequence of bases in the protein's blueprint.

One kind of base will join only with one other kind of base. In this way, a complementary copy of a precise sequence of these bases is made.

The first step in making a protein is to obtain such a copy of the particular sequence of bases in DNA that encodes the directions to make that protein. This copy is made in the nucleus of the cell and is known as messenger RNA.

The messenger RNA moves out of the nucleus into the cytoplasm, and attaches itself to a ribosome, the site of protein synthesis. As the triplets of bases are "read" on the messenger RNA, the corresponding amino acids are delivered via transfer RNA, and the amino acids are connected. When the entire messenger RNA is read, the newly-formed protein is released from the ribosome.

Our dietary protein requirement provides the amino acids necessary for protein synthesis. For adults, the dietary protein requirement is generally that amount needed to maintain the body's proteins. Relative to body weight, children and pregnant women need more protein because they are adding—rather than just maintaining—body proteins. Nursing mothers also need additional protein in order to make milk protein.

Athletes do need a little more protein, but typically the protein in their diets alone far exceeds their need. When protein intake is excessive, the excess isn't stored. Rather, the amino acids are converted to fat or carbohydrate-like compounds, and are then broken down to produce energy or are stored as body fat. Because protein-rich foods are generally expensive, such uses of protein are economically wasteful.

The RDA for protein, like the RDA for other nutrients, is generous. The average protein intake in the United States is well above the RDA.

Many of the vegetarians in the U.S. include dairy products and/or egg in their diet (lacto and/or ovo vegetarians), so can easily get adequate amounts of vitamin B-12, calcium, and high-quality protein. Strict vegetarians (vegans) have to be more vigilant, especially in getting vitamin B-12, because B-12 isn't found naturally in plant foods.

In many developing countries, severe protein deficiency is common. The protein deficiency is usually accompanied by deficiencies of other nutrients and inadequate calories. Inadequate calories makes the protein deficiency worse, be-cause the body's first priority is fulfilling energy needs—the body will break down amino acids to meet the need for energy rather than using the amino acids to make protein. This manifests itself in large numbers of children with the ills of protein-energy malnutrition.

Breastfeeding can be a matter of life or death for the infants—breast milk can be their only dependable source of high quality protein and other essential nutrients.

Moderation is a key to good nutrition. Protein intake is no exception. Animal sources of protein are generally high in protein, but have no fiber, and are generally high in fat. Since the typical American diet is high in protein and fat and low in fiber, our diet could be improved by eating smaller portions of meats and high-fat dairy products, and eating larger portions of whole grains, vegetables, and fruit.

Part 4

Fats–Mysteries and Simplicities

Chapter 8

Fats Seen and Unseen

If the carbohydrates have had a sinister image, fats have been portrayed as downright evil. Of course the very word fat *has had unpleasant associations even beyond the modern obsession with slimness; the word has traditionally suggested inferiority, as in "fat head" and "fat chance." But now it has an additional burden to bear in our national consciousness, as we hear of the dangers of too much fat in our food.*

As our major health concerns have shifted to chronic diseases, we have increasingly received messages about dietary fats. Are the fats in our diet bad? Should we give them up completely?

Once again we come back to the nutrition goals of balance and moderation—hardly soul-stirring battle cries, but profoundly important. As the facts of dietary fat are examined, the true perspective of the good and not-so-good of this essential nutrient become clear, and we take another step toward becoming our own nutrition expert.

The old-timers of the Hudson's Bay Company, who knew the Arctic north very well, called it "rabbit starvation." Anthropologist explorer Vohjalmur Stefansson, who left Harvard in 1906 to live and hunt with Arctic tribes, described the problem as "fat hunger." He tells us that: *"After the last scrap of fat is gone from the diet of a hunting people, headache and diarrhea will start. Fur traders believed that death from fat starvation would come in from four to eight weeks..."*[1]

Stefansson also reports that, while this problem was common among these Indians, it was rare among the inland Eskimos because the inland Eskimos: *"... bought pokes of seal oil from the coastal people which they carried with them in case of shortage."*[1]

The true nature of the "fat hunger" is obscure. But there is the clear reminder that fat is an essential nutrient.

To understand the role of fat in the diet, we must know some basic principles of fats in nutrition. We begin by looking at the nutritive values of dietary fats, and then look at the various types of fats—relating their chemistry to their physical properties as food, and to their functions in the body.

Fat is Not Evil

There has been a lot said about the dangers of eating too much fat. There are good reasons for focusing attention on dietary fat. But for the unwary, these dire warnings can be misleading. For the evils associated with dietary fats are related to excessive use, not to harm in fat itself. In fact, fat is an essential nutrient.

The Essential Fatty Acids

We really do not know whether the Arctic Indians suffered from fat starvation because their game grew scarce and lean. We do know, however, that certain fats are required for health. These fats are called *essential fatty acids*, and there are two—*linoleic acid* and *linolenic acid*. Like essential amino acids, these fatty acids are required in the diet—they are needed in the body, and the body cannot make them.

Figure 8-1: Fat-soluble nutrients accompany fats in food.

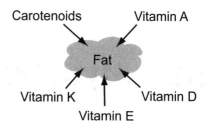

Although our need for essential fatty acids is very basic (for such tasks as forming cell membranes and for the synthesis of some fundamental chemicals), our total need for them is small. Deficiencies of these essential fatty acids are rare, generally occurring only in cases of medical problems severely affecting fat intake or fat absorption.

| The two diet-essential fats: | • linoleic acid |
| | • linolenic acid |

Special medically administered diets, using liquid formula diets or intravenous feedings with little or no fat, have resulted in deficiencies. Linoleic acid deficiency can retard infant growth and cause scaly skin lesions. Symptoms of linolenic acid deficiency include blurred vision and numbness and pain in the legs.

The essential fatty acids come mainly from plant and fish oils. They are scarce in most meats. Game tends to have far less fat than domesticated-animal meat. And hungry game has even less fat. So perhaps the Arctic Indians—when they had only some very lean meat and little access to plant foods—did suffer from some sort of shortage of dietary fat. In contrast, the Eskimos consumed whale, seal, and fish oils, which are rich in essential fatty acids.

Fats Carry Vitamins, Too

Another speculation about the Arctic Indian illness stems from the fact that when the game were short of feed, plant foods would have been scarce for the Indians as well. Thus there could have been shortages of a number of other nutrients commonly found in plants, such as vitamin C, folate, magnesium, and potassium. On the other hand, even assuming there were adequate plant food sources of such nutrients, the leanness of their diet alone may have deprived the Indians of some vitamins. Four vitamins (A, D, E, K) are *fat-soluble vitamins.* That is, they accompany fats in foods (see Fig. 8-1).

Fat and Pleasure

Fat not only carries the fat-soluble vitamins, but gives certain desirable properties to food. Fat satisfies hunger longer, gives a smooth texture to foods, and carries fat-soluble flavors. When cookies are described as so delicious that they "melt in your mouth," it is the fat in those cookies (as well as the fat in any chocolate chips) that melts.

Fat makes foods tender, moist, and flavorful—as in the porterhouse steak marbled with fat, and in the croissant baked with layers of butter. When food is put into hot fat, it cooks quickly (*fast food*) as the fat browns, flavors, and crisps the outside—thus the ever-popular fried chicken and French fries.

So when the Indians were deprived of fat, we can expect that they were deprived of much of the pleasure of eating as well. This may have led to a loss of appetite that could have aggravated any malnutrition.

While we have no sure answers about the Arctic Indian malady, we have seen how the nutritional role of fats could easily have been a critical factor. And we begin to see how fats in appropriate amounts are anything but dietary villains.

What is a Fat?

Fats are a group of chemical compounds which do not dissolve in water, but do dissolve in organic solvents (solvents which have a chemical backbone of carbon, such as ether or chloroform). To put it simply, fat added to water floats to the top, as on the surface of chicken soup (thus the classic statement that oil and water do not mix). Similarly, if we dribble gravy on our clothing, water will not sponge it away. Instead, we use cleaning fluid (an organic solvent) to remove it.

Figure 8-2: Structure of Triglycerides.

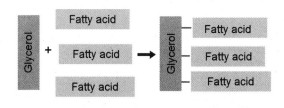

Glycerol and 3 fatty acids ⟶ 1 Triglyceride

Triglycerides

There are various kinds of fats, but when we speak of fatty foods, or body fat, or salad oil—or just plain fat—we are generally referring to triglycerides. Triglycerides comprise 98% of fat in food and are the storage form of fat in our body. A triglyceride derives its name from its structure—three *fatty acids* linked to *glycerol* (see Fig. 8-2).

Glycerol is a fairly familiar substance, with the household name of glycerin. Indeed, it is probably more common in the lives of most consumers than they suspect, since glycerol/glycerin is one of the most basic ingredients of the creams and lotions that are rubbed into so many hands and faces, mixed with colors and spread on the lips, or worked into hair for "styling."

Fatty acids make up the bulk of triglycerides. Because glycerol is always the same, differences between triglycerides are accounted for by differences among the fatty acids. Since all triglycerides have three fatty acids in their structure, the differences in triglycerides are the result of different combinations of fatty acids.

Fat and oil are both triglycerides, but we think of fat as oil when it is liquid (e.g., salad oil). But some oils (e.g., palm and coconut oils, some fish oils) are solid. As a rule, fats from plants and sea animals (e.g., fish, seal) are called oil, and fats from land animals are called fat. Contrary to popular belief, liquid oil has as many calories—and as much fat—as solid fat.

Chemically, the structures of fatty acids are somewhat similar to carbohydrates—made of carbon (C), hydrogen (H), and oxygen (O). Let us compare glucose (a carbohydrate) and caproic acid, a fatty acid found in butter and coconut oil.

Look carefully, and we see some distinguishing differences. The most striking difference is that the fatty acid has very little oxygen. (The "acid carbon" at the one end of the fatty acid is the only part that carries oxygen. This is the part that attaches to the glycerol in a triglyceride.)

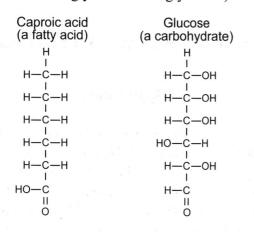

Caproic acid (a fatty acid)   Glucose (a carbohydrate)

Fat as a Concentrated Source of Calories

Since it is the carbon portion of fat or carbohydrate that is "burned" as fuel, the lesser amount of oxygen in the fatty acid's structure makes fat a concentrated source of fuel (concentrated carbon). Witness the crude oil lamps used in so many cultures for millennia, really nothing much more than dishes of oil and a wick. From Aladdin, to the Roman catacombs, to Colonial America, these were the basic lighting utensils.

Recall that the burning of fuel is a process of oxidation—the addition of oxygen. With so little oxygen in its structure to begin with, the carbons in fat can take on more oxygen before becoming fully oxidized to carbon dioxide. In contrast, a carbohydrate starts out with more oxygen in its structure—its carbons are already partially oxidized.

The fact that fat excludes water makes fat an even more concentrated source of calories. In other words, water does not mix with fat to dilute its caloric value, as it does with protein and carbohydrate.

Salad oil, for example, is 100% fat, and thus has an energy value of 9 calories per gram (120 calories/tablespoon). In contrast, carbohydrate and protein hold about three times their weight in water. As examples, potatoes, bananas, and the non-fat portion of meat are about 75% water and 25% carbohydrate or protein. The 4 calories per gram of dry carbohydrate and protein have thus been diluted to only 1 calorie/gm of potato:

$$4 \text{ cal}/(1 \text{ gm dry carbohydrate or protein} + 3 \text{ gm water})$$
$$= 4 \text{ cal}/4 \text{ gm} = 1 \text{ cal/gm}$$

Thus in realistic terms, the caloric differences between fats on the one hand, and proteins and carbohydrates on the other, are much greater than the 9 calories/gm for fats and 4 calories/gm for protein and carbohydrate. As normally found in food (and in our own tissues), water-holding carbohydrate and protein actually have an energy value of 1 cal/gm compared to fat's 9 cal/gm. This striking difference has important implications.

If you add just 1 tablespoon of butter to ½ cup cooked rice, you will double the calories, since each contains about 100 calories (see Table 8-1). One can see why a high-fat diet easily becomes a high-calorie diet—and why many people in developing countries, where fat is a luxury item, suffer from a lack of calories.

Fat has 9 cal/gm (calories per gram) versus 4 cal/gm for carbohydrate and protein.

When a diet is low in fat, it is "bulky." Consider a child who needs 1,800 calories a day and only has low-fat plant food to eat. That child would have to eat about 26 cups of carrots or 17 bananas or 15 boiled potatoes or 8 cups of rice to get those 1,800 calories.

When American school children are asked, "When is chocolate candy nutritious?," they are stumped. They aren't accustomed to thinking of candy this way. And when they dawdle over the vegetables at dinner, and their parents say, "think of the poor starving children in the world," chances are they would be glad to send their vegetables overseas. But in fact, chocolate bars (rich in fat, a chocolate bar provides about 150 calories per ounce) would be better to send—these are more nutritious to starving children than vegetables (a dilute source of calories).

Table 8-1: Fat, Water, Calorie of Some Foods.

	Calories	% Water*	% Fat*	Cal/gram
One Tablespoon:**				
Salad oil	120	0	100	9
Butter, margarine, mayonnaise	105	15	80	7
Table sugar (sucrose)	45	0	0	4
Honey	60	15	0	3
Jam, jelly	55	30	0	3
Sour cream	25	70	20	2
Catsup	15	70	0	1
Mustard	10	80	5	1
2 oz. almonds	355	0	55	6
2 oz. chocolate bar	300	0	35	5
1 saltine cracker	15	5	10	4
1 slice bread	70	35	5	3
½ cup cooked rice	105	75	0	1
1 banana	105	75	0	1
1 orange	65	80	0	0.5
1 egg white	15	90	0	0.5
½ cup watermelon	25	95	0	0.3

* % Water by weight and % Fat by weight, rounded to the nearest 5%

** 1 tablespoon (T) of foods has different weights, e.g., 1 T sugar weighs less than 1 T honey or jam.

Fat serves as a concentrated source of energy in our body as well. It enables us to store excess calories without adding much bulk. A 150-pound person of normal weight might have about 15 pounds of stored expendable fat. To store this many calories (more than 60,000) as carbohydrate would require about 120 pounds.

Birds that migrate long distances accumulate fat to store the large amount of energy needed for the flight. If they stored it as carbohydrate, they would have trouble even getting off the ground. Plants—"stuck" in the ground as they are—can effectively store the bulk of their energy as carbohydrate. Note, however, that many seeds of plants are rich in fat (e.g., sesame seeds). This gives the seeds a lightness (a mobility of sorts) that allows them to be more easily dispersed, and provides a compact source of the initial energy the seed needs to sprout.

Fat Substitutes: Fat being such a concentrated source of calories, the calorie-conscious among us may wonder: How can we indulge in the pleasures of fat-laden foods without taking in so much fat and calories? It is a billion-dollar question that food companies race to answer.

Simplesse, the fat substitute used in the 1990s to make the imitation ice cream *Simple Pleasures,* is based on protein (from egg and milk) shaped into tiny spheres. Because protein holds water, it's a low-calorie (1 cal/gm) substitute for fat (9 cal/gm). The protein sphere was designed to give the slippery "mouth feel" of fat. Simplesse doesn't work in products that must be heated (e.g., cookies and crackers) because this changes its shape (i.e., denatures the protein) and thus its feel.

What is "juicy" about a hamburger patty is its fat. A lean hamburger patty tends to be quite dry. How does one get a hamburger that is both lean and juicy? In McDonalds' McLean Deluxe burger (dropped from the menu because it didn't sell), lean beef was mixed with carrageenan, a soluble fiber derived from seaweed. Carrageenan, like all dietary fibers, holds water—and thus provides "juiciness" to a lean hamburger patty.

The juiciness in McDonalds' Mclean Deluxe burger came mainly from water rather than fat. More fat in a food means less water in the food—and more calories.

What about the condiments that can add to the fat content of the burger? The McLean Deluxe came without cheese and without the mayonnaise-type dressing. It was dressed only with low-fat condiments of lettuce, tomato, ketchup, mustard, onions, and pickles. Although the McLean Deluxe weighed about the same as a Big Mac and weighed more than a Quarter Pounder, it had fewer calories (320) and much less fat (10 gm) than either the Big Mac (540 cal, 29 gm fat) or the Quarter Pounder (410 cal, 19 gm fat).

What about French fries? As yet, there are no fat-substitutes that are approved for frying foods other than chips. Awaiting government approval

Fig 8-3: Structure of Olestra. Olestra adds the "juicy" quality of fat, but is not digested.

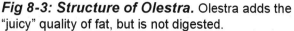
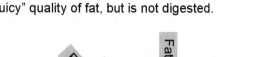

for use in frying is olestra (Olean®). Olestra is a very versatile fat substitute because it is, in fact, a fat—yet calorie-free. How can this be?

Instead of having 3 fatty acids attached to a glycerol backbone (as a triglyceride has), Olestra has a sucrose (*table sugar*) backbone with 6 to 8 fatty acids attached (see Fig. 8-3). This makes olestra indigestible by humans—and *calorie-free*. Olestra is approved for use in salty snacks (e.g., "Light" or "Wow" potato chips), but not for use in frying foods like French fries, or in foods like salad dressing or cookies.

The technical name of olestra is sucrose polyester. The properties of sucrose polyester can be changed by changing the number and kinds of fatty acids attached to the sucrose backbone.

One concern was that olestra could act as a laxative. Being indigestible, it becomes part of the stool and might make it "slippery." (Some people take mineral oil as a laxative—to make the stool "slippery.") Many consumers complained of diarrhea and such, but a double-blind study showed diarrhea, stomachache, "gas," etc., to be the same, whether or not olestra was consumed.[3]

At a Chicago Cinemaplex, 1123 volunteers ages 13-88 were randomly given regular or olestra potato chips. Followed-up for 4-10 days, symptoms and episodes of GI upsets were similar in both groups, with no relationship to the number of chips eaten.[3]

Because olestra is chemically a fat, fat-soluble substances dissolve in olestra (but only when eaten about the same time), and can be lost along with olestra in the stool. To compensate for this, the fat-soluble vitamins A, D, E, and K are added to products made with olestra.

Saturated vs. Unsaturated Fats

Back to triglycerides. At room temperature, certain fats are liquid and others are solid. This reflects a basic difference in the kinds of fatty acids that are attached to glycerol in a triglyceride. Solid fats, as in bacon, are predominantly *saturated fatty acids*. Liquid fats, such as salad oil, are predominantly *unsaturated fatty acids*.

Of course, every shopper knows about unsaturated fatty acids—or was it polyunsaturated? And that there is something good—or was it bad?—and more expensive about them. They are why, if we really love our families, we buy the corn oil margarine—or was it safflower? Anyway, they have something to do with the oil floating on top of old-fashioned peanut butter—or does it? And the magazine article said that polyunsaturated fat is better for you—or was it worse?

Happily, the basic chemistry of saturated and unsaturated fatty acids is not so complicated. A saturated fatty acid is one in which all the positions for hydrogen (H) are filled: the carbons in the fatty acid are saturated with hydrogen. *Stearic acid*, common in beef *(steer)*, is an example (see Fig. 8-5a).

An unsaturated fatty acid is one which does not hold all the possible hydrogen—it is unsaturated with respect to hydrogen. *Oleic acid*, common in olive oil, is an example (see Fig. 8-5b).

Let us look at these two structures carefully. We see that both molecules have 18 carbons, and in most other ways are exactly alike. The key difference is that the unsaturated oleic acid is missing two hydrogens. This seemingly trivial difference is important in its effects in the body (as we shall see in the next chapter). It also determines whether the fat in food is liquid or solid. If the oleic acid (with two missing hydrogens) predominates in the triglyceride—as it does in olive oil—it is liquid at room temperature. But if stearic acid (with all its hydrogens) predominates—as in beef fat—the fat is solid.

In unsaturated fatty acids, hydrogens are missing in twos, causing the adjoining carbons to form

Figure 8-4: Unsaturated fats do not stack compactly and are liquid at room temperature. Saturated fats stack tightly and form solids.

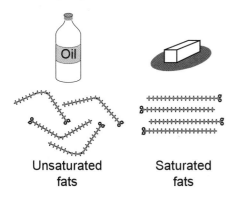

Unsaturated fats   Saturated fats

Figure 8-5: Chemical Structure of Some Fatty Acids

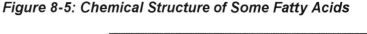

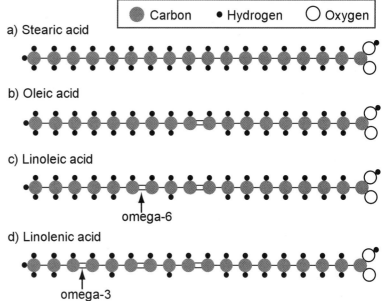

a) Stearic acid

b) Oleic acid

c) Linoleic acid

omega-6

d) Linolenic acid

omega-3

an extra bond—a double bond. Thus, oleic acid is called *monounsaturated* because it has one double bond—one (mono) place where it is unsaturated (can take on more hydrogen).

A polyunsaturated fatty acid has more than one double bond. An example is the essential fatty acid *linoleic acid*, with two double bonds (see Fig. 8-5c). The other essential fatty acid *linolenic acid* also has 18 carbons, but contains three double bonds (see Fig. 8-5d).

As has been said, the number of double bonds in the fatty acids affects whether a fat is solid or liquid at a given temperature. Triglycerides contain mixtures of fatty acids (see Table 8-2), so whether the fat is solid or liquid depends on which ones predominate. For example, corn oil is richest in linoleic acid (2 double bonds), and olive oil is richest in oleic acid (1 double bond), and both are liquid at room temperature. But if you put these oils in the refrigerator, olive oil partially solidifies, whereas corn oil (with more double bonds) does not.

All fats and oils contain a variety of fatty acids.

Beef fat is solid at room temperature because its fatty acids are mainly saturated. In contrast, fats from plants are usually liquid because their fatty acids are mainly unsaturated.

Fish contain fatty acids that are particularly polyunsaturated (contain many double bonds) since their fat-containing tissues need to be limber in their cold environment. For example, one fatty acid found in fish contains five double bonds. When fish migrate to waters of different temperature, they change the number of double bonds in their fatty acids to keep the same degree of fluidity in their tissues. If fish had the fatty acids of cows, they would be too stiff to swim. On the other hand, if cows had the fatty acids of fish, more than their tails would swish.

It's warmer in the Tropics, and the oil in tropical plants—such as coconut and palm oils—are more saturated, keeping the same degree of fluidity at a warmer temperature.

Omega Double Bond: Unsaturated fatty acids not only differ in the number of double bonds, but differ also in the location of the double bonds.

In order to describe the location of double bonds, the carbons in the fatty acid are numbered starting from the far end (the CH_3 end)—the omega end—of the fatty acid. The number of the carbon holding the first double bond is the *"omega number."* Linoleic acid, for example, has its first double bond between the 6th and 7th carbon *(omega-6)*. This makes linoleic acid an omega-6 fatty acid. Linolenic acid is an omega-3 fatty acid since its first double bond is located between the 3rd and 4th carbon.

Table 8-2: Fatty Acid Composition of Fats Common in the American Diet

	% of Total Fatty Acids		
	Satu-rated	Mono-unsaturated	Poly-unsaturated
Plant Source:			
Canola oil	6	62	32
Safflower oil	8	13	78
Corn oil	14	28	58
Soybean oil	15	23	61
Olive oil	16	72	11
Peanut oil	17	49	34
Palm oil	51	39	9
Cocoa butter	60	35	3
Coconut oil	91	6	2
Animal Source:			
Salmon fat	19	55	26
Chicken fat	31	48	20
Lard (pork)	41	47	12
Tallow (beef)	52	44	4
Tallow (lamb)	59	35	5
Butterfat	65	31	4

> Omega is the last letter—the far end—of the Greek alphabet. The omega number designates the location of the first double bond, counting from the far end. Omega-3 and omega-6 fatty acids are essential fatty acids.

The location of the first double bond—the omega number—is important because the body can add double bonds or more carbon atoms only beyond that first double bond. In other words, the structure of a fatty acid up to that first double bond is fixed. The body needs linoleic acid for its omega-3 structure, and linolenic acid for its omega-6 structure—making them essential nutrients.

Hydrogenated Fats

Food manufacturers can take polyunsaturated salad oils and add hydrogen to them. In other words, fatty acids are made more saturated. (Hydrogen gas is used along with high temperature, high pressure, and a catalyst to speed the reaction.) This process is called *hydrogenation* (see Fig. 8-6).

When the list of ingredients on a food label includes *partially hydrogenated corn oil*, this means that some, but not all, of the double bonds in the fatty acids in the oil have had hydrogen added to them (converting double bonds to single bonds).

Shortening, such as Crisco, can be made by partially hydrogenating vegetable oil, thereby turning a clear liquid into a white solid. Margarine can be made in the same manner from vegetable oil; nutrients and flavoring added; and colored with carotenoids (a plant pigment) to simulate the vitamin content and color of butter. Margarine sold in cubes (*stick margarine*) is usually more hydrogenated (harder) than margarine sold in plastic containers (*tub margarine*).

In the same way, hydrogenating the oil in peanut butter solidifies the oil so it won't float to the top. This makes the peanut butter smooth and consistently spreadable from the top to the bottom of the jar. Sometimes, more hydrogenated oil is added—more peanut butter without more peanuts. The oil in "old-fashioned" peanut butter is not hydrogenated, and the oil floats to the top.

It should be noted that when vegetable oils are hydrogenated, they don't contain the same fatty acids they had originally. If, for example, linoleic acid (2 double bonds) is completely hydrogenated, it becomes stearic acid instead. In other words, hydrogenated oils no longer have the fatty acid composition shown in Table 8-2.

In practical terms, this means that when you choose between margarines made from corn oil or safflower oil, for example, choose by price, flavor, etc., since the fatty acid composition of both margarines will be somewhat similar if they are similar in softness. So a margarine label that says, "made from 100% corn oil," is correct but misleading because the implication is that the margarine contains the same fatty acids as corn oil. As noted earlier, hydrogenating the oil to make margarine changes its fatty acid content.

> Hydrogenation adds hydrogen to double bonds, making fat more saturated and more solid.

Because different vegetable oils can be hydrogenated to be similar in physical properties (e.g., hard/soft, "melts in the mouth"), companies that

Figure 8-6: Oxidation and Hydrogenation of Unsaturated Fatty Acids. Hydrogenation lessens the chance of oxidation, increasing the product's shelf-life.

Oxidation:
Oxygen splits an unsaturated fatty acid at a double bond.

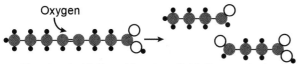

Unsaturated fatty acid   Oxidation products

Hydrogenation:
Adding hydrogen across the double bond of an unsaturated fatty acid produces a saturated fatty acid.

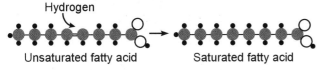

Unsaturated fatty acid   Saturated fatty acid

Figure 8-7: Cis vs. Trans Fatty Acids

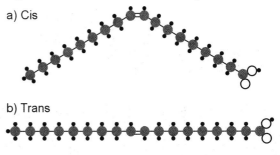

a) Cis

b) Trans

make cookies, crackers, etc., generally buy whatever oil happens to cost the least at the time. The ingredient list will then say, for example, "contains one or more of the following hydrogenated oils: soybean, cottonseed..." so that the label won't have to be changed depending on which oil is used. Buying the least expensive oil for this purpose makes economic sense. If one oil is more unsaturated than another, it can simply be hydrogenated more to achieve the same physical properties (e.g., firmness) desired in the food product.

Also, by hydrogenating the oils (or by using coconut or palm oil, which are naturally rich in saturated fatty acids), food companies can extend the shelf-life of their products. This is because double bonds in fatty acids are more easily broken by oxidation (see Fig. 8-6), making the oil disagreeably rancid ("go bad"). By hydrogenating the oil used in a food product, the product tastes fresh longer (has a longer shelf-life) because there are fewer of the susceptible double bonds,

---
Hydrogenating fat extends the product's shelf life.

Bacteria in the rumen of cows and sheep can hydrogenate fatty acids. For this reason, fat in beef and lamb is more saturated than fat from animals without a rumen (e.g., chickens). The extent of saturation of the fat can also be affected by the saturation of the fat in the animal's diet.

Trans fatty acids are a by-product of partially hydrogenating unsaturated fatty acids—whether by food companies or in an animal's rumen. This relates to the "shape" of a fatty acid wherever there is a double bond.

A double bond in an unsaturated fatty acid creates a distinctive bend in the fatty acid—a cis arrangement (see Fig. 7). The process of partially hydrogenating a fat can flip the arrangement around the remaining double bonds—a trans arrangement. Removing that distinctive bend makes it resemble a saturated fatty acid (see Fig. 8-4). Trans fatty acids are more solid than a cis fatty acid of the same length and with the same number of double bonds. Also, as we shall see in the next chapter, "trans fat"—like saturated fat—can raise our risk of heart disease.

Before 2006, partially hydrogenated fat was used extensively in food products (crackers, cookies, etc.) and to fry foods (French fries, fried chicken, etc.). The listing of trans fat on food labels has been required since 2006. Before, only the amounts of total fat and saturated fat were required. Because consumers recognized trans fat—like saturated fat—as "bad fat," marketers knew that products labeled as having trans fat could lose market share, and that "trans fat free" touted on labels would have market value.

In 2003, Frito-Lay started frying their Lays and Ruffles potato chips in corn oil instead of hydrogenated fat, to eliminate trans fat. In 2006, they switched to NuSun™ sunflower oil, a brand that has less polyunsaturated fat (to extends shelf life), less saturated fat, and more monounsaturated fat.

Food manufacturers found ways to eliminate partially hydrogenated fat (and its trans fat) by substituting tropical oils, substituting a mixture of

Figure 8-8: Phospholipid.

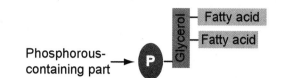

Figure 8-9: Cross section of a sphere of phospholipids, such as lecithin in water.

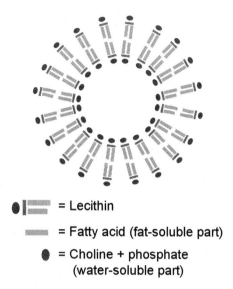

●▐ = Lecithin

▭ = Fatty acid (fat-soluble part)

● = Choline + phosphate (water-soluble part)

completely hydrogenated fat and polyunsaturated fat, etc. Why didn't they do this before trans fat was required on the label? For one, tropical oil costs more than partially hydrogenated oil. For another, the trans fat in partially hydrogenated oil made the fat more solid, yet wasn't a saturated fat—making the fat more solid with lower amounts of saturated fat to list on the label. The companies could go back to using the original polyunsaturated oils, but this shortens shelf life (see Fig. 8-6).

Not All Fats Are Triglycerides

Although triglycerides are what we generally speak of when we speak of fats, there are two other fats—*phospholipids* and *cholesterol*—that play essential roles in the body. These represent a very small part of dietary fat and are not required in the diet because the body can make them. In other words, phospholipids and cholesterol are required in the body but not in the diet.

Phospholipids

Phospholipids are similar in structure to triglycerides. They differ from triglycerides only in that a phosphorus-containing substance replaces one of the three fatty acids (see Fig. 8-8). There are several kinds of phospholipids—the phosphorus-containing portion can vary, as can the kinds of fatty acids.

> Lipid is the scientific name for fat. Hence the name phospholipid (phosphorus-containing fat).

Lecithin is the most common phospholipid in our body and in food. Its phosphorus-containing portion contains a substance called choline. Lecithin is a fairly familiar name on food ingredient lists, and provides a good example for a discussion of phospholipids.

Lecithin is used as an emulsifier in food preparation. An emulsifier suspends small particles of fat in a watery fluid. In effect, it allows fat and water to "mix." It does this by acting as a bridge between fat and water—the fat-soluble part of lecithin (the fatty acids) dissolves in fat, and the water-soluble part (the phosphorus-containing part) dissolves in water.

Classic mayonnaise is made of salad oil, egg yolk, and a small amount of lemon juice or vinegar. The lecithin in egg yolk is responsible for the suspension of oil in mayonnaise. In making mayonnaise, the egg yolk and lemon juice are mixed vigorously while the oil is added slowly. The oil is thus finely divided and kept suspended in this emulsion by the egg lecithin. Hollandaise sauce and béarnaise sauce are made in a similar fashion, except butter is used instead of salad oil.

> Soy lecithin is in soybeans, egg lecithin in eggs, etc. Lecithins vary in their fatty acids. It's the lecithin in egg yolk that keeps the fat suspended in mayonnaise and hollandaise sauce.

In the body, phospholipids like lecithin make up the membranes of cells because of the same chemical properties that make them useful as an emulsifier. If lecithin is put into water, the choline part dissolves in the water, whereas the fat-soluble part repulses water and attracts the fat-soluble parts of other lecithin molecules. In doing this,

Figure 8-10: Cholesterol and Some of Its Products.

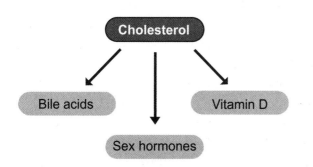

Table 8-3: Cholesterol and Total Fat Content.

	*mg Cholesterol	*gm Fat
1 egg or egg yolk	215	6
Meats:		
3 oz. fried liver	410	7
3 oz. lean broiled hamburger patty	75	18
3 oz. lean roasted leg of lamb	75	7
3 oz. roasted chicken breast	75	3
3 oz. (3 slices) bologna	45	24
3 oz. canned ham, roasted	35	7
Fish:		
3 oz. canned shrimp	130	1
3 oz. baked salmon	60	5
3 oz. baked sole or flounder	50	1
3 oz. tuna, canned in water	50	1
Dairy products:		
1 cup whole milk	35	8
1 oz. Cheddar, American, or cream cheese	30	9
½ cup ice cream	30	7
½ cup cottage cheese (4% fat)	15	5
½ cup low-fat cottage cheese (2% fat)	10	2
1 tablespoon butter	10	11
1 tablespoon sour cream	5	2
Plant food (no cholesterol):		
1 tablespoon salad oil	0	14

*1,000 mg (milligrams) = 1 gm (gram)

the lecithins automatically arrange into spheres, much like globes filled with and surrounded by water (see Fig. 8-9).

Since the fluid of blood and tissues is water, cell membranes form "naturally" from phospholipids. It's an ideal cell membrane in that it has a center layer of fat (see Fig. 8-9) which serves as a selective barrier to keep substances out—or in—a cell. Many substances can't dissolve in fat (i.e., they aren't fat-soluble) and thus can't cross this "fat barrier" by themselves. Also, this cell membrane is ideal in that the cell can insert proteins by "simply" pushing them between the phospholipid molecules.

Cholesterol

Cholesterol is found in all cell membranes in the body and helps regulate the fluidity ("softness") of these membranes. Flat in structure, it fits easily between the phospholipid molecules that form cell membranes. Cholesterol has many important functions in the body—it's needed to make such essential substances as sex hormones, and the bile acids used in digestion (see Fig. 8-10).

Since cholesterol is an integral part of cell membranes of all animals, all animal tissues contain cholesterol. But plants do not. (Plants have cell walls made mainly of fiber.)

If a particular brand of margarine, shortening, or salad oil, or indeed any plant food product is labeled "cholesterol free," don't be fooled into thinking that cholesterol was removed. Coming from plants, there wasn't any cholesterol in them to begin with.

The cholesterol content of some foods is listed in Table 8-3. The total fat content is also listed in this table, to emphasize the point that a food's cholesterol content is independent of its total fat content. Hamburger, lamb and chicken have different amounts of fat, but the same amount of cholesterol. Shrimp has more cholesterol, but much less fat. Salad oil is 100% fat, but has no cholesterol.

Cholesterol has a basic structure of carbon, hydrogen, and oxygen, but the body can't break it down to carbon dioxide and water, as it can triglycerides, phospholipids, carbohydrates, and proteins. Thus, when people eat—or their bodies make—excess cholesterol, their bodies can't readily dispose of it. As we shall see in the next chapter, large excesses can form deposits in the arteries and lead to coronary artery disease.

Summary

Dietary fat is important in several ways:

- It contains the essential fatty acids linoleic acid (an omega-6 fatty acid) and linolenic acid (an omega-3 fatty acid). These are the only fats known to be required in our diet, and deficiencies are rare.

- It carries the fat soluble vitamins A, D, E, and K.

- It makes food more pleasurable—carrying fat-soluble flavors and making foods more tender, smooth, and juicy.

- Fat is a very concentrated source of calories—compared to carbohydrate or protein, it doesn't have much oxygen in its structure, and excludes water.

Fat, by definition, doesn't dissolve in water, but dissolves in organic solvents such as ether or chloroform. Triglycerides, phospholipids, and cholesterol are three different types of fat, but when we speak of fat or fatty foods or salad oil, we are generally referring to triglycerides. Triglycerides make up 98% of the fat in our food, and is the storage form of fat in our body. Phospholipids and cholesterol generally are referred to specifically by name.

A triglyceride is made up of three fatty acids attached to a backbone of glycerol. Since the glycerol portion is a constant, and there are always three fatty acids, triglycerides differ only in having different fatty acids. When one speaks of saturated or unsaturated fats, one is referring to the kinds of fatty acids in the triglyceride.

A fatty acid can be thought of as a chain of hydrogen carrying carbons. It can vary in the number of carbons in its chain (fatty acids with 16-18 carbons predominate in our diet) and also in the number and location of double bonds in that chain. The terms omega-3 and omega-6 refer to the location of the first double bond in the chain.

Fatty acids that don't have any double bonds in their carbon chain are called saturated fatty acids. Fatty acids with one double bond are called monounsaturated, and those with more than one double bonds are called polyunsaturated.

Saturated means that a fatty acid is holding all the hydrogens it possibly can hold—it's saturated with hydrogen. In contrast, an unsaturated fatty acid can take on more hydrogens wherever there is a double bond between two of its carbons.

A predominance of saturated fatty acids makes a fat solid at room temperature, whereas a predominance of unsaturated fatty acids makes a fat liquid. Fats from land animals generally predominate in saturated fatty acids, whereas fats from plants and sea animals generally predominate in unsaturated fatty acids and are called oils.

By a process called hydrogenation (adding hydrogen to unsaturated fatty acids), food companies can take vegetable oils and make them more solid. The extent of hydrogenation can be adjusted to get the desired "softness," etc. Oils treated this way are described on food labels as "partially hydrogenated oils." A by-product of partially hydrogenating oils is trans fatty acid, where the arrangement around a remaining double bond changes to where it is more like a saturated fatty acid in shape and function.

Phospholipids are similar in structure to triglycerides, except that one of the positions on the glycerol backbone holds a phosphorus-containing substance rather than a third fatty acid. Phospholipids (e.g., lecithin) are used as an emulsifier in foods. In the body, phospholipids form the basic structure of our cell membranes.

Cholesterol is quite unlike the structures of triglycerides and phospholipids. It can't be broken down in the body, and therefore excessive amounts can be a problem. It's used in our body in cell membranes and to make essential substances. Cholesterol is found only in animal tissues. Phospholipids and cholesterol are made in our body and aren't essential in the diet.

Chapter 9

Fat and the Doctor's Dilemma

Food advertisers get a lot of mileage out of fat (including cholesterol). "One-third less fat!" or "No Trans Fat!" seems to herald a multitude of products, and they must be effective. Yet we hear that our eating habits are generally lousy. Why aren't these wondrous fat-reduced products making a difference?

The general message is that we eat too much fat. But how much is too much? Are we asking for trouble if we don't make drastic changes—and how do we know which changes to make?

How about over-the-counter supplements such as fish oils and niacin? Do they work to prevent heart disease, and if so, how much do we need?

Fat in the diet is indeed an important factor affecting our health, but much of what we hear is confusing if not misleading. Looking at the facts behind the claims can help a lot.

A major dietary concern in many developed countries is the relationship between heart disease and dietary fats. In the United States, heart disease is the leading cause of death for both men and women. Our high-fat diet is related to heart disease, and other major health problems as well.

As a concentrated source of calories, a high-fat diet increases the risk of obesity which, in turn, increases the risk of various other diseases, such as diabetes and gallbladder disease. Our high-fat diet is also associated with an increased risk of certain kinds of cancer. In the United States, cancer is the second leading cause of death, and the leading cause of death for those under age 65.[1]

While there are many unanswered questions about the relationships between dietary fat and health, there are some practical matters of food choice which are quite clear. We begin by looking at some of the diseases themselves and then their relationship to dietary fat. From this, we can appreciate the basis of dietary advice regarding these diseases, and look at ways to put the recommendations into practice.

Narrowing and Blocking of Arteries

When researchers look at heart disease, strokes, complications of diabetes, and even senility, they see them mainly as the result of a single underlying disease—*atherosclerosis.* Atherosclerosis is a disease characterized by damaged and narrowed arteries, the blood vessels that carry oxygen-rich blood to every part of the body.

Atherosclerosis is first seen as fatty streaks in the inner lining of an artery. Over time, increased fatty deposits damage the cells that line the arteries, and fibrous scar tissue leads to progressive narrowing (see Fig. 9-1). This process can begin early in life. Early stages of atherosclerosis are commonly seen in autopsies of young American men killed in war or accidents.

Since arteries carry oxygenated blood, severe narrowing can cause blood-and-oxygen starvation to that part of the body the artery feeds. If the arteries feeding the heart (coronary arteries—see Fig. 9-2) don't deliver enough oxygenated blood,

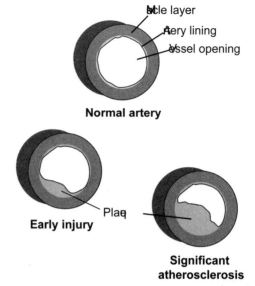

Figure 9-1: Cross Section of Arteries in Atherosclerosis.

Muscle layer
Artery lining
Vessel opening

Normal artery

Plaque
Early injury

Significant atherosclerosis

it's felt as chest pain, and is called angina pectoris ("anger of the breast") or simply *angina.*

Angina is commonly triggered by physical activity and relieved by rest. The physical activity causes the heart to beat faster to provide more oxygen to the muscles. The more rapid heart beat increases the heart's own need for oxygen, but this need can't be met if the coronary arteries are severely narrowed.

In the brain, the effects of an insufficient supply of oxygenated blood will depend on which part of the brain is served by the narrowed artery. Possible effects include slurred speech, confusion, weakness, and loss of vision.

Narrowed arteries are not the only problem caused by atherosclerosis. As atherosclerosis progresses, the thickened and damaged lining of the artery becomes rigid, often with a rough surface. The rigidity lessens the artery's elasticity, and the fibrous scar tissue that characterizes advanced atherosclerosis can rupture, causing a blood clot that can block the artery. A blocked artery shuts off the flow of oxygenated blood to the body tissue served by that artery, leading to the death of those cells in a very short time.

When such a blockage occurs in the heart muscle, it is called a "heart attack." If a significant portion of the heart muscle is damaged in this way, the heart can't contract, causing sudden death. When the blockage occurs in the brain, it is called a stroke. The brain damage also could be

Figure 9-2: Coronary Arteries Nourish the Heart. They encircle the heart "like a crown."

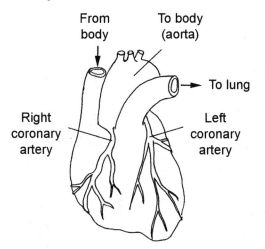

Figure 9-3: Lipoprotein composition and size. LDL is bigger and contains more cholesterol.

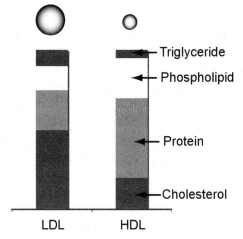

immediately fatal, or it could cause paralysis, loss of speech, loss of memory, or coma.

Stroke can also be caused by a rupture of an artery in the brain—a hemorrhagic stroke. It's often preceded by an outpouching of the arterial wall, usually due to a weak spot and/or high blood pressure. The effect is similar, whether the stroke is due to a blockage or rupture of an artery. In both cases, the flow of oxygen to the brain is interrupted.

Blood Cholesterol

The fatty deposits in atherosclerosis are rich in cholesterol. This is no coincidence. Generally speaking, the higher the level of cholesterol in the blood, the greater the risk of atherosclerosis (see Fig. 9-6). But there's a confounding aspect, related to how the cholesterol is transported. Cholesterol uses different chemical vehicles for transport, which affects cholesterol's destination, which in turn affects the risk of atherosclerosis.

Cholesterol Transport

Because fat and water don't mix, fat (lipid) is transported in the blood in combination with protein. These lipid-protein packages are appropriately called *lipoproteins,* and are classified according to their density. Since fat is less dense (lighter) than protein, the density of a lipoprotein indicates the relative amounts of fat and protein (see Fig. 9-3). The two kinds of lipoproteins that are im-

portant in cholesterol transport are *low-density lipoprotein (LDL)* and *high-density lipoprotein (HDL).*

Low-Density Lipoprotein (LDL) is mostly cholesterol and delivers cholesterol to the cells for use in making cell membranes, sex hormones, etc. When LDL in blood is excessively high, some of it is taken up by scavenger cells in the lining of arteries. As a result, excessive amounts of LDL can lead to deposits of cholesterol in the arterial lining. For this reason, the cholesterol transported in LDL (*LDL-cholesterol*) is called "bad" cholesterol. (Again, however, what's "bad" isn't the LDL-cholesterol itself. Rather, it's an excessive amount that's "bad.")

High-Density Lipoprotein (HDL) is mostly protein, but also contains a fair amount of cholesterol. HDL generally takes cholesterol from cells and to the liver, where the cholesterol can be made into *bile acids* and secreted into the intestine. (Bile acids are used in digestion, and will be discussed in the next chapter.)

To remember whether it's "bad" or "good," think of LDL-cholesterol as Lousy—high levels raise the risk of atherosclerosis. HDL-cholesterol is Healthy—high levels protect against atherosclerosis.

Although most of the bile acids in the intestine are reabsorbed back into the bloodstream, some of it gets trapped by dietary fibers in the intestine and is lost in the stool. The loss of cholesterol via bile is about the only way in which the body can rid itself of cholesterol. The cholesterol in HDL

(*HDL-cholesterol*) is thus called "good" cholesterol. A high level of HDL-cholesterol in the blood
protects against atherosclerosis.

It should be emphasized that the cholesterol itself is the same whether it is being transported
in LDL or HDL. In other words, the description
of cholesterol as LDL ("bad")-cholesterol or HDL
("good")-cholesterol refers to the lipoproteins carrying cholesterol in the blood. Sometimes people
are confused in thinking that there are two types
of cholesterol in the diet—"good" cholesterol and
"bad" cholesterol. Cholesterol is cholesterol.

Risk Factors

A risk factor is a condition or circumstance
that increases the chance of developing a disease
or injury. There are many risk factors for atherosclerosis, the primary ones being genetic predisposition, aging, male gender, smoking, high LDL-
cholesterol, and high blood pressure. Diabetes also
increases the risk. Of course, the more risk factors
one has, the higher the risk of atherosclerosis

Metabolic Syndrome—a cluster of risk factors
occuring together, e.g., high blood pressure,
low HDL-cholesterol—markedly increases
the risk to both diabetes and heart disease.[3]

High Blood-Cholesterol: The Expert Panel
of the National Cholesterol Education Program
recommends that everyone age 20 and older have
their blood cholesterol measured every 5 years.
Total cholesterol should be less than 200 (mg/100
ml), and HDL-cholesterol more than 40. The
target level of LDL-cholesterol is less than 160 for
those at low risk of heart disease. Target levels are
lower, the more risk factors you have.[2]

Genetic Predisposition ranges from the
subtle to the substantial. A family history of heart
disease or stroke suggests a genetic predisposition
to atherosclerosis, especially if heart disease or
stroke occurred in one's father or brother before
age 55, or one's mother or sister before age 65.
Keep in mind, however, that such relationships
may be influenced by other factors; families not
only share genes but also tend to share eating,
smoking, drinking, and exercise habits.

*Figure 9-4: Death Rate in 2005 for Heart
Disease and Stroke in Black and White Men
and Women by Age.[1]*

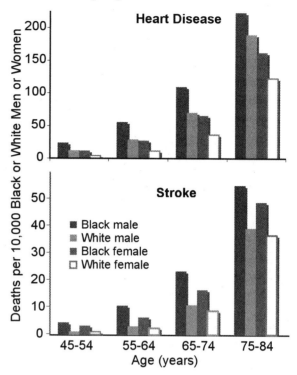

A genetic predisposition is usually reflected
in high levels of LDL-cholesterol in the blood.
Fortunately, the high levels—and thus the risk of
atherosclerosis—can be lowered by diet and/or
medication.

Male Gender: Men of all ages have a higher
death rate from atherosclerosis-related diseases
than women of the same age and race (see Fig.
9-4), perhaps because women have higher HDL-
cholesterol than men. The female sex hormone estrogen raises HDL-cholesterol, whereas the male
sex hormone testosterone lowers it.

Smoking: Smoking increases the risk of a
heart attack—particularly sudden death from
heart attack—even more than it increases the risk
of lung cancer. Smoking reduces the amount of
oxygen the blood can carry, causes constriction
of the blood vessels and damage to the vessel lining, raises blood pressure, and increases the risk
of blood clots.

Aging: In this country, the risk of suffering
or dying from heart disease or stroke increases
progressively and dramatically after age 45 among
men and black women, and after age 55 among
white women (see Fig. 9-4).

Figure 9-5: Age-Adjusted Death Rate for Heart Disease and Cancer (1950-2005).[1]

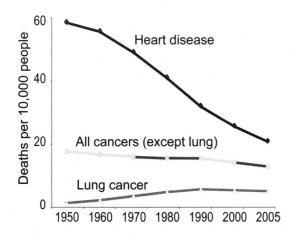

However, the age-adjusted death rate from these diseases has fallen dramatically in this country since the 1950s (see Fig. 9-5). A combination of factors, including less smoking by men, improved treatment of high blood pressure and heart disease, and dietary changes have all contributed.[2]

> Age-adjusted death rates adjust for changes in the proportion of elderly in a population. Otherwise, increased death rates can simply be due to the elderly making up a greater portion of the population.

High blood pressure (140/90 mm Hg or higher) increases the risk of heart attack and stroke. High blood pressure can cause damage to the lining of arteries and can be a determining factor in the formation and rupture of outpouchings of blood vessels in the brain *(hemorrhagic stroke)*. High blood pressure is much more common among blacks than whites in this country.

The 140 in the 140/90 mm Hg blood pressure reading is the pressure in the arteries when the heart contracts (beats). The 90 is the arterial pressure between heartbeats.

Keeping the Pipes Open

Although we can't change our gender or genetic predisposition, we can alter other risk factors. Because atherosclerosis develops over many years, even a modest reduction in its rate of progression can delay significantly the onset of symptoms. For example, dietary changes beginning in

young adulthood to lower LDL-cholesterol levels could possibly slow the progression of atherosclerosis so that a heart attack or stroke that might have occurred at age 60 might be delayed to age 75 or older.

Do Not Smoke

It seems that much of the smoking-caused damage to the arteries can be reversed by quitting smoking. Some of smoking's immediate effects, such as constriction of blood vessels (from tobacco's nicotine), and reduced oxygen in the blood (smoke's carbon monoxide displaces oxygen), are reduced quite fast. Studies indicate that smoking's added risk of heart attack and stroke falls markedly within a year after quitting. But it doesn't seem to disappear entirely for a number of years, depending on how long and how much a person had smoked.

Prevention or Early Treatment of High Blood Pressure

Maintaining normal blood pressure (less than 80/120) can help prevent heart attacks and strokes. Everyone should have their blood pressure checked periodically. The exact cause of high blood pressure in most cases is not known, but genetic factors are involved. Regardless of cause, there are effective treatments.

Medications to lower blood pressure have to be taken continually. A barrier to this is that high blood pressure itself doesn't make you feel bad (so you don't feel any better taking the pills), yet there can be side effects, such as impotence and blood pressure falling to where one feels faint. Changes in dose or medication are made to avoid or lessen such side-effects.

High blood pressure also increases the risk of other diseases such as kidney and heart problems. So early treatment of high blood pressure helps prevent these diseases as well.

Body Weight: If a person with high blood pressure is overweight, weight reduction to a normal weight may, in itself, normalize blood pressure. If one can't reach a normal weight, any weight loss—or at least not gaining more—can help.

Weight loss can also lower risk in other ways. Among those genetically susceptible, obesity can cause a type of diabetes that is generally reversible upon return to a normal weight. The progression of atherosclerosis is accelerated in diabetics—diabetes increases by more than three-fold the risk of dying from diseases related to atherosclerosis.

Psychological Stress can result in high blood pressure in those who are genetically susceptible.

Salt Intake: Some people can lower their blood pressure by limiting salt in food, but a high-salt diet doesn't always cause high blood pressure. Many people don't develop high blood pressure despite a salty diet, presumably because they don't have the genetic predisposition. However, since most of us don't know if we're genetically susceptible, and there's no known advantage to consuming excess salt, the general advice is to avoid eating a lot of salty foods.

Sodium is thought to be the culprit in high-salt diets, but there's some evidence that the chloride in salt may be a contributing factor. Low dietary calcium might also play a role.

The salt intake in the typical American diet is estimated to be about 10-12 grams per day—about 2 teaspoonfuls. The 2005 Dietary Guidelines for Americans recommends keeping sodium to less than 2300 mg sodium (less than a teaspoonful).

Salt (sodium chloride) = 40% sodium
1 tsp salt (5000 mg) = about 2,000 mg sodium.

Alcohol intake shouldn't be excessive. More than two drinks a day tends to increase both blood pressure and the risk of a hemorrhagic stroke independently of high blood pressure.

"Moderate drinking" is up to 1 drink a day for women, and up to 2 drinks a day for men. "One drink" has about a half-ounce of pure alcohol, e.g., a 12-oz. can of beer or wine cooler; a 5-oz. glass of wine; $1\frac{1}{2}$ oz. (jigger) of gin, rum, whisky, or vodka.

Reducing High Levels of LDL-Cholesterol

To lower LDL-cholesterol levels, the Dietary Guidelines Advisory Committee established by U.S. Dept. of Agriculture and the U.S. Dept. of Health and Human Services has dietary recommendations for the general U.S. population, except for children under 2 years old. A program of such magnitude is said to be warranted because:

- Even if blood-cholesterol is at the recommended level, lowering LDL-cholesterol seems to reduce further the risk of heart disease (see Fig. 9-6).

- Since LDL-cholesterol generally goes up we age, a life-long "prudent diet" may help maintain blood cholesterol at recommended levels.

- For those who have atherosclerosis, it appears that lowering LDL-cholesterol can partially reverse the atherosclerotic process by reducing the size of fatty deposits already formed in arteries.

Some people's LDL-cholesterol levels can be modified by diet within a few weeks. But there's a wide variation in how people's bodies respond to diet, since the body's own cholesterol-producing processes are involved.

Three main components of the diet can potentially affect LDL-cholesterol levels:

- Saturated and unsaturated fats
- Cholesterol
- Fiber

Of these, the amount of saturated fat (plus trans fat—see Chap. 8) in the diet has the greatest effect. Trans fat acts like saturated fat in raising LDL-cholesterol, and is a bit worse in that it also lowers HDL-cholesterol slightly.

Saturated vs. Unsaturated Fat: As discussed in the last chapter, triglycerides make up most of the fat in our diet, and are called saturated, mono-unsaturated, or polyunsaturated fat, depending on which fatty acids predominate.

High amounts of saturated fat (and/or trans fat) in the diet tend to increase the LDL-cholesterol levels in the blood (possibly by interfering with the cells' ability to take in LDL-cholesterol from the blood). This LDL-raising effect of saturated fat is fairly common, although some people are much more sensitive than others.

The "typical American diet" contains a lot of saturated fat in such favorite foods as meat, high-fat dairy products, and pastries. The recommendation to eat less saturated fat to lower LDL-cholesterol means cutting down on such foods.

Eating more unsaturated fats generally lowers LDL-cholesterol. Again, some people are more responsive than others.

The American diet contains more saturated fat than either monounsaturated or polyunsaturated fat, so fat consumption in general tends to increase LDL-cholesterol. However, since the total amount of fat in the American diet is high, the aim should not be to eat more unsaturated fats, but rather to eat less saturated and trans fats (and thus less total fat and fewer calories for the overweight).

The recommendation is to eat as little saturated and trans fat as possible "while consuming a nutritionally adequate diet.[5]" One might, for example, replace fatty cuts of meat with poultry, fish, or lean cuts of meat; drink non-fat or low-fat milk instead of whole milk; and eat sherbet, ice milk, or frozen low-fat yogurt instead of ice cream.

Dietary Cholesterol: The amount of cholesterol in the diet generally has much less effect on LDL-cholesterol than the amount of saturated fat. On the other hand, individuals respond very differently to changes in dietary cholesterol. Some can lower their LDL-cholesterol by reducing their cholesterol intake, whereas others cannot.

Since cholesterol in the diet is unnecessary, and many people can benefit from eating less cholesterol, a *2005 Dietary Guidelines for Americans* (see Chap. 18) is to restrict dietary cholesterol to an average of less than 300 mg per day.

The recommendation focuses particularly on egg yolks, since other rich sources of cholesterol (such as organ meats, e.g. liver, brain) are not widely consumed. In practical terms for most people, following the advice means limiting egg yolks to 3 or 4 per week. Other animal foods provide the remainder of the cholesterol "allotment."

One egg yolk has about 215 mg cholesterol. Egg white is virtually fat-free and has no cholesterol.

There is some concern that restriction of eggs in the diet may be a hardship for some people. Eggs are inexpensive, keep a long time in the home refrigerator, and are tasty and easy and quick to cook. Also, the softness of eggs makes them

Figure 9-6: Lower risk of heart disease with Lower LDL-cholesterol e.g., for every rise (or fall) of 30 in LDL-cholesterol, the risk of heart disease rises (or falls) by 30%.[3]

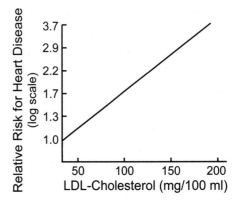

desirable for people with missing teeth or ill-fitting dentures. These are significant considerations for many people, especially the poor and elderly. For many of these people, eggs are a major source of several nutrients.

As a general proposition, it's important to remember that foods contain a variety of nutrients, and individual foods have their pluses and minuses. Although dietary recommendations for prevention of atherosclerosis are important, they shouldn't be viewed in isolation.

For a healthy person whose LDL-cholesterol is raised by dietary cholesterol, reducing or eliminating eggs can, on balance, be beneficial. Yet, there are those whose LDL-cholesterol is not affected by cholesterol in the diet. For those who don't have much money to spend on food or have trouble chewing, etc., the reduction or elimination of eggs could have a negative effect on their diet and health.

Fiber: *Soluble fibers* (see Chap. 4) can help lower LDL-cholesterol. As discussed earlier, soluble fiber can promote the excretion of bile acids (which are made from cholesterol), and can interfere with the intestinal absorption of dietary cholesterol. Furthermore, some breakdown products of certain fibers (broken down by bacteria in the colon) are absorbed into the blood from the colon and may inhibit cholesterol production by the body.

Foods that are particularly rich in soluble fibers include oats, beans, and fruits. Dietary fiber—soluble or insoluble—is not found in animal foods.

Niacin: One particular form of the B-vitamin niacin—nicotinic acid—is used in huge doses 1,000-9,000 mg/day) to lower LDL-cholesterol. It functions as a drug, rather than a vitamin (adult RDA = 14-16 mg/day), when taken in such huge doses. Nicotinic acid is called niacin to avoid confusion with nicotine, the addictive drug in tobacco. Another form of niacin, known as nicotinamide or niacinamide, doesn't have the same effect as nicotinic acid in lowering LDL-cholesterol.

Because nicotinic acid is a vitamin, it can be purchased without prescription. However, huge doses should be taken only under the supervision of a physician. Milder side-effects include itching and hot flushes in the skin, and digestive upsets. More serious side-effects include irregular heartbeats and liver damage. Physicians generally prescribe liver-function tests when treating patients with large doses of nicotinic acid.

Maintaining Normal Levels of HDL-Cholesterol

A blood HDL-cholesterol of less than 40 is associated with increased risk of atherosclerosis. Smoking, lack of exercise, and obesity all tend to lower HDL-cholesterol. Thus, quitting smoking, exercising, and losing excess weight lowers risk by increasing HDL-cholesterol.

> Some people are genetically endowed with unusually high HDL-cholesterol. This protects them against atherosclerosis, and they tend to have a family history of longevity.

A moderate intake of alcohol (up to 2 drinks per day for men; up to 1 for women) is associated with higher HDL-cholesterol. But it can be unwise to start drinking simply to raise HDL-cholesterol. Even moderate amounts of alcohol can cause problems for some people and, as noted earlier, excessive alcohol tends to increase both blood pressure and the risk of hemorrhagic stroke. Also, alcohol slightly raises the risk of breast cancer.

Some people who hear repeatedly through the mass media that exercise increases "good cholesterol" are misled into thinking that more and more exercise will lead to such high HDL-cholesterol that other risk factors become insignificant. It's better to focus on the other side of the coin—that

low HDL-cholesterol is associated with increased risk of atherosclerosis. Where it's stated that a sedentary lifestyle lowers HDL-cholesterol, people may be more likely to conclude simply that moderate exercise is a good idea.

Added exercise (beyond moderate exercise) doesn't proportionately raise HDL-cholesterol. Furthermore, low HDL-cholesterol isn't as important a risk factor as is high LDL-cholesterol, smoking, or high blood pressure. While regular exercise can be important in lowering risk of atherosclerosis, its importance shouldn't be either underestimated or overestimated.

Fish in the Diet

Eating fish is associated with a reduced risk of atherosclerosis. It is thought that the omega-3 fatty acids (see Chap. 8), found mainly in fish, are what reduce risk.

The native Eskimo diet, which includes large quantities of fish, seal, and whale, is very rich in omega-3 fatty acids. Eskimos have a low incidence of heart disease even though their diet is high in cholesterol.

Omega-3 fatty acids are used in the body to make substances that are to reduce the dangers of heart attack and stroke, by dilating arteries, reducing the ability of the blood to clot, lowering blood pressure, and increasing the amount of a substance in blood that helps dissolve clots.

> Nosebleed is a side effect of a high intake of omega-3 fatty acids. Eskimos eating a native diet are more prone to hemorrhage and hemorrhagic stroke; one suspects an excessive intake of omega-3.

Extensive studies have shown that men who eat fish regularly have a lower rate of death from cardiovascular disease than those who don't. But the studies, do not conclusively show that omega-3 fatty acids alone reduce risk. Other protective factor for the fish eaters (and the Eskimos) might be other substances in fish, or something different about fish-eaters, other than eating fish.

Eating fish about twice a week is also linked to a lower chance of dying suddenly from a heart attack. The sudden lack of oxygen to heart muscle in a heart attack can cause the heart to quiver (fibrillate) instead of beat. Omega-3 fatty acids in fish are incorporated into heart tissue, and this may help stabilize it in a heart attack, lessening the chance of sudden death.[6]

Defibrillators are available in many public places to shock the heart into resuming its beat. Best place to have a heart attack? Casinos have their eye on you and can get a defibrillator to you very fast.[7]

The American Heart Association does not recommend taking fish-oil supplements or capsules of omega-3 fatty acids, except under the supervision of a physician. Fish-oil supplements (and other dietary supplements) are classified as a food rather than as a drug, so they are not subjected to the strict regulations (for content, safety, purity, dosage, etc.) established for drugs.

Cancer

Although Heart Disease is our leading cause of death, it has fallen so much that cancer is now the leading cause of death for those under age 85.[8] (Those over age 85 are three times more likely to die of heart disease than cancer.)[8]

Since "getting older" is a risk factor for cancer (about 77% of cancers are diagnosed in those 55 and older[9]), cancer rates rise as the average age of the population rises. When one adjusts for an aging population and excludes lung cancer, the death rate from all other cancers combined has decreased over the past 50 years (see Fig. 9-5).

In looking at death rates from various causes, keep in mind that if we do not die of one thing, we will eventually die of something else. When fewer people die of heart attacks, other causes fill the gap. For example, over 65% of prostate cancers are diagnosed in men age 65 and older.[9] The fact that fewer middle-age men die of heart disease may be at least partially responsible for greater numbers of older men—middle-aged men who live longer—getting and dying of prostate cancer.

Lung cancer is the leading cause of cancer death in both men and women (see Fig. 9-7). About one-third of all cancer deaths is attributed to exposure to tobacco products.[11] Smoking cessation lowers the risk of both cancer and heart disease.

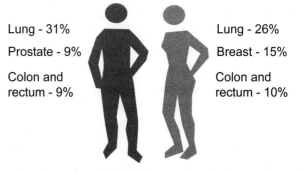

Figure 9-7: Cancer deaths *(estimated % of total cancer deaths in 2007).*[9]

Lung - 31%

Prostate - 9%

Colon and rectum - 9%

Lung - 26%

Breast - 15%

Colon and rectum - 10%

Another one-third of cancer deaths is attributed to diet, physical activity, and being overweight.[11] Cancer of the colon, prostate, and breast is associated with diets high in animal fats, but studies have not shown fat itself to be the culprit.

Diets high in animal fats tend to be low in plant foods and fiber, and high in protein, saturated fat, cholesterol, and calories. Animal studies support the relationship of this general dietary pattern to cancer. For example, animal studies have shown that tumors are more common in animals fed high-fat diets, that diets low in protein and calories suppress the development of tumors, and that certain plant constituents protect against cancer.

Obesity is also more common in populations with high-fat diets. Thus, obesity represents another variable along with the various dietary factors. Many variables are clustered, however. A diet high in fat and calories, for example, coupled with inactivity leads to excess calories and overweight.

Breast Cancer

Breast cancer is more common than lung cancer, but fewer women in the U.S. die of breast cancer—it's detected earlier and is less fatal than lung cancer. Nearly 90% of breast cancer patients (but only 15% of lung cancer patients) live 5 or more years after diagnosis.[9]

The causes of breast cancer are not known, although there are some known risk factors. Genetic susceptibility is a factor (inheriting "breast cancer genes" BRCA-1 and 2 account for 5-10% of breast cancers).[9] Women with mothers or sisters with premenopausal breast cancer have a significantly higher risk.

A woman's reproductive history also affects her risk, presumably through the timing and duration of various female hormone levels. This includes first menstruation before age 12, prolonged use of birth-control pills, no children or having the first child after age 30, menopause after age 55, prolonged hormone-replacement therapy after menopause—all involve long stretches of uninterrupted high-estrogen levels.

Diet-related risk factors include being overweight after menopause,[11] and alcohol intake (more risk with more alcohol).[12] Alcohol raises estrogen levels, as does excess body fat in postmenopausal women. (Estrogen falls at menopause, making body fat a major source of estrogen production.)

There is a wide variation in the frequency of breast cancer throughout the world. Countries with higher fat diets have higher rates of breast cancer. When women move from countries with low-fat diets and low breast cancer rates, to countries with high-fat diets and high breast-cancer rates, their rate of breast cancer rises. In animal studies, a high-fat diet produces more mammary (breast) tumors.

Because of the number of variables present in population studies, however, it's hard to determine whether a specific dietary component (e.g., animal fat) promotes breast cancer. To get groups of women that are comparable in terms of race, socioeconomic level, etc., the control and experimental groups are best drawn from the same population. But when this is done, the diets are usually fairly similar. Also, diets assessed at the time of the study may not be as important as the diet in earlier years.

We've been left to rely on international comparisons to get large differences in diet. Studies comparing breast cancer rates in Japan with rates in the United States are especially noteworthy, because the countries are comparable in industrialization, yet have dramatically different rates of breast cancer.

Age-adjusted death rates for breast cancer are much lower in Japan than the U.S. In 2002, the age-adjusted death rate (deaths/100,000 women) for breast cancer was 19 in the U.S. and 8 in Japan.[10] If genetics were a determining factor, Japanese-Americans would be expected to have rates similar to their racial counterparts in Japan. Japanese-Americans, however, have higher rates (though not as high as Caucasian-Americans). As Japanese in Japan and the U.S. have become more "Americanized," their breast cancer rates have gone up.

It is important to emphasize that proof of a link is not proof of cause-and-effect. As noted earlier, a high-fat diet tends to be high in calories, etc., so it's difficult to fault one dietary component. There are also protective dietary factors to consider. For example, substances in soybeans (prominent in the Japanese diet) might affect the risk of breast cancer. There are also non-dietary factors to consider. For example, breast-feeding is more common in Japan than the U.S., and the use of birth-control pills and post-menopausal hormone-replacement therapy is much less common.

Japan's changing social factors and dietary patterns are giving us more clues. Fish, rice, and soy are staples in the traditional Japanese diet. As Japan's diet has become more Americanized—more meat, fat, fast-foods, sweets, etc.—breast cancer and obesity have become more common.

Healthy Eating

Dietary advice to lower risk of heart disease and cancer are part of the dietary recommendations for a healthy diet, discussed in Chapter 18. A healthy diet includes eating a lot of vegetables and fruits—one of the strongest and most persistent links to less cancer and heart disease.

Lycopene gives tomatoes a red color and is linked to a lower risk of prostate cancer. Guys who can't stay away from fries, can at least drown them in catsup!

Since fat has been a focus of this chapter and the previous one, let's look at lowering fat in the diet. By lowering fat intake, one tends to follow other dietary recommendations as well. A diet lower in fat tends to be higher in plant foods and fiber, and lower in saturated fat, salt, cholesterol, and calories.

Because fat is such a concentrated source of calories, a low-fat diet helps prevent obesity. Obesity, as we have seen, tends to raise blood pressure and

Figure 9-8: Recommended fat intake as a percent of total calories.

Saturated fat (10%)

Total fat intake (20-35%)

1 cup whole milk (3.5% fat by weight) has 8 gm fat and 150 calories:
8 gm fat x 9 cal/gm = 72 cal from fat
72 cal from fat ÷ 150 total cal) x 100
= 48% of total calories from fat

Whole milk

1 cup reduced-fat (2%) milk (2% fat by weight) has 5 gm fat and 120 cal:
5 gm fat x 9 cal/gm = 45 cal from fat
(45 cal from fat ÷ 120 total cal) x 100
= 33% of total calories from fat

2% Low-fat milk

1 cup low-fat (1%) milk (1% fat by weight) has 2 gm fat and 105 cal:
2 gm fat x 9 cal/gm = 18 cal from fat
(18 cal from fat ÷ 105 total cal) x 100
= 17% of total calories from fat

1% Low-fat milk

1 cup of non-fat milk (0% fat by weight) has 0.5 gm fat and 85 cal:
0.5 g fat x 9 cal/g = 4.5 cal from fat
(4.5 cal from fat ÷ 85 total cal) x 100
= 5% of total calories from fat

Non-fat milk

lower HDL-cholesterol, thereby increasing the risk of atherosclerosis. Obesity also raises the risk of diabetes and certain cancers.

Fat Content as a Percent of Total Calories

The 2005 Dietary Guidelines for Americans recommends that 20-35% of the calories in our diet come from fat (see Fig. 9-8). Such advice is too precise to be of practical use to the ordinary consumer—most consumers don't know whether their fat intake is 25, 30, or 40% of their energy intake. Practically speaking, this recommendation is best followed by knowing how the "% of calories from fat" calculation is made, and using these values as a gauge in making food choices.

Comparisons are easiest when fat content is expressed as a percent of total calories rather than as a percent of total weight. When the fat content is expressed as percent of total weight, comparisons are distorted by the amount of water in the food.

For example, fat from dairy products is a major source of saturated fat in our diet. Whole milk contains 3.5% total fat by weight, lower-fat milk is 1–2% fat, and non-fat milk is almost fat-free. It's not readily apparent that switching from whole milk to lower-fat milk would make much difference in total fat, much less saturated fat. Milk, however, is mainly water, so its fat content, by weight, is low and misleading.

To calculate the percent of calories from fat, only two numbers are needed—the grams of fat (or the calories from fat) and the total calories in the food, numbers which are found on food labels and in food composition tables.

About **50%** of the calories in whole milk comes from fat, while it's **35%** of the calories in reduced-fat (2%) milk, **15%** of the calories in low-

fat (1%) milk, and **5%** of the calories in non-fat milk. Looking at fat content this way, the advice to switch from whole milk to lower-fat milk is more convincing.

In another example, consider the meaning of 80% *fat-free* on the label on a package of frankfurters. One wonders if 80% *fat-free* means that 80% of the fat was taken out of this particular brand of frankfurters, making them low in fat. Looking more carefully at the label, one finds that a frankfurter of 100 calories has 8 grams of fat. Since each gram of fat represents 9 calories, 72 (9 x 8) of the 100 calories (72%) comes from fat:

8 gm fat x 9 calories/gram = 72 calories from fat
(72 calories from fat ÷ 100 total calories) x 100 = 72% of total calories from fat

The label is misleading. But it's technically correct because the percentage of fat was calculated as a percentage of total weight, and over half of the frankfurter is water. The label says that each frankfurter weighs 45 gm and contains 8 gm of fat. This means, that *by weight,* the frankfurter is 18% fat [(*8 gm fat/45 gm total weight) x 100 = 18% fat by weight*]. The other 82% of the frankfurter is fat free! It would be more to the point to state, "More than 70% of the calories come from fat," but this, of course, would be disastrous for sales.

U.S. government standards allow a maximum of 30% fat (by weight) in frankfurters. If there is less fat than this, one can expect this to be emphasized on the label. A label stating *33% less fat,* for instance, means that the frankfurters contain 20% fat by weight instead of the allowed 30%.

Going back to the example of switching to lower fat milk, the switch also helps in the Dietary Guidelines to keep cholesterol to less than 300 mg, and saturated fat intake to less than 10% of total calories. 1 cup of whole milk has 33 mg cholesterol and 30% of its calories from saturated fat; the numbers are 18 mg and 22% for 2% low-fat milk, 10 mg and 17% for 1% low-fat milk, and 4 mg and 5% for non-fat milk.

As a final note, keep in mind that there aren't any forbidden foods in a healthy diet. The point is to eat foods rich in saturated fat and cholesterol in smaller amounts and/or less frequently.

Summary

Heart disease is the leading cause of death in the United States. The underlying cause of most heart disease is atherosclerosis, a disease in which arteries are narrowed and damaged. Atherosclerosis not only affects the arteries that feed the heart but other arteries as well. For this reason, atherosclerosis can be the underlying cause of other diseases such as stroke and kidney disease. One of the greatest concerns is that a clot might form in the blood and completely block a narrowed artery leading to the heart or brain. This could lead to sudden death or disability from a heart attack or stroke.

The major risk factors for atherosclerosis are a high LDL-cholesterol, diabetes, genetic predisposition, male gender, smoking, aging, and, high blood pressure.

To maintain normal blood pressure, we're advised to be a normal weight, and avoid excess salt and alcohol. To avoid raising blood levels of LDL ("bad")-cholesterol, we're advised to eat a diet low in saturated (and trans) fat and cholesterol, and a diet rich in soluble fiber. Although extremely high amounts of nicotinic acid (a form of niacin, a B-vitamin) also lowers LDL-cholesterol, taking such amounts is not recommended, except under the supervision of a physician. To maintain normal blood levels of HDL ("good")-cholesterol, one should avoid smoking, lose weight if overweight, and get regular exercise.

We're also advised to eat fish twice a week, since this dietary pattern is associated with a lower risk of dying suddenly from a heart attack. Fish is a rich source of certain omega-3 fatty acids, and it's thought, but not proven, that it is these fatty acids in fish that reduce risk.

Cancer is the second leading cause of death in the U.S. and the leading cause among those under age 65. Lung cancer is our leading cause of death from cancer, and is mostly due to smoking. Our next most common fatal cancers—colon, breast, and prostate cancers—are all associated with a diet high in animal fats. It is important to keep in mind, however, that such a diet tends to be high in cholesterol and calories, and low in plant foods and fiber. The relationship between diet and cancer is not as well understood as the relationship between diet and atherosclerosis, but a diet rich in vegetables and fruit is linked to less cancer in countries throughout the world.

The percent of calories from fat in a food gives a more realistic picture of a food's fat content, and can be calculated from the grams of fat and total number of calories. These two values are found on food labels, as well as in tables of food composition.

Although there are various dietary recommendations to lower risk of atherosclerosis and cancer, it is simplest to focus on lowering the amount of saturated and trans fat. A diet low in these fats tend to be low in cholesterol, salt, and calories, and tends to be high in plant foods and fiber—a diet plan that emphasizes principal dietary recommendations.

Guest Lecturer: Peter D. Wood, DSc, PhD

A Runner's High—HDL

We runners are a dedicated bunch. In the early 1960s, however, we weren't a very big bunch. One evening after work, I was running around Lake Merritt in Oakland, California, in my running shorts. It was dark, cold, and raining. A police car pulled alongside, and the officer asked suspiciously what I was doing running around in my underwear. After I explained myself, there was a long pause before he said, "Well, you have to admit, this is not normal!"

Running is more normal now, but not normal enough. Physical activity is important to one's health, and it has been my good fortune to combine this message and my love of running with my scientific endeavors.

One of my earliest studies on the effects of exercise, published in 1965, was on how certain fatty acids in the blood differ in how they are taken up by working muscles during vigorous exercise (e.g., running a mile in about 5 minutes).[1] In going on to study lipoproteins in blood, I noted that I had a lot of a particular kind—HDL (High-Density Lipoprotein). Indeed, runners have higher HDL.

In comparing a group of long-distance runners (43 women, 41 men), matched for age and sex with a larger control group, my colleagues and I found that the runners not only had higher HDL-cholesterol, but lower LDL-cholesterol.[2] Low HDL-cholesterol raises the risk of cardiovascular disease, as does high LDL-cholesterol.

	Runners	Controls
Women's HDL	75	56
Men's HDL	64	43
Women's LDL	113	124
Men's LDL	125	139

HDL-cholesterol can also be raised by losing excess weight. In one study, we randomly divided 131 overweight sedentary men into 3 groups. A diet-only group was put on a low-calorie diet with no change in physical activity; an exercise-only group was put on an exercise program (mainly running) without lowering calorie intake; and the third group was the control group. At the end of the year-long study, both the diet-only and exercise-only groups lost weight and increased their HDL-cholesterol.[3]

The diet-only group lost more weight (-17 lbs) than the exercise-only group (-10 lbs), but a greater portion of the weight loss was from lean body mass in the diet-only group (27% vs. 15%). In other words, the men lost weight and raised HDL-cholesterol by diet alone or exercise alone, but exercise helped prevent the loss of lean body mass. A good combination, of course, is to eat less and exercise more, because the calorie-restriction and increased exercise can be more moderate, making it easier to stick to the weight-loss plan.

The risk of having low HDL-cholesterol is greater in those who also have a high LDL-cholesterol and are older. We took 180 postmenopausal women (age 45-64) and 197 men (age 30-64) who had this combination of risk factors and randomly assigned them to four groups: aerobic exercise, diet moderately low in fat and cholesterol, exercise plus diet, and control. At the end of the year-long study, all groups had lower LDL-cholesterol, but only the diet+exercise group had a big enough drop to reach statistical significance. For HDL-cholesterol, the exercise group had the biggest rise, but the intra-group variations were so large that there were no statistically significant differences in HDL-cholesterol between the groups.[4]

The studies are complex, but they all point to the simple message that physical activity is important to one's health. Exercise not only lowers the risk of obesity, heart disease, and some cancers, it also adds to the quality of life. I run for the joy of running; the higher HDL and other health benefits are but a bonus.

Studies Cited

1. Wood, P, Schlierf, G, Kinsell, L. 1965. Plasma free oleic and palmitic acid levels during vigorous exercise. Metabolism 14:1095-1100.

2. Wood, PD, Haskell, WL, Stern, MP, Lewis, S, Perry, C. 1977. Plasma lipoprotein distributions in male and female runners. Annals of the New York Academy of Sciences 301:748-763.

3. Wood, PD, Stefanick, ML, Dreon, DM, Frey-Hewitt, B, Garay, SC et al. 1988. Changes in plasma lipids and lipoproteins in overweight men during weight loss through dieting as compared with exercise. New England Journal of Medicine 319:1173-1179.

4. Stefanick, ML, Mackey, S, Sheehan, M, Ellsworth, N, Haskell, WL, Wood, PD. 1998 Effects of diet and exercise in men and postmenopausal women with low levels of HDL cholesterol and high levels of LDL cholesterol. New Eng. J. of Med. 339:12-20.

Dr. Wood did research in England and Australia before coming to California. He was part of the research faculty in the Stanford Heart Disease Prevention Program for more than 20 years. In addition to his extensive scientific work, he was on the Science Advisory Board of *Runner's World* magazine for more than 10 years, and is now chairman of the Science Advisory Board of *Marathon & Beyond* magazine. He has run more than 100 marathons, placed 35th in the 1968 Boston Marathon (2:49:40), ran in the first 5-boroughs New York Marathon in 1976 at age 47 (3:05:52), and still runs marathons at age 78.

Part 5

Fueling the Body

Chapter 10

The Digestive System

Digestion is often thought of in a negative context—as in indigestible, and indigestion. We don't think much about it unless something goes wrong. We take for granted that we can put a great variety of substances in our mouths, of which a certain amount of leftovers will exit the digestive tract—and the body will somehow make use of what disappears in between.

We give little thought to how the body can accommodate a tremendous variety of foods, in many different circumstances, and extract and make use of what it needs without generally being aware of anything going on—unless something reminds us of our digesting innards. But even then we tend to think only of the sensation that has our attention.

As a matter of fact, the digestive process is an amazing cooperative enterprise that involves a variety of substances, and processes what we consume in an orderly and efficient way, day in and day out, throughout our lives. It makes a good story, one that answers a lot of questions we seldom think to ask.

The essential purpose of digestion is so simple that it's been correctly understood for thousands of years. It's expressed by the old Latin word *digestio*, which means "a breaking down." Even before the time of the Roman Empire, classic Greek physicians realized that digestion served to break down food so that its nutritive values would be made available to the body.

But for some twenty centuries following the time of Hippocrates, physicians sought in vain to learn how the process worked. Again and again, they studied what went into the body at one end and what came out at the other. But they found no real clues to what was happening in between.

This chapter begins with a short narrative of some early discoveries of the digestive process. We then proceed—from mouth to colon—to what we know today.

The Mechanical Theory of Digestion

Through the generations, endless explanations of digestion and its relationship to health were advanced. Endless diets and other digestive treatments were proposed. But essentially, they all followed the oldest idea—that the digestive process was mainly mechanical.

In this view, the teeth tore and ground food into small fragments, which proceeded into the core of the body. There, the body somehow squeezed out a kind of nutritive juice. Most physicians thought this juice held a single nutritive factor, from which a life force came.

Long before the first clues to the truth appeared, human innards were studied, those of the living through wounds and those of the dead through post-mortem studies. But all those early researchers saw was a muscular bag (the *stomach*) followed by a long, twisted muscular canal (the *intestines)*. Squeezing seemed to be about its only possible function. After all, what else could this tangled tube do? Why else would the stomach and the tube be so muscled? These studies of human anatomy seemed to confirm the old idea that some vital juice was squeezed out of food.

The Chemical Principle of Digestion

There's no telling how long this mechanical view of digestion might have persisted if it hadn't been for a pet bird and a wounded trapper. Between the two, they opened the way for our modern understanding of digestion.

The Pet Bird

The bird (a kite, relative of the owl), came along toward the end of the 1700s, the beloved pet of French scientist Rene de Reaumur. It had eating habits which, while repugnant to some, were fascinating to Reaumur.

The bird would gobble down its food in gluttonous chunks—then later spit up parts of the food, such as bones. To Reaumur, who was familiar with the mechanical ideas of digestion, it was another of nature's ways of separating the nutritive from the non-nutritive. But as he looked closely at what was regurgitated, he had another impression. Some of it seemed to be decomposed, rather than just broken up or torn apart. Could something more than mechanical be happening in the bird's stomach?

Actually, this observation wasn't unique. Too many people had seen food returned after being partially digested. After all, the Roman wealthy had vomitoria adjacent to their dining rooms, in order to enable banquet guests to keep eating long after normal capacity had been reached. It was perfectly clear that such returned food had changed. But how—and why?

Reaumur had an idea. He put meat into a bit of metal tubing fastened to a string, lowered it into the bird's stomach, and after an interval, pulled the tube up again. The meat had deteriorated.

Again and again, he experimented and was able to extract some kind of stomach juice from the meat. The juice was acid. When this juice was mixed with meat in a test tube, the meat began to disintegrate.

Word of Reaumur's work intrigued others, who—stringing tubes and sponges—trapped the stomach juice of many kinds of animals and verified Reaumur's discovery. Scientists even went so far as to fashion a perforated little metal ball which they used to get substances in—and out of—peoples' stomachs. It became clear that the body had a ***chemical means of digestion,*** which caused food to be broken down and absorbed. But beyond this, the process remained a mystery.

The Wounded Trapper

The work of Reaumur and his colleagues seemed to have reached a dead end until 1822, when a severely wounded Canadian trapper named Alexis St. Martin was brought into the primitive surgery of young Dr. William Beaumont. Beaumont was the military surgeon of a frontier U.S. Army post on MacKinac Island, Michigan. St. Martin had been shot accidentally in the stomach.

With great care and skill, Beaumont managed to save the trapper, who was overwhelmingly grateful. But during convalescence, it appeared that St. Martin would retain a curious kind of souvenir. In healing, the wound formed a tube of flesh and muscle, following the path of the shot, from the skin of the belly into the stomach.

The surrounding abdominal muscles closed this odd hole, but Beaumont could open it and actually peek in to see the stomach at work. He was fascinated and asked permission to perform some experiments. The grateful St. Martin agreed—at first. Beaumont took the trapper into his home and provided financial support, but the experiments— eventually, over a hundred of them—dragged on for years.

As one can imagine, it became a constant struggle to get St. Martin to cooperate. (The repeated peeping into his stomach did no apparent harm. The trapper went on to father 17 children, and lived to the ripe old age of 86.)

Beaumont's meticulously recorded observations opened up many new avenues of research. For example, copious amounts of acid juices seemed to come out of the stomach wall whenever food came through the trapper's mouth. Yet, these digestive juices didn't appear when Beaumont put food directly into the stomach through St. Martin's special opening.

Beaumont also was fascinated to find that the appearance of the stomach was changed by thoughts and emotions—whether a fantasy of dinner or anger or fear. Thoughts and emotions also

Table 10-1: Nutrients and Digestive Products.

Nutrient:	Digested to:
Carbohydrate	Glucose, other single sugars
Protein	Amino acids
Fat	Fatty acids, monoglycerides

seemed to change the blood supply, the secretion of juices, and the activity of the stomach.

The extent of the stomach's activity surprised Beaumont. Far from being a passive sack, the stomach somehow twisted and kneaded, slowly churning food with the digestive juice. Liquids went through the stomach fairly quickly. Solid foods took much longer. The food seemed only to break down in the stomach, and not to be absorbed there into the body. With each stomach contraction, Beaumont noted that a small amount of partially broken-down food was pushed down into the intestine.

Beaumont's observations led to further study of what happened in the intestine. By the middle of the 19th century, scientists perceived some dim outlines of the digestive truth.

The most active chemistry of digestion appeared to go on in the intestine. But little was then known of human nutrient needs—beyond some general ideas about carbohydrate, fat, and protein. It was evident that the digestive process had to proceed until it had refined the nutrients in some way. Indeed, scientists had a glimmer that even a refined nutrient had to be broken down further before it could be absorbed into the body. They even theorized about catalysts that would enable this ultimate digestion to take place.

Digestion breaks down food into a form that can be absorbed. Absorption is the process of taking substances from the digestive tract and into the body.

Today we understand how far digestion must go in refining nutrients from foods. Starch, for example, must be broken down into glucose before it can be absorbed into the body. This extreme of refinement is the real purpose of our body's system of digestion and absorption.

The processes of digestion and absorption are far more subtle and complex—and involve much more of the body—than Beaumont ever imagined.

Table 10-2 Some Digestive Enzymes

Location	Nutrient Digested	Enzyme
Mouth	Starch (amylopectin)	Salivary amylase
	Fat (lipid)	Lingual lipase
Stomach	Fat	Gastric lipase
	Protein	Pepsins
Small Intestine	Starch	Pancreatic amylase
	Fat	Pancreatic lipase
	Protein	Trypsin, Peptidases
	Maltose	Maltase
	Sucrose	Sucrase
	Lactose	Lactase

Digestive Enzymes

Vitamins, minerals, alcohol, and cholesterol can be pretty much absorbed "as is" (i.e., without the need for digestion), but the bulk of our food—carbohydrate, protein, and fat—must first be digested (broken down) into simpler components. Starch and double sugars (disaccharides) must be broken down to single sugars (monosaccharides), proteins to amino acids, and triglycerides must have at least two of its three fatty acids removed (see Table 10-1). Digestive enzymes are what make this breakdown possible. (Enzymes were discussed in Chap. 4.)

A wide variety of enzymes are used in digestion (see Table 10-2). The mechanical actions of digestion—chewing, liquefying, mixing, and moving the food along—aid the enzymatic digestion by bringing food into intimate contact with its digestive enzymes.

The Mouth—The First Chamber of Digestion

The digestive tract—almost 30 feet long in an adult—can be envisioned as a series of chambers (see Fig. 10-1). Each chamber is a processing unit separated from the next by a muscular ring which opens to let the digesting food pass through and then closes to keep it from going back.

The lips could be seen (quite unromantically) as a muscular ring leading to the mouth. Lips are made of a special tissue which is highly sensitive, especially to heat and pressure. They give us information about prospective food. Along with the help of the eyes and nose—under which approaching food must first pass—we learn enough decide whether or not to open our lips to let the food enter.

To watch the system in action, offer a new food to a small child. The head snaps back to let the eyes focus. Then the lips purse tight (backed up by the tightening of powerful jaw muscles) until the nose can sniff. That sniff carries aroma high into the nose where much of our tasting ability resides. Finally, the tip of the tongue protrudes to sample, and at last the mouth may open. But if the taste doesn't live up to the advance billing, how quickly the food comes back out.

The mouth holds an intricate system for responding to food. Salivating is an initial response. The aroma, or even the thought of food, triggers the release of saliva from the salivary glands.

Saliva provides the moisture and lubrication needed for food to slip comfortably through to the stomach. Taste and perception of texture may cause the release of still more saliva, as in the case of very dry food, or when a strong acid is perceived and more saliva is needed to dilute it. The next time you taste a vinegar (acid) salad dressing, note how quickly your saliva flows. Or simply think about biting into a lemon. The mere memory of acidity is enough to flood the mouth.

Throughout the digestive tract, there's a pattern of preparing for what's coming. Seeing, smelling, even thinking about food brings saliva into the mouth, ready for the anticipated food. Indeed, this same stimulation may even begin the secretion in the stomach of a hormone which starts the stomach's production of acid. This triggering of saliva in the mouth and acid in the stomach is but one part of a complex cascade of chemical messages and responses triggered during digestion. Many of the chemical messages are transmitted by hormones. Some of these hormones and their actions are listed in Table 10-3.

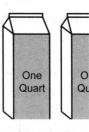

Daily Saliva

Figure 10-1: Mouth to Anus Pathway.

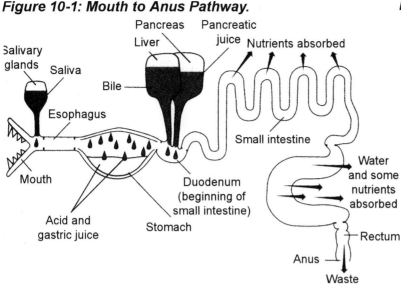

Predominant tastes on the tongue.

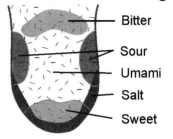

Saliva contains a number of substances, including a digestive enzyme (salivary amylase) that begins the digestion of starch, and a lubricant (mucin) that makes the food "slippery." We secrete about a quart-and-a-half of saliva a day.

As the food enters the mouth, the jaw begins to move—forward and back, up and down, side to side—to work the cutting-and-grinding edges of the teeth. Meanwhile, the muscular tongue and cheeks help to churn the food and keep returning it to the teeth for more cutting and grinding, while mixing it with saliva.

A Matter of Taste

The old idea that we taste only with our tongue was disproven long ago. Taste buds are tiny receptor organs buried in the surface of the tongue and are almost closed over except for individual small open pores. A few taste buds aren't even on the tongue but in the lining of the mouth and at the back of the throat.

Plentiful as they are, these organs recognize only five basic "tastes"—sweet, salty, sour, bitter, and umami. All other "tastes" are really smelled. We acknowledge this when we bemoan the taste-lessness of food when we have a "stuffy nose."

Aromas from food are perceived by a small colony of smell receptors high up in the nose. Attached to these smell receptors are nerves that connect to the brain and report on the odors of food. Typically, *smell receptors* are much more

numerous in other animals than in man, explaining why a St. Bernard dog can do a much better job of sniffing things out than we can.

Taste receptors for all five basic tastes are all over the tongue, but sweetness and saltiness are a bit better perceived at the tip of the tongue, sourness at the sides, and bitterness at the back. This pattern may have emerged by evolution from an ancient need to differentiate between nutritious foods and noxious ones. Tasting sweetness at the tip of the tongue encourages selecting sweet and nutritious foods like fruit. Poisons are often bitter, and as the food goes towards the back of the tongue, it's the last chance to spit it out.

Umami is the Japanese word for savory/delicious, and is the taste of certain amino acids, like the glutamate in MSG (monosodium glutamate). It has a "meaty" flavor and drives a "craving" for protein-rich foods.

Tastes can be perceived only when "tasty" chemicals are dissolved. When your mouth is very dry, it's hard to taste the saltiness of a potato chip—a dry crystal of salt is too large to fit into a taste bud. As the salt dissolves in the saliva, it becomes small enough to fit.

Aromas are really combinations of a number of smell sensations detected by the smell receptors in the nose. The process of recognition is subtle and complex. The brain assembles a combination of scent signals, and refers the particular combination to its memory bank for interpretation. Imagine the refinement of learning necessary for a wine taster to take a sip, bubble air inwardly from the lips to lift the aromatics to the smell receptors high in the nose, and say, "Definitely a claret..., French..., Chateau Margaux 1976."

Table 10-3: Some Gastrointestinal Hormones.

Production Site	Hormones	Trigger	Target	Action at Target
Stomach	Gastrin	Stretching stomach	Stomach	Secrete acid, pepsin
	Ghrelin	Low calorie intake	Brain	Increased appetite
	Obestatin	Unknown	Brain	Decreased appetite
Small Intestine	CCK (cholecystokinin)	Protein, fat	Gallbladder	Contract to release bile
			Pancreas	Secrete enzymes
	Secretin	Stomach acid, protein	Pancreas	Secrete bicarbonate
			Stomach	Inhibit acid secretion
	GIP (Glucose-dependent insulinotrophic peptide)	Glucose	Pancreas	Secrete insulin
	PYY (Peptide YY)	Eating	Brain	Decreased Appetite

Many other factors influence taste and aroma. Temperature is one. Note how much sweeter ice cream tastes melted than when frozen. Tastes are also interactive. A dash of salt enhances the sweetness in a food—which explains why some people sprinkle salt on their watermelon. Salt cuts down the sour taste of certain acids, such as vinegar. In turn, certain acids make salty tastes more pronounced. Salad dressings often include both vinegar and salt. A popular fast food (particularly in Canada and England) is fish and chips sprinkled with salt and vinegar.

Durian, a fruit from Southeast Asia, is known for its horrible smell ("smelly socks," "sewage") and its exquisite taste ("rich almond-flavored custard").

All the senses enter into the final perception of what we call "taste." We find food appealing by touch ("the crust on the roll feels crisp"), temperature ("an ice cold beer"), color ("a lovely ripe tomato"), sound ("crunchy celery"), and even the sensation of "melting" ("cookies so delicious they melt in the mouth"). All these qualities have much to do with which foods we take into our mouths.

Swallowing isn't as simple as it seems. The process starts with a closing of the lips and a voluntary push of the food towards the throat by the tongue. This act touches off a series of reflexes that close off alternate routes for the lump of food about to be swallowed into the esophagus.

The soft palate (a rearward extension of the roof of the mouth) rises to close off the nasal passages to prevent the food from going up into the nose. Simultaneously, the windpipe is blocked by the epiglottis, located at the top of the windpipe, which moves upward and forward to close the flap over the windpipe. This produces the familiar movement of the "Adam's apple." If food should accidentally enter the windpipe, the body uses violent coughs—sharp expulsions of air from the lungs—to try and blow the intruding matter away.

These patterns help explain some familiar experiences—why you may choke if you're talking or laughing while eating; why it's hard to swallow with your mouth open—as when you try to swallow the saliva that collects while the dentist works in your mouth; and why you can't keep drinking without pausing for breath—as a baby can.

Babies can breathe and swallow at the same time, as when they are nursing or sucking a bottle. The baby's short lower face causes the epiglottis (the flap that sits up over the windpipe) to extend above the level of the soft palate (the rearward extension of the roof of the mouth) and into the back of the nasal cavity. Thus, the windpipe doesn't have to be shut off when the baby swallows because it's already protected. The milk can just go around the epiglottis and down the esophagus.

Beyond the Mouth

In a very simplified way, the digestive tract beyond the mouth can be seen as a kind of tube. And this is how early investigators saw it—a long, simple tube of uneven width made up of four

Figure 10-2: The Digestive Tract.

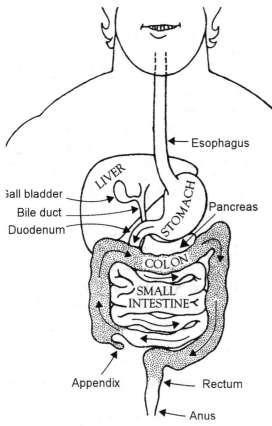

major chambers: the *esophagus, stomach, small intestine,* and *colon* (large intestine). But this "tube" isn't so simple (see Fig. 10-2).

The digestive tube is multilayered. It not only has the layer of cells that make up the intricate and absorptive inner lining, but also layers of muscles—circular muscles that provide a squeezing motion and longitudinal muscles that contract lengthwise. The coordinated contraction of these muscles results in "waves" of motion (peristalsis) that propel the contents of the digestive tract steadily downward from esophagus to anus.

The squeezing motion of the circular muscles also performs the important task of mixing the food being digested. This mixing aids the chemical reactions of digestion, and increases the contact of the digestive products with the absorptive surface of the tube.

Peristalsis: Wave-like contractions of digestive tract muscles that move the digestive material downward.

The digestive tract's movement, blood flow, and secretions are coordinated by its own nervous system containing about 100 million nerve cells.[1] Disruptions in this system cause a variety of digestive problems, as can happen in diabetes, for example.[2]

The Esophagus—
Just a Swallow Away

The esophagus is straight and relatively short (about nine inches long and about 1 inch wide), and the time in the esophagus is brief—about one or two seconds for liquids and six to seven seconds for solids. Even if you ate or drank standing on your head, the food would progress to your stomach because of the muscular contractions of the esophagus. It's not so for some life forms—especially birds, who must tilt their heads back to get food to go down. (Circus sword-swallowers must also tilt their heads back—to get the sword to go straight down the esophagus. Their talent is their ability to suppress the normal gag reflex.)

The esophagus isn't actually essential to digestion or life—as an Irish-American patient known only as Tom demonstrated. In 1895, the nine-year-old took a huge gulp of scalding-hot soup and permanently damaged his esophagus. The doctors created a permanent opening to his stomach—much like that of the trapper, Alexis St. Martin. Thereafter, Tom chewed his food and spit each mouthful into a funnel that led to the discrete opening in his belly. He did this in private—until over 30 years later, when he accidentally injured the opening while working on a labor crew and needed medical attention.

Accidental damage to the esophagus still occurs among children, mostly from swallowing caustic chemicals like household drain openers.

Tom's special opening caught the attention of Dr. Stewart Wolf, a young resident at a New York hospital, who saw Tom as a unique opportunity for study and hired him as a lab assistant. And for 20 years thereafter, into the 1950s, Tom provided Dr. Wolf with a wealth of information on the effects of stress on the lining of the stomach. One particularly interesting observation was that, minute by minute, the color of Tom's stomach reflected the emotional color of his face. When Tom was pale from fear, the lining of his stomach was pale also. And when Tom's fear was relieved, the color returned to both his face and stomach.

The Churning, Acid Stomach

Once food reaches the bottom of the esophagus, it passes through a circular band of muscle called the ***cardiac sphincter*** (located near the heart) and into the stomach. The stomach is about 10 to 12 inches long and about 4 inches in diameter, a kind of muscular elastic bag, capable of stretching when food enters and then later returning to its normal size.

The stomach is the widest part of the digestive tract. It looks quite different than the esophagus, but it's fairly similar in structure. As we shall see with respect to each digestive chamber, the layers of tissue are modified to enable each chamber to do its special work.

Sphincter: A ring-shaped muscle that can open or close to let substances pass—or not pass.

Two of the most common complaints one hears about the stomach are that it's "acid," or that distress makes it "churn." But the fact is that these characteristics refer to the normal state of the stomach during digestion. Necessarily so.

In addition to its ballooning shape, the stomach differs from the esophagus in two other major ways. One is a dramatic increase in muscularity.

In addition to the ***circular*** and ***longitudinal muscles***, the stomach has ***diagonal muscles*** which make it possible for the stomach to twist and churn. This kneading effect actually breaks up food.

The second key change is in its lining. In the esophagus, this lining did little more than supply mucus, both to ease the food along its way and to protect itself from physical damage. In the stomach, the lining gets much thicker, and multitudes of glands appear.

In all, there are about 35 million glands in the folded, velvety lining of the stomach. These glands secrete numerous substances, including ***digestive enzymes, hydrochloric acid, mucus***, and a protein called ***intrinsic factor***. Intrinsic factor is necessary for the absorption of vitamin B-12. It attaches to B-12, and the complex is absorbed later in the lower part of the small intestine.

The stomach secretions total about 3 quarts

The Stomach. Food from the esophagus (a) enters the stomach (b), goes to the curved duodenum (c), the site of most ulcers, and into the small intestine (d) from which most nutrients are absorbed. At the right, the stomach as it looks in action, with churning peristaltic waves mixing the food with digestive juices, at the same time moving it along.

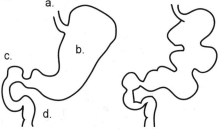

per day, and the hydrochloric acid makes the mixture very acid. Food, in effect, goes through an acid bath. The acid is strong enough to eat into meat—and strong enough to kill large numbers of bacteria. In this sense, the stomach is the disinfecting organ of digestion.

Very little absorption of nutrients occurs in the stomach. But alcohol can be absorbed here. It only needs to make contact with the lining of the stomach and intestine. Therefore, alcohol's effects are felt sooner when it's consumed on an empty stomach.

Alcohol is first broken down to acetaldehyde, which is normally broken down quickly by a second enzyme (aldehyde dehdrogenase). Many asians have a genetic variation of this enzyme that's less efficient, causing higher levels of acetaldehyde.[4,5] This results in flushing ("red face"), a more severe hangover—and less alcoholism.

The stomach secretes an enzyme (alcohol dehydrogenase) that breaks down alcohol. Women have less of this enzyme in their stomach than men.[3] This, plus their smaller body size and having more body fat, means higher blood-alcohol levels and an increased risk of damage to the liver (the only other organ with this enzyme) and heart.

Excess Acidity

Contrary to popular belief, acid foods have little to do with excess acidity in the stomach. By the time acid foods such as citrus fruits have been diluted by saliva and mixed with other foods, they aren't acid enough to increase the acidity of the stomach. In treating ulcer patients, physicians used to prescribe an "ulcer diet" that avoided certain acid foods. Studies have since shown that most of the prohibitions of that diet were unwarranted. Today, physicians commonly limit the "avoid list" to coffee and alcohol (these stimulate acid production by the stomach).

The pain associated with stomach acid isn't usually experienced in the stomach at all, but rather in the lower end of the esophagus. Here the strong muscular squeezing of a full stomach, or an excess of stomach gas, may splash stomach acid up past the cardiac sphincter (the muscular ring between the stomach and esophagus) onto the lining of the esophagus. This splashing of acid can cause pain because the esophagus isn't as well protected as the stomach against acid.

Because the lower esophagus is near the heart, the pain is described as "heartburn." Heartburn is really "esophagus burn."

When this happens, the sphincter isn't doing its job of preventing this back-tracking. The stretching of the stomach by a large meal and/or a high-fat meal can cause the sphincter to relax inappropriately. Thus, heartburn often can be avoided by eating smaller, lower-fat meals, and not lying down after eating. Heartburn is especially common among those who eat a small breakfast and lunch, and a large high-fat dinner.

GERD (Gastroesophageal Reflux Disease) is the chronic (more than twice a week) backing up of acid. It can cause abnormal cells in the esophageal lining, which sometimes results in cancer of the esophagus. It's important to get GERD treated by a physician.

A self-prescribed, over-use of antacids is unwise. The advice is to not use an antacid product for more than two weeks without consulting a physician. A continuing need for an antacid suggests a problem that should be investigated by a physician.

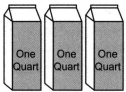

Stomach acid secreted daily

Vomiting

Vomiting brings up the contents of the upper digestive tract (usually from the stomach up, but sometimes from as far down as the duodenum). The vomiting reflex is relayed through a vomiting center in the brain, and involves a squeezing of the stomach by a downward movement of the diaphragm together with a contraction of the abdominal muscles.

Its strongest triggers are irritation and marked stretching of the stomach. But other things such as motion sickness, the morning sickness of early pregnancy, or a blow to the head can cause vomiting. Even emotional upsets can cause it.

An empty stomach is more susceptible to vomiting, so eating a little can help ward it off. Prolonged vomiting can cause serious problems, especially for infants and the elderly.

Vomiting can be induced by initiating the gagging reflex, as it often is by those suffering from the eating disorder bulimia (see Chap. 3).

Burps and Belches

Gas from the stomach is a common concern, at least as a social embarrassment. The usual cause has nothing to do with digestion at all, but the harmless result of swallowing air. We swallow air not only with our food, but with two other substances that we swallow almost continually—excess saliva (especially if we feel nervous or hungry) and mucus from the nose. We swallow about 2,400 times a day.

The nose is protected by a thin blanket of mucus. This mucus originates near the start of the nasal passages, descends down the back of the throat, and is swallowed. Among other things, this nasal flow washes away bacteria that, when swallowed, can be killed by the stomach acid.

When enough gas has accumulated—from air-swallowing or from chemical reactions of gastric secretions and food—and when the pressure from the filling of the stomach or from muscular churning is great enough, the bubble of gas breaks upwards into the esophagus. And we burp.

Small Intestine— Where the Action Is

The first 12 inches of the small intestine is the duodenum [from the Latin "twelve (fingers breadth) each." It's given a separate name, distinguishing it from the rest of the intestine, because so much happens here.

As the stomach churns the digesting food, the contractions squirt a little of the now-liquefied food (called *chyme)* down into the duodenum. The muscular ring between the stomach and small intestine only opens when the food has been liquefied into chyme and only allows it to pass through in small and steady squirts. The duodenum isn't as well protected as the stomach against acid, but it does get some chemical protection from some nearby alkaline secretions.

The duodenum is a common site of painful craters (ulcers), which can become so damaged as to bleed. But pain isn't a dependable warning sign. Many people diagnosed with duodenal ulcers don't report pain as a symptom. Sometimes the discomfort of an ulcer is misinterpreted as hunger, which can unwittingly lead to overeating and weight gain. When there isn't pain, a bleeding ulcer is often discovered by blood in the stool, or anemia resulting from blood loss.

Surgical removal of part of the stomach was once a common treatment. (When part of the stomach is removed, less acid is produced.) Later, drugs (e.g., cimetidine/Tagamet) that reduce the stomach's acid production replaced surgery as the standard treatment.

It's now known that most duodenal ulcers are caused by *H. pylori* bacteria. (Most of the other cases are caused by "nonsteroidal anti-inflammatory agents," like aspirin and ibuprofen.) *H. pylori* infection can be diagnosed by a blood or breath test, and cured with a precise combination of medications that includes antibiotics.

H. pylori infection is thought to occur by close person-to-person contact and by exposure to vomit of an infected person. A vaccine is being developed.

Ulcers can also occur in the esophagus or stomach, but these are much less common than duodenal ulcers. H. pylori-related stomach ulcers raise the risk of stomach cancer, but this doesn't seem to be the case with duodenal ulcers.

Chyme from the stomach isn't all that enters at the duodenum; there are also secretions from the *pancreas* and *liver.*

From a meal, carbohydrates and proteins leave the stomach first (after two hours or more), and then fats—the last fat not leaving for perhaps four or five hours. (Fats tend to be the last to leave the stomach on the downward, digestive journey because characteristically they float to the top of the watery mixture.)

This doesn't mean that all carbohydrates or all fats follow tidy, distinct schedules. Remember that the stomach has worked hard to make an intimate mix of small particles. The entry of chyme into the small intestine triggers a flurry of activity and a medley of individual digestive processes.

The digestive fluids of the pancreas, liver, and *gallbladder* enter the small intestine by way of small tubes (ducts) that converge into a single duct (the *bile duct)* which empties into the duodenum. Like vicious animals awaiting their prey, the *digestive enzymes, bile,* and *bicarbonate* rush through the bile duct and into the small intestine to literally pounce on the incoming chyme.

Digestive Secretions from the Pancreas

The pancreas is about 6 inches long and about 1 inch thick and lies horizontally behind the stomach. It's a lumpy sort of organ, resembling blobs of whitish flesh. In fact, its name comes from two Greek words which mean "all flesh." If you've ever eaten sweetbreads, you're acquainted with the pancreas of the cow. (A good many people who get a look at the lumpy cow pancreas go to some lengths to avoid eating it.)

The digestive duty of the pancreas is to make sodium bicarbonate ("baking soda") and digestive enzymes, and secrete them into the duodenum. The bicarbonate is alkaline and neutralizes the acid chyme coming from the stomach. Pancreatic enzymes include those necessary to digest starch, protein, and fat (see Table 10-2).

As discussed in Chapter 5, the pancreas also makes insulin and glucagon, the hormones that regulate blood sugar.

Digestive Secretions from the Liver

The liver lies just below the diaphragm and weighs about three pounds. Its role in digestion is to make and secrete bile. Bile isn't an enzyme but, rather, an *emulsifier* that divides dietary fat into very small particles (see Fig. 10-3).

From the moment that fat enters the digestive tract, it presents a special problem because it doesn't dissolve in water—a characteristic that's not compatible with much of body chemistry. The digestive system, along with most of the body's chemistry, is a watery system.

We have a similar problem when we want to wash dishes. We can't deal with the grease of dirty dishes with water alone. So we add detergent. Detergents don't really make fats dissolve in water. They divide the fat into very small particles so that they can be carried away.

Emulsification is the process of finely dividing the fat so that it's suspended in a water-based fluid. It's analogous to the homogenization of whole milk, in which the fat (cream) is finely divided so that it stays suspended in the non-fat portion of milk, rather than rising to the top. But in homogenization, the fat particles are made smaller by mechanical means (i.e., forced through a small nozzle), whereas an emulsifier such as bile has chemical properties that finely divide the fat (see Fig. 10-3).

Finely dividing the fat markedly increases its surface area. This is crucial for fat digestion because the fat-digesting enzymes are in a watery solution and can't penetrate the fat. The fat-digesting enzymes can only reach and digest the fat that lies exposed on the surface of a fat particle.

Bile is made up of bile acids, bile pigments, cholesterol, and other substances—all dissolved together in an alkaline solution. The bile acids are made from cholesterol, and the bile pigments are made from breakdown products of hemoglobin (the oxygen-carrying molecule in red blood cells). Bile contains both red and green pigments, and the two can form a color range from yellow to green to varying shades of brown, effectively changing the color of the feces.

Lacking true explanations, changes in the color of bile were used for centuries to explain illness

Figure 10-3: Bile salts emulsify fats into small droplets.

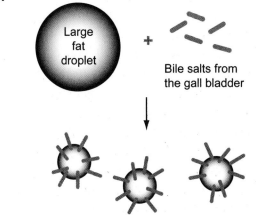

and changes in mood. Recall a part of the 12th century poem quoted in Chapter 1:

"Peaches, apples, pears...engender black bile and are enemies of the sick."

Abraham Lincoln's young son Willie died from what was diagnosed as "bilious fever" (probably typhoid or malaria). Even today, we describe an ill-tempered person as bilious.

Bile is made steadily by the liver—about a quart a day. But since the need for it isnt constant, the bile is shunted aside into the gallbladder, where it's stored until needed.

The Gallbladder

The *gallbladder* is a pear-shaped organ about 3 or 4 inches long that serves as a reservoir for the bile produced by the liver. Here the bile is concentrated and sits at-the-ready, to be released into the intestine to do its job of emulsifying fat.

The release of this bile is triggered by the entry of chyme into the small intestine. The intestine responds to this chyme by producing a hormone, which travels via the bloodstream to the gallbladder and causes the gallbladder to contract and squirt bile into the duodenum.

The gallbladder isn't an essential organ. Many people have their gallbladder removed without serious consequences. Without a gallbladder, bile enters the duodenum directly from the liver in a steady and less concentrated amount. Thus, even after a gallbladder has been removed, most fatty foods are still tolerated, unless they're eaten in particularly large amounts.

The usual reason for removing the gallbladder is the painful presence of gallstones. In the United States, gallstones are very common, and their incidence increases with age. Cholesterol is a normal component of bile and is the major component of most gallstones. Cholesterol tends to form stones because it doesn't readily dissolve in bile fluid.

Precisely why gallstones form isn't known, but they are more common among women, the overweight, Native-Americans, Mexican-Americans, those eating a western diet, and those with a family history of gallstones. A stone can cause pain and inflammation if it blocks the flow of bile in the gallbladder itself or in the bile duct leading to the duodenum. The gallbladder is removed if this stone can't be passed, broken up by ultrasound, or dissolved by medication.

The Incredible Lining of the Small Intestine

The adult small intestine is about 1¹/₂ inches wide and about 20 feet long when relaxed (about 10 feet long when contracted). It's the main site of *digestion* and *absorption.*

The ancients were puzzled by its great length. If the stomach, as they believed, was where digestion took place, what use was all this coiled tubing? Today we understand that the stomach does relatively little digesting and absorbing of nutrients. The stomach is more of a churning, acid place of preparation for digestion and absorption, and as a muscular reservoir of food that squirts out disinfected chyme onto the luxurious carpet of the small intestine.

The lining of the small intestine is truly remarkable. In much the same way as a wadded terry-cloth towel is used to quickly absorb a spill, the absorptive surface of the small intestine is expanded by folds and loops (see Fig. 10-4). The folds in the lining are covered with tiny upraised fingers (villi) which are densely packed, like very expensive carpet. Each of the villi, in turn, is

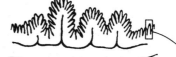

Figure 10-4: Inner Surface of the Small Intestine.

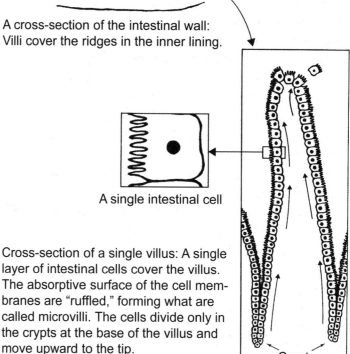

A cross-section of the intestinal wall: Villi cover the ridges in the inner lining.

A single intestinal cell

Cross-section of a single villus: A single layer of intestinal cells cover the villus. The absorptive surface of the cell membranes are "ruffled," forming what are called microvilli. The cells divide only in the crypts at the base of the villus and move upward to the tip.

Crypts

covered with a brush-like set of projections of its own—the microvilli. It's been estimated that the inner surface area of a person's small intestine (including all the villi and microvilli) is about 1800 square feet—about the floor space of a three-bedroom house.

The microvilli also contain digestive enzymes such as lactase (which splits the "milk sugar" lactose) and sucrase (which splits the "table sugar" sucrose).

This lining is only one cell thick and is continually renewed. There's a completely new lining about every three days. New intestinal cells are born at the base of the villi, and they migrate to the tips of the villi where—at the "old age" of three days—they come off.

Imagine the chyme squirted into the small intestine, being immediately mixed with the rich digestive fluid coming from the bile duct, and continually pushed against an active and extensive absorptive surface that aids and abets rapid digestion and absorption. This process is so effective that virtually all the nutrients have been completely absorbed by the time the digestive material reaches the lower part of the small intestine. But not all: Vitamin B_{12} combined with intrinsic factor is absorbed in this lower segment. Bile acids are also absorbed here so they can be recycled to the liver and made into bile again.

The remarkable efficiency of the small intestine is exemplified by a rather bizarre weight-loss scheme—surgically bypassing most of the small intestine so that a person can overeat and still lose weight. Mainly in the 1970s, this desperate procedure was performed on morbidly obese patients. To achieve the malabsorption necessary for rapid weight loss, all but about two or three feet of the small intestine was shunted aside. Rapid weight loss was a result—along with massive amounts of smelly stool.

Once the desired weight loss was achieved, the patient's intestinal bypass could be undone. But, as one would expect, unless the old dietary habits had changed, the lost weight returned. The popularity of this procedure faded when serious side-effects, such as liver failure, became a recognized complication.

The Colon

The undigested material moves out of the small intestine and into the colon (large intestine). The colon is only about 5 feet long and its width averages about $2^{1}/2$ inches. Its lining is far more simple than that of the small intestine—it has much less to do. Its main job is to absorb the excess water from the digestive residue and store the feces that form.

The lining of the colon has no villi and few of the folds that characterize the small intestine. No digestive enzymes are secreted here. Indeed, after all the furious activity of the small intestine, the colon is rather like a quiet pool after churning rapids. But just as was seen in peeking into Tom's stomach, the colon can react to emotion. This was shown vividly in an experiment in which a healthy medical student's colon was being monitored as it was implied that he had a tumor there (even pretending to take a biopsy)—and then told that this wasn't true (see Fig. 10-5).[6]

Figure 10-5: Stress and the Colon.

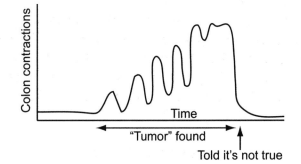

Life in the Colon

Just as life's more prolific in the pool of a mountain stream than it is in the tumbling rush of the rapids, so is there more life in the colon—bacterial life. In fact, bacteria make up about 30% of the dry weight of stools.

The bacteria alter bile pigments to make the stool brown, and alter certain residual amino acids to give stool its characteristic odor. The bacteria also synthesize some vitamins, such as vitamin K, which are then absorbed.

The bacteria need nutrients to sustain themselves, and they use all they can get from whatever comes their way. Bacteria produce gaseous by-products when they "eat" substances such as certain indigestible polysaccharides in beans.

Some of this gas is absorbed in the colon and discharged in the breath. The rest is expelled through the anus. The expulsion of gas (flatus) through the anus is called flatulence—useful information for those seeking an alternative word.

Vitamin K deficiency is uncommon because of bacterial production of vitamin K, but can occur when the colon bacteria are markedly cut back, e.g., when a person has taken antibiotics for a long time. A vitamin K injection is routinely given to newborns in this country as a preventative measure, since there are no bacteria in the colon at birth.

Ingesting pills of "starch blockers" (which inhibit the activity of the starch-digesting enzyme amylase) was once a popular short-term money-maker. *Popular,* since its pitch was irresistible ("Eat all the pasta and potatoes you want without gaining weight!"); *short-term,* since its inhibition of starch digestion was trivial. And a *money-maker* for the ever-present hucksters who keep telling people what they want to hear.

Actually, those who ingested starch blockers along with their pasta and rice should have been grateful that the pills didn't work. The bacteria in the colon would have had a feast on all that starch coming their way. The gaseous result would have been "explosive."

Lactose Intolerance

The reduced ability to digest lactose *(lactose intolerance)* is very common among adults. We're born with high levels of *lactase* (the lactose-digesting enzyme) in our small intestine, which supports digestion of the ample lactose in milk, our first food. But as the intestine matures, the amount of lactase normally declines to low levels, and the ability to digest lactose declines accordingly.

Recall that lactose is a double sugar (glucose + galactose), and only single sugars can be absorbed. Lactase splits lactose into glucose and galactose.

When lactose is consumed in amounts larger than can be fully digested, the undigested lactose proceeds to the colon, where the bacteria make a meal of it. The person hosting this meal may suffer the consequences, in the form of diarrhea, gas, and abdominal cramps.

Many who think they are lactose intolerant might not be. A double-blind study of people who said they were severely lactose-intolerant found that the gastrointestinal symptoms of those given regular milk didn't differ from those given milk with "predigested" lactose.[7]

Describing adult populations as lactase deficient is misleading because it implies an abnormality. In fact, about 75% of adults, worldwide, have low levels of lactase. The high level of lactase found in some populations (such as Northern Europeans and the pastoral Fulani tribe of Nigeria) is an anomaly, probably due to a selective mutation thousands of years ago that conferred a nutritional advantage to members of dairying cultures. Low levels of lactase in adults are found in about 90% of Asians and about 75% of American Blacks and Native Americans. In contrast, less than 20% of Caucasian adults of Northern European origin have low levels of lactase.

Milk is the only food that naturally has lactose. But since milk is made into and added to other foods, lactose is found in a variety of food products. In practical terms, adults with low levels of lactase are concerned with the amount of milk and milk products they can comfortably consume. This is best determined by a person's own eating experience. Some adults with low lactase levels, for example, can't tolerate gulping down a glass of milk on an empty stomach but find no discomfort in drinking a glass of milk leisurely throughout a meal.

Some people have sucrose intolerance, resulting from low levels of sucrase enzyme. The condition is analogous to lactose intolerance.

Yogurt and "acidophilus milk" are better tolerated because the added bacteria *(Lactobacillus acidophilus)* have "predigested" some of the lactose. Cheese and ice cream are also better tolerated because they're high in fat and contain relatively little lactose. The high fat content of these foods slows the passage of the lactose from the stomach to the intestine. (Also, the high fat content ordinarily limits how much we eat.)

Leaving the Digestive Tract

The slow, kneading contractions in the colon move the fecal matter toward the rectum (the last five inches of the digestive tract). More or less regularly, this leisurely pattern of motion is replaced by a powerful set of waves, accompanied by a series of muscular actions.

This pushes the feces into the normally-empty rectum, and the resulting distention triggers the defecation reflex. The muscles of the abdominal wall contract, and the muscular ring called the anus relaxes. The result, of course, is a bowel movement—unless we prevent it. We can voluntarily tighten the anus and begin a pattern of shallow breathing until the rectum accommodates to the mass.

Frequently, eating or drinking triggers this urge to defecate ("gets the intestines moving"). Infants usually defecate after a meal. But adults, often suppress or ignore this defecation reflex.

Constipation

The blocking of the normal defecation reflex is thought to be the most common cause of constipation. Commonly, the chronically constipated person has learned to break the defecation reflex. Such willful breaking of the reflex makes matters worse. As the feces remain overlong in the colon and rectum, more and more water is extracted, and the feces become hard and dry—and harder to pass.

A common American response to habitual constipation is to take a *laxative*. The person who blocks the defecation reflex (usually unconsciously) and then uses laxatives, is caught in a vicious cycle. The intestines become dependent upon artificial stimulation and won't function properly without it. This is often spoken of as laxative addiction.

People often seek to explain constipation by laying the blame on what they've eaten. It's true that some foods, such as low-fiber foods, tend to slow intestinal motility. It's also true that modest amounts of fiber can help prevent constipation by holding water, thereby making the stools bulkier, softer, and easier to pass. (Fiber, in this way, can also help prevent diverticulosis, discussed in Chap. 5). But an ordinary mixed diet causes neither constipation nor diarrhea.

It's a popular belief that a daily bowel movement is essential to health—a belief so strong that many people worry if they miss a day. But there is usually nothing to worry about if one is "irregular." In fact, it's quite normal to be irregular. Three times a week—or twice a day—are both well within normal. If given a chance, the bowel is normally self-regulating.

One shouldn't be unduly concerned with bowel movements, but a physician should be consulted if there's blood in the stool or a marked change in the usual pattern of bowel movements or in the appearance of the stool. A change to a very light color, for instance, might be a result of fat malabsorption due to inadequate bile production, or a change to a black color might be due to blood from a bleeding ulcer.

Diarrhea

There are many diseases that cause *diarrhea*. In developing countries, a common cause is disease-causing bacteria (usually from sewage) that have contaminated the drinking water. Because water's lost in diarrhea, severe diarrhea can cause severe dehydration. This is, in fact, a major cause of infant death in developing countries.

When we eat contaminated food, the body's natural reaction is to get rid of the irritant, often by vomiting or diarrhea. It doesn't take a great deal of vomiting or diarrhea to get rid of the food that causes the problem, but once started, these expulsive reactions may last longer than we'd like.

Though diarrhea, nausea, and vomiting are protective, and perhaps usefully prolonged when one's digestive state isn't capable of handling a meal just then, there are limits to how long such reactions are useful. In a matter of hours, vomiting or diarrhea can dehydrate the body and rob it of essential salts. If vomiting or diarrhea continues until it causes weakness, or there's much pain, call your doctor.

Some diarrheas aren't related to disease, but caused by emotional upset or, as we have seen, lactose intolerance. Ingesting large amounts of sugar alcohols such as sorbitol and mannitol can also cause diarrhea. Sugar alcohols are commonly used as sweeteners in sugarless gum and dietetic foods, but are only slowly absorbed; some may remain unabsorbed and proceed to the colon and produce diarrhea—and gas.

Psychological or Emotional Effects

Aside from specific medical problems, the vast majority of upsets of the digestive system appear to be of psychological or emotional origin. As many of us know, even worrying about end-of-the-semester exams can cause a "nervous stomach," indigestion, and diarrhea. Recall how peeking into those two famous stomachs and the medical student's colon revealed that they mirrored the emotions. So closely linked are digestion and emotions that merely believing that a food will cause distress usually guarantees that it will.

Imagine you're the house-guest of an eccentric host. For breakfast, you're served a glass of hot orange juice and a cup of cold coffee with salt added. The main dish is a chocolate donut smothered with clams in a bit of peanut butter sauce, garnished with chopped liver and marshmallows.

Automatic indigestion? Quite possibly. But not because of the food or your digestion. If this breakfast makes you ill, it's because you think it will. There's no other reason why it should trouble you. A basic tenet of digestion is that any two foods that may be eaten separately may also be eaten together.

In general, it can be said that when the healthy person is made ill by uncontaminated food, it isn't usually the food that's at fault, but the emotional response to the food or to one's life situation. Much of the rest of indigestion is the result of contaminated food, or of grosser abuses such as excessive alcohol.

Occasional gas, heartburn, diarrhea, or constipation is so common as to be relatively normal. Even when the cause isn't emotional, there's little to worry about unless the discomfort persists or is chronic. Bacterial contamination of food being rather common, we may all expect an attack now and then, especially if we eat out a lot.

Letting the Digestive System Do Its Job

From what we've seen of digestion and absorption, we can understand why they're so important to nutrition and health. But it's equally true that the normal digestive tract neither needs, nor can use, much help beyond the avoidance of obvious kinds of abuse.

There's a common misconception that we need to fast occasionally or eat special diets to "cleanse" or "detoxify" our digestive system. This is nonsense. The normal digestive tract is self-regulating—and self-cleaning. That's what's happening when it spontaneously reacts—often violently—to toxins by causing vomiting and/or diarrhea.

Summary

Digestion is the process of breaking down food into a form that can be absorbed from the digestive tract into the body. Carbohydrates must be broken down to single sugars (monosaccharides),

Mouth	Receives food; some starch digestion
Esophagus	Passageway
Stomach	Holds food; acidity kills bacteria, denatures protein; some protein digestion
Small Intestine	Digestion; absorbs nutrients and water
Bile duct	Provides entry at top of small intestine for bile and pancreatic secretions
Pancreas	Provides digestive enzymes, and sodium bicarbonate to neutralize acid chyme from stomach
Liver	Provides bile to emulsify fat
Gallbladder	Stores bile
Colon	Absorbs water; holds indigestible remains
Rectum	Defecation

proteins to amino acids, and triglycerides (the predominant dietary fat) must have at least two of their three fatty acids removed before they can be absorbed. Most vitamins and minerals don't need to be digested since they're usually consumed in an absorbable form.

Digestive enzymes catalyze the chemical reactions of digestion. The digestive tract aids these chemical reactions by breaking up, liquefying, mixing, and moving the food so that it will be constantly accessible to the digestive enzymes and to the intestinal lining, where nutrients are absorbed.

The mouth breaks up the food and mixes it with saliva so it easily slips through the esophagus to the stomach. The ample secretions and the churning of the stomach acidify and liquefy the food into a fluid called chyme. The chyme is gradually delivered in squirts to the small intestine.

Most digestion and absorption occurs in the small intestine. The pancreas contributes sodium bicarbonate to neutralize the acidity of the chyme, and contributes enzymes that digest protein, fat, and carbohydrate. The liver secretes bile, which emulsifies fat and makes fat more accessible to the fat-digesting enzymes. The small intestinal lining also has some digestive enzymes within its absorptive surface. Most of the nutrients are completely absorbed by the time the digestive material reaches the lower part of the small intestine.

The colon's main job is to absorb water from the digestive residue and store the feces that form.

Chapter 11

Metabolism and the Vitamin Key

Have you ever wondered about the first snake oil salesman? (Probably in the Garden of Eden after the unfortunate affair about the apple.) It's hard to imagine a human society without someone promoting a product to 'pep you up,' 'get rid of that tired run-down feeling.' It used to be tonics sold door-to-door or at carnivals. Now it's one dietary supplement or another.

If there was a logic to a theory supporting dietary supplements for people on ample balanced diets, it might well have come from some of the history of vitamin deficiencies—where people have suffered from terrible weakness when their diets did not provide enough of one or more vitamins. If too little makes you weak, a lot will bring extra vigor, right? Well, no.

It all comes back to that basic fact that energy comes from the sun, and to humans through food, not from vitamins themselves. Once one understands the process by which vitamins help make that energy source available, it is easy to see what foods effectively do provide energy, and how to choose those that will indeed make us energetic.

As the 19th century neared its close, nutrition science began a search for "the balanced diet." This search confronted scientists with the most basic of nutrition mysteries: How does the body use nutrients it digests and absorbs from food, to sustain life?

It seemed then that it should not take long to determine the ideal diet. After all, the scientists were sure that there were only four nutrients to balance—fat, protein, carbohydrate, and "ash." However, the scientists soon found that these four nutrients alone do not sustain life.

The term *ash* is still used in food analysis. It refers to what remains when a food is burned completely, and consists of the minerals in food.

As we saw in Chapter 2, scientists discovered that there was something in a water extract of food that was essential to life (now known as water-soluble vitamins). Using fat solvents, they extracted from food the remaining missing nutrients (now known as fat-soluble vitamins).

But what, they wondered, was in these extracts? What role did they play in the chemistry of life? How could they miraculously enable protein, fat, carbohydrates, and ash to sustain life? The unraveling of the answers to these questions—and some of the answers themselves—are recounted in this chapter.

The Microbes that Couldn't Be Found

At about the same time that scientists first puzzled over their food extracts, some physicians were at work on similarly vexing problems, which at first seemed unrelated to nutrition. One line of research had started in the 1880s, sparked by an epidemic of **beriberi** that had broken out when the Dutch were taking over Indonesia. Though beriberi was long familiar to medical science (it had been identified by Chinese physicians thousands of years before), its cause remained a mystery.

Beriberi was characterized by weakness, which worsened as the disease progressed. In fact, the very name means "I cannot." This weakness would be accompanied by various kinds of

physical degeneration, commonly resulting, for example, in the inability to walk. The course of the disease was like a slow, painful, and helpless surrender to death.

The Dutch administrators pleaded for help with the mounting plague. Besides humane considerations, it was politically embarrassing. They had set up hospitals and medical care for people in the areas of Indonesia under their control, and even built fine, modern rice mills for their inhabitants. Yet, it was in these regions that the beriberi struck hard. In contrast, there was little beriberi in the lands held by rebels who fought against Dutch sovereignty.

The Dutch Crown responded by sending physicians, chief among them, Dr. Christiaan Eijkman. It happened that at that time, Europe was enthralled by the exciting new knowledge of how microbes caused disease. Predictably, Eijkman was instructed to find the microbe that caused beriberi, halt the epidemic, and heal the infected.

Pretty Rice, Beriberi, and the Puzzling Chicken Cure

At his hospital in Java, Eijkman kept an experimental colony of chickens. In an attempt to infect them, suspecting that perhaps food was the carrier of the "beriberi microbe," he ordered that they be fed on the rice from the new government mills. The chickens began to weaken. Soon they were clearly victims of polyneuritis (a multiple inflammation of the nerves), the bird version of beriberi. The rice must carry the infection, Eijkman thought.

Certainly there could be nothing wrong with the rice itself. It was the best available, finely polished white by the modern mills to remove all traces of the brown hull. Yet Eijkman could find no bacteria from the rice under his microscope.

Then inexplicably, the chickens began to get well. Confused, Eijkman checked to see if there had been any change in their care. He learned that the caretaker, appalled that chickens were being fed the beautifully polished white rice, had switched them to the cheap, brown rice from the native mills.

Suspecting something of the truth, Eijkman fed the brown, native rice to his beriberi patients. They, too, began to recover. After many experiments, Eijkman had to conclude that infection was not the problem. Instead, there was something in the hulls, something that was missing from the lovely white rice. He had no idea what it was, but he was sure that it was the difference between beriberi and good health.

Upon returning home to his university post, Eijkman entitled his first lecture, "The Truth Need Not Necessarily Be Simple."

Pigeons, Beriberi, and the Curative Extract

In 1910, a 26-year-old Polish biologist named Casimir Funk arrived at London's Lister Institute and set up a colony of pigeons. Preoccupied with the reports of both Eijkman and the scientists who were making food extracts, he was convinced, as were many others, that the two lines of research were connected.

With a diet of refined grain, Funk soon induced beriberi in his pigeons. Then he made an extract from the sweepings of a grain mill—the hulls left on the mill floor—using hundreds upon hundreds of pounds of sweepings to make ounces of extract. He gave the extract to the dying pigeons. Within hours, they were on their feet, pecking for food.

The world thrilled to Funk's announcement of his findings. He had found a new key to curing disease, the missing essence of nutrition captured in a bottle. What cures might not be on the way?

Goldberger, Pellagra, and the Deepening Mystery

Only a year after Funk's announcement, the U.S. Public Health Service sent Dr. Joseph Goldberger into the American South. His mission: to find the microbe which was disabling, and eventually killing some 200,000 southerners, with a disease called *pellagra*.

The name pellagra came from Italy. It means *rough skin,* referring to the fact that the first signs were rashes on sun-exposed areas of the body, rashes which developed into sores and then fis-

sures. Then diarrhea began, and with it pains in the back, and then throughout the body. With the pain, came exhaustion, sleeplessness, and extreme irritability of the whole nervous system. In the end was madness, then death.

Healing Pellagra with Food

The more Goldberger studied pellagra, the more he was convinced that there was no infection link among victims. The main arguments for the belief that pellagra was infectious were that most patients were poor and lived under substandard sanitary conditions; the disease seemed to cluster in poverty-stricken areas and institutions.

Like Eijkman, Goldberger could find no microbes. But he did find certain living patterns common to the areas and institutions where pellagra was rife. Especially, he found certain dietary patterns.

He found that those with pellagra typically had enough to eat. Checking diets against the known nutrients, Goldberger saw that they got carbohydrates from corn, rice, sweet potatoes, greens, and sweet syrups. They got enough fat, particularly from fried foods and the gravy served with the corn and rice. But Goldberger was unsure about protein. Corn was the protein staple. Hadn't corn been the protein staple in pellagra outbreaks in Italy, too? And elsewhere?

He set up an experiment in a pellagra-ridden orphanage. Curiously, all the children in the orphanage were not afflicted with pellagra. The infants were well, but they got milk. And the children over 12 were also free of pellagra, but they had heavy work to do, so they were given beans and meat. The children in between had pellagra.

So Goldberger, using federal funds, supplemented their diets with meat four times a week, peas and beans all winter, and an egg a day. The pellagra disappeared. The plan also worked in controlled tests in prisons and elsewhere.

Microbe or Malnutrition? Goldberger's Test

The Public Health Service and many local physicians still were not convinced that pellagra was not an infectious disease. So on May 7, 1915, at the U.S. Pellagra Hospital in Spartanburg, South Carolina, Goldberger took a final step. He had shown that he could prevent or cure pellagra with food, and that he could induce it with a restricted diet. Now he had to prove that it wasn't infectious.

To develop this proof, Goldberger, his wife, and a few other hardy volunteers made themselves the guinea pigs. They took some of the stool from a pellagra patient and stirred it into some flour. To this they added skin scales from the sores of other pellagra patients. Then each of the human guinea pigs swallowed some of this noxious mixture. Finally, they injected one another with blood from a pellagra patient.

Surely, if pellagra were an infectious disease, they would soon get pellagra. But they remained healthy. Goldberger had been right. Pellagra was not caused by a microbe. Rather, it was caused by a nutritional deficiency.

The Missing Link of Nutrition— Vitamins

Although the vitamin pioneers could change the diet or use food extracts to heal, they understood little of either why the disease occurred, or why it was healed. In fact, those pioneering scientists were uncovering more scientific problems than they were solving.

Consider beriberi, what we now know is a thiamin-deficiency disease. Thiamin wasn't purified until 1926, 14 years after Funk's announcement that his crude extract of rice hulls cured beriberi. And it wasn't until 1936 that the chemical structure of thiamin was known and synthesized. As for what thiamin had to do with nutrition, real understanding had to wait for the 1940s and the 1950s. Even today, some puzzles remain.

Regarding pellagra, Goldberger's discoveries were for some years thought to be a matter of protein nutrition. He had cured pellagra, but he had no idea that the disease was really the result of a particular *vitamin deficiency.* He was never to know. It was 1937 before niacin was identified and recognized as the long-sought, anti-pellagra factor.

An Early Vision of Vitamin Subtlety

Soon after Goldberger's first reports on pellagra, it was becoming apparent that the role of vitamins was complex, and that vitamins were intricately related to all the nutrients. Goldberger's team wanted to know exactly why the corn-based diet led to pellagra, and why adding other protein-containing foods could cure and prevent the disease.

Several other researchers had been exploring the world of amino acids and showed that some were essential in the diet. They began giving individual amino acids to pellagra patients. In 1921, they thought they had proved that pellagra was caused by a deficiency of the amino acid *tryptophan.*

The solution seemed very tidy. The protein of corn has limited amounts of two amino acids, lysine and tryptophan. The reasoning ran that it was the low level of tryptophan in the corn-based diet that led to pellagra.

Then came disappointment and confusion. For other researchers reported that they, too, had cured pellagra, but with an amino-acid-free extract of yeast. Thus it seemed that tryptophan wasn't the deficiency that caused pellagra. But then why should tryptophan and improved protein diets cure the disease? What made the yeast extract work? Was a vitamin involved? If so, what had the vitamin to do with tryptophan? Even later, when niacin was identified in 1937 as the substance that prevented pellagra, the puzzle of tryptophan was still unsolved.

> The body can convert the amino acid tryptophan to the B-vitamin niacin.

It was finally solved in 1945, when it was found that the body can convert tryptophan to niacin. Pellagra had become prevalent in the South among the poor and institutionalized because of a double dietary failure of their corn-based diet: It was low in niacin, and the corn protein was also low in tryptophan.

But even if Goldberger had somehow known this, he wouldn't have had a glimmer of how it all worked. An understanding of vitamin chemistry had to wait for the revelation of some of the basic chemistry of life—at the level of the cells and the molecules of which we are made.

Eijkman, the beriberi pioneer, was right in saying that "the truth need not necessarily be simple." Despite what you see in popular nutrition books, in magazines and advertisements, the truth of how the body uses the vitamins and other nutrients it takes from food is not simple.

Each vitamin performs an essential function in its own way. But the most common role of vitamins is to assist in the reactions of metabolism.

Vitamins as Coenzymes in Metabolism

The chemical reactions that occur in cells are collectively called **metabolism.** The very word comes from the Greek term for *change.* And even the early Greek physicians saw that change was the essence of life, the difference between life forms and the inanimate.

Metabolism includes both the energy-releasing reactions in which larger molecules are broken down, and the energy-requiring reactions in which larger molecules are made.

To understand what vitamins are and what they do, scientists need to know the fine details of energy metabolism. Here was the great stumbling block for the vitamin pioneers. Lacking this knowledge, they had no insight into how, for example, a shortage of thiamin could cause the weakness of beriberi victims. They didn't know that thiamin serves as a **coenzyme** ("cooperates with enzymes") in the chemical reactions that the body uses to release energy from carbohydrate, fat, and protein.

We've seen how the body breaks foods down to the simpler chemical fuels and building materials of life (e.g., starch into glucose). And we've seen how the body manufactures some of its components (e.g., amino acids into protein). Both of these processes—the breaking down (catabolism) and the building up (anabolism)—involve a series of intricate chemical reactions, each **catalyzed** by an **enzyme.**

Catalysts are substances that markedly increase the speed of chemical reactions. Enzymes are biological catalysts. Without enzymes, very few of the body's chemical reactions could take place

---

Coenzymes are crucial accessories to enzymes, usually acting as carriers—carrying a product of one chemical reaction to be used in another chemical reaction. Niacin, for example, is a part of a coenzyme that picks up the hydrogen released in one reaction, and ferries it to be used in another reaction.

The eight B-vitamins are: thiamin, riboflavin, niacin, vitamin B-6, folate, vitamin B-12, biotin, pantothenic acid (see Table 1-1).

Each of the eight B-vitamins is an essential component of different coenzymes. A single B-vitamin deficiency can have widespread effects for several reasons:

- One coenzyme is usually used in a variety of chemical reactions. (An enzyme, in contrast, is very specific and usually catalyzes only a single reaction.)

- One B-vitamin can be a component of more than one coenzyme. Thiamin, for example, is an essential component of several coenzymes.

- The coenzymes are needed in the chemical reactions that release energy from food—reactions that are basic to the function of cells throughout the body.

The Energy Balance of Life

Some of the earliest as well as some of the most modern advances in nutrition science deal with parts of the same puzzle—how the body takes energy from food. Understanding this process, and the role that vitamins play in it, can give us insight into the chemical basis of all nutrition.

Let's go back to the beginnings of food. In Chapter 4, we noted that all the energy of life begins with the sun. And we saw that the energy

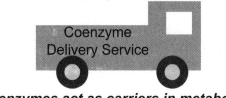

Coenzymes act as carriers in metabolism.

Figure 11-1: We use the energy that the plants get from the sun.

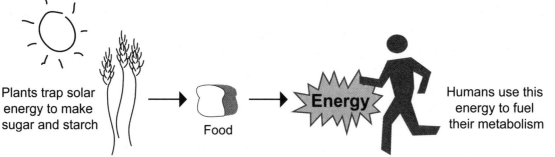

of the sun was trapped by plants. That entrapment was carried out by using solar energy to join two of the earth's most basic molecules—carbon dioxide and water—by what is called ***photosynthesis***.

When plants assemble the molecules that become our food, the spark of the sun doesn't magically make the atoms jump into the appropriate positions. They are precisely assembled by enzymes and coenzymes (which the plants also make from scratch). The plant energy, taken from the sun, is used to make the bonds that hold the atoms together in a molecule.

Plants make their own vitamins. And we (or the animals we eat) must consume the plants to get the vitamins we need for our own coenzymes.

The general description of photosynthesis, and of the process by which the trapped energy was used by animals, were really the two fundamental pieces of knowledge which opened the way to nutrition science and to much of our understanding of medicine and biology.

If we put these processes in a nutritional perspective, one way to express the meaning is: Plants take up energy from the sun and store it by making food. The food holds that energy in a chemical form. To get the energy, the cells of animals such as humans must take apart the food chemicals. When they do, the energy is released and can be used by the cells for the activities of life. (See Fig. 11-1.)

The Release of Energy in Metabolism

Earlier, in looking at how the body gets energy, we saw that it wasn't a matter of direct burning. We don't use our food fuel as a car does, by an explosive combining of the fuel with oxygen.

Instead, although some of the energy is released as heat, the body takes energy from food in what is essentially a chemical form. It does this through ATP.

The making of ATP is the primary objective of our energy metabolism. It is to this end that our cells so laboriously break down the energy-supplying nutrients.

We saw in Chapter 2 that the fires of life—of each individual cell—burn continuously, or life stops. And the energy demands of life are far from constant. The fires burn brightly when we run, slowly when we sleep. Each individual cell has its own surges and resting phases. An intestinal cell has a lively bout of action after a meal. A white blood cell must suddenly do battle with a microbe at the site of a splinter.

Plainly, the mechanisms of getting energy from food must be closely controlled, not only for the body as a whole, but also for each individual cell. Thus, an extremely sophisticated system for energy use must exist. And it does. It makes the most elegant, electronic, automotive fuel-injection system look as simple as a kerosene lamp.

Only the specialist needs to understand all the intricate details of these chemical reactions. We only need to explore the outlines of how our cells are able to use and control the energy from our food to see that the cell's use of nutrients is the essence of how foods sustain life.

Sugar Begins to Yield Energy by Glycolysis

It's in the ***cytoplasm*** ("cell fluid") of individual cells that glucose enters the first phase of metabolism. It's here that glucose begins to yield energy which we can use.

Enzymes and coenzymes within the cytoplasm go to work. They begin by taking the glucose apart, generally reversing the process by which the plant's enzymes and coenzymes put it together in the first place:

Plant Cells:
Carbon Dioxide + Water + Solar Energy = Glucose + Oxygen

Animal Cells:
Glucose + Oxygen = Carbon Dioxide + Water + ATP Energy

The first energy from glucose is extracted when glucose is broken in half. The process is known as **glycolysis** (meaning, logically enough, *breaking sugar)*. From a single molecule with a skeleton of six carbon atoms, glucose is broken into two separate molecules, each with three of the carbons. These two smaller molecules are called **pyruvate**.

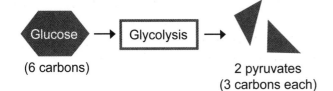

Glucose (6 carbons) → Glycolysis → 2 pyruvates (3 carbons each)

Although the breaking apart of glucose to pyruvate—along with a release of some of its energy—is essentially a simple idea, the process is not simple.

It isn't done directly, say, as one would cleave two pork chops apart. Glycolysis involves ten distinct chemical reactions, precisely engineered by an array of enzymes and coenzymes, as well as some other special chemicals—"simply" to convert glucose to pyruvate.

A Vitamin Role in Glycolysis

At one point in the breaking down of glucose to pyruvate, a vitamin becomes essential. Without this vitamin, the process will stop after a few steps—indeed before any energy at all has been extracted from the glucose.

The vitamin is niacin. It's the anti-pellagra factor which Goldberger sought. And it's an indispensable part of a coenzyme needed in energy metabolism.

In fact, if you were to look closely at the chemistry of glycolysis, you would see that until the niacin-containing coenzyme enters the picture, the cell actually spends ATP energy. But once the niacin-containing coenzyme does its job, the energy balance changes, and glycolysis stops costing energy and begins to release energy. Thus, once we know that this essential coenzyme can't be made without niacin, it's easy to see why people who suffer from pellagra (a severe lack of niacin) feel weak.

They *are* weak. They are hampered in their ability to release energy from food. This isn't the only reason why niacin deficiency produces pellagra symptoms, for the vitamin has other roles, too. But it shows dramatically why vitamins are defined as essential.

Energy Metabolism Without Air

The reactions of glycolysis are **anaerobic** (**an**[without] **aerobic**[air]), meaning that oxygen isn't needed or used in these reactions. In other words, glycolysis enables ATP to be made in the absence of oxygen.

In weight lifting, for example, the strong muscle contractions squeeze the capillaries in the muscles, temporarily cutting off the muscles' supply of oxygen through the blood. Through glycolysis, ATP is made despite the lack of oxygen, fueling the strong muscle action needed for the lift and hold.

Muscle has a short-term back-up for ATP needed for bursts of intense anaerobic muscle action—a bit of phosphocreatine to replenish ATP. Our bodies make creatine, and also get it in meat and fish (animals have creatine in their muscles for the same reason we do). Some athletes take creatine supplements, which may help in "explosive" anaerobic events, e.g., sprinting, weight-lifting.

But the anaerobic production of ATP energy can only fuel sudden energy needs for a very short time. For a sustained source of energy, the body must use an **aerobic** energy pathway.

A Turning Point—and Emergency Energy

The end product of glycolysis—pyruvate—can go in one of two directions (see Fig. 11-2). The normal pathway is to enter the aerobic (oxygen-re-

Figure 11-2: Glycolysis breaks glucose into pyruvate, releasing ATP energy in the process.

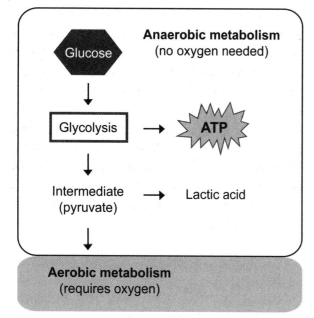

Run Now and Pay Later

When the need for energy becomes greater than the supply of oxygen to burn fuel, pyruvate is stopped from going onto the aerobic phase of energy metabolism. Instead, it gives up some of its energy by being converted into a compound called ***lactic acid***.

Detour for getting more ATP energy without oxygen: Pyruvate → Lactic acid

---

When the action is either very vigorous or very prolonged, the lactic acid accumulates. Such accumulation might contribute to muscle ache and fatigue.

Meanwhile, the failure of pyruvate to proceed along the normal energy pathway because of lack of oxygen sends a constant stream of messages to the heart and lungs—demands for a faster heart beat and more rapid deep breathing. This state, called ***oxygen debt***, is tremendously stressful. Your heart hammers, your lungs ache, you gasp and feel faint.

The term *oxygen debt* is a very real one. For in effect, by using this detour, you're merely deferring the need for oxygen. Eventually, oxygen must be used to deal with the lactic acid. Until your oxygen debt is paid, the pounding of your heart and your heavy breathing will continue, even after your vigorous physical activity has stopped.

Physical fitness extends the time one can exercise vigorously before becoming short of oxygen. Success in endurance events, for example, is very much dependent on how fast blood (which carries the needed oxygen) is delivered to the muscles. Endurance training (aerobic exercise) increases the heart's pumping capacity by increasing the amount of blood pumped with each beat. Since the heart can only beat so fast, this means faster delivery of blood—and oxygen—to the muscles.

Aerobic Metabolism and the Mitochondria

It doesn't matter which nutrient—carbohydrates, proteins, or fats—one begins with. The vast majority of its energy is extracted in the same unifying process of aerobic energy metabolism

quiring) phase of metabolism that takes place in the ***mitochondria*** of the cell (see Fig. 7-2). This aerobic metabolism is the means by which we ordinarily release some 90% of the energy in our food.

But there's a possible detour. And virtually all of us have experienced what it feels like to use it. Understanding this detour for pyruvate helps us to know what really happens when a football halfback breaks through the line and sprints for a long touchdown. It helps to explain what we feel when we race desperately down a seemingly endless corridor for a departing airplane. We feel muscularly exhausted.

The burning of fuel—whether in a car, furnace, or in our body—takes place mainly through the (aerobic) oxidation of fuel. In the body, when all-out extremes of activity go on for more than a few seconds, the demands for oxygen quickly outpace the body's ability to restore oxygen supplies by breathing and circulation.

Both the halfback and the late passenger, in going all out, quickly outpace the body's oxygen-delivery system. So if the action is to continue, the detour for pyruvate must be taken—whether the activity is a 50-yard dash in a track meet or a terrified run from a burning building.

Figure 11-3: ATP production comes mostly from aerobic metabolism in the mitochondria.

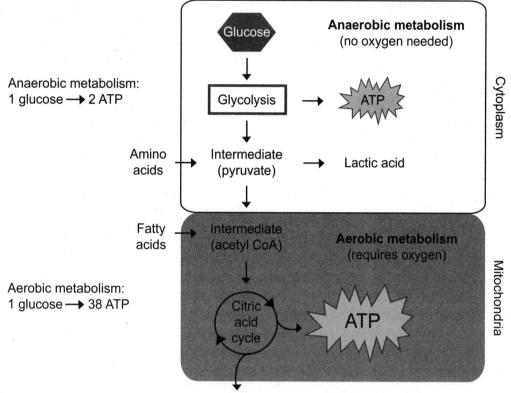

Anaerobic metabolism:
1 glucose → 2 ATP

Aerobic metabolism:
1 glucose → 38 ATP

Carbon dioxide + water + heat

that takes place in the mitochondria of cells (see Fig. 11-3).

Hans Krebs discovered this aerobic phase of metabolism, for which he received a Nobel Prize in 1953.

In a typical cell, there are 1,000 to 4,000 mitochondria. These mitochondria are the power plants of life. For it's inside them that most of the energy from nutrients is released. For example, the use of oxygen enables a net production of 38 molecules of ATP from one molecule of glucose. In the absence of oxygen, net production is only 2 molecules of ATP. Because oxygen-requiring reactions (aerobic metabolism) take place only in the mitochondria, it's clearly advantageous in terms of energy production for cells to contain mitochondria.

Each of these energy-providing nutrients has its own special path to reach this aerobic core of energy metabolism. Although the paths are intricate, the outlines are really quite simple.

Just remember that the energy of food is stored originally by photosynthesis—the joining of carbon dioxide (carbon, oxygen) and water (hydrogen, oxygen). And then more energy is stored as

the resulting building blocks (compounds of carbon, hydrogen, and oxygen) are assembled into more and more complicated molecules which become the substance of our food.

Mitochondria as "Ancient Microbes"

It's thought that mitochondria were once microbes that hundreds of millions of years ago permanently infected certain cells. Uninfected cells would have been unable to use oxygen, and limited to the energy produced by glycolysis (anaerobic metabolism). When the supply of nutrients was limited, cells "infected" with mitochrondria could make more ATP energy, giving them evolutionary advantage by enabling greater growth, movement, and synthesis of complex molecules.

True, other elements are added to the carbon-hydrogen-oxygen compounds along the way. But though these processes add complexity, the over-all process remains simple. When we try to understand energy metabolism, we shouldn't be distracted from the cell's central purpose.

Fundamentally, the cell's energy objective is a primitive one—as old as the first stirrings of life. It is, in effect, to reverse the process of chemical building. It is to tear apart the chemicals which

ATP Production

Anaerobic metabolism:

1 glucose → 2 ATP

Aerobic metabolism:

1 glucose → 38 ATP

1 fatty acid → 129 ATP

make food, and keep tearing them apart, releasing the energy with which they were put together, until there's nothing left but the original carbon dioxide and water.

In the aerobic phase of energy metabolism, this final resolution is achieved. All the stages of preparation which lead to this phase serve to filter out the substances that can't participate, and to end with only a small, single molecule (acetic acid) made of carbon, hydrogen, and oxygen.

In energy metabolism, all the energy-providing nutrients—carbohydrate, fat, protein—are broken down to the same small molecule (acetic acid).

It's this little molecule—still holding much of the energy of the big molecules of food—which finally become carbon dioxide and water again, yielding food energy to the mitochondria and to life.

Let's see how carbohydrate, fat, and protein, eventually reach this point, starting with carbohydrate.

Coenzyme A and the Final Preparation of Glucose

Carbohydrates are absorbed from the intestine as single sugars, predominately glucose. (Other single sugars are, for the most part, immediately converted to glucose upon absorption.)

As we have seen, glucose is converted to pyruvate (see Fig. 11-2). Only one chemical step then remains to change the pyruvate into the molecule that goes into the aerobic phase of energy metabolism. That small molecule is *acetic acid*—more commonly known as vinegar.

While the conversion of pyruvate to acetic acid is straightforward, the execution is intricate. It involves some large and complicated coenzymes that contain some vitamins as part of their structure. The process is worth looking at to see some of the ways in which vitamins are needed by the body.

First, the pyruvate combines with a coenzyme called thiamin pyrophosphate. From the name, we correctly surmise that the coenzyme includes thiamin (the B-vitamin missing in beriberi). In a series of changes which follow, three more B-vitamins become involved. A coenzyme containing niacin (the B-vitamin missing in pellagra) and a coenzyme containing riboflavin (another B-vitamin) are also needed to convert pyruvate to acetic acid.

Finally, the acetic acid is attached to coenzyme A, which contains pantothenic acid (another B-vitamin), This acetic acid and coenzyme A combination is called *acetyl CoA*.

The end result of all this is that glucose is broken down to acetyl CoA, which is what enters the aerobic phase of metabolism (see Fig. 11-3). In other words, coenzyme A carries the acetic acid made from glucose into the final phase of energy metabolism—the aerobic, high-energy-yielding phase that converts acetic acid to carbon dioxide and water.

While the details of this aerobic core of energy metabolism are complex, the essence of what's happening may be envisioned in a simple way.

Remember that when glucose was made from carbon dioxide and water by photosynthesis, oxygen was freed. If the process is to be reversed, the oxygen must be restored. This is why this release of energy from food is referred to as oxidation or aerobic (air-dependent) energy metabolism. Oxygen is restored to the carbons in acetic acid, forming carbon dioxide and water—and ample amounts of ATP energy (see Fig. 11-3).

How Fats Yield Their Energy

As discussed in Chapter 8, the fat in our fat stores and most of the fat in our diet come as triglycerides. For use in energy production, the fatty acids in these triglycerides are let loose.

Like glucose, fatty acids are compounds of carbon, hydrogen, and oxygen. The difference, we might recall, is partly that fatty acids hold a good deal less oxygen. Compared to glucose, fatty acids join with more than twice as much oxygen to produce carbon dioxide and water. And this is why fats (9 calories/gram) have more than twice the energy potential of carbohydrates (4 cal/gm).

The fatty acids—whatever the length of their carbon chains—are broken down to acetic acid, and join Coenzyme A to become acetyl CoA. They thus enter aerobic metabolism, indistinguishable from the acetyl CoA that came from glucose (see Fig. 11-3).

For his part in discovering the chemical reactions that break down fatty acids to acetic acid, Feodor Lynen won a Nobel Prize in 1964.

It should be noted that energy isn't released from fatty acids until after they enter aerobic metabolism as acetyl CoA. The energy-releasing metabolism of fatty acids doesn't include glycolysis. The anaerobic release of energy by glycolysis is unique to carbohydrates (and a few amino acids). In other words, oxygen is essential for energy production from fatty acids.

How Amino Acids Enter Energy Metabolism

As we saw in Chapter 6, the amino acids that make up proteins are also built primarily from carbon, hydrogen, and oxygen. But they are characterized by the addition of nitrogen, in the form of the amino group (NH_2).

In order to be used for energy, amino acids must first have their amino groups removed. As discussed in Chapter 7, the amino groups removed from amino acids are a liability, since they can be converted to ammonia, which is toxic even in fairly low concentrations. To prevent this toxic effect, the amino groups are used to make urea, which can be tolerated at much higher concentrations (see Fig. 11-4). Then, the urea is excreted in the urine.

Once the amino acids are stripped down to their carbon-hydrogen-oxygen structure, they become suitable for the energy-releasing reactions of metabolism.

The carbon skeletons of amino acids, however, are a lot more varied than those of glucose or fatty acids. Depending on its structure, an amino acid is converted to either pyruvate or acetic acid (acetyl CoA). In doing so, the amino acids become indistinguishable from the pyruvate that came from

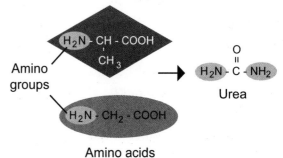

Figure 11-4: Amino groups removed from amino acids form urea, which is disposed in the urine.

glucose or from the acetyl CoA that came from glucose and fatty acids.

We see here a model of efficiency in the energy-releasing reactions of metabolism. All energy-providing nutrients funnel through acetyl CoA in releasing their energy while breaking down to carbon dioxide and water (see Fig. 11-3).

A coenzyme that contains vitamin B-6 is needed for the conversion of amino acids to acetic acid (acetyl CoA).

Take note of the two waste products that result once the energy has been freed—carbon dioxide and water. The system has gone full circle. And the atoms which formed our food have not themselves been changed or used. The food molecules have merely served as energy carriers—with solar energy being used in plants to put and hold the atoms together, and energy being released in our cells when the atoms are separated again.

Athletic Performance

Athletes are useful examples in explaining anaerobic and aerobic energy production, because in their training and competition they attempt to push ATP production to its limits. Athletic events can be roughly divided into two groups, based on whether the fuel used in the event is mainly fatty acids (endurance events) or glucose (strength-and-power events) (see Table 11-1).

Endurance athletes need a steady production of ATP over a long period of time, and they need more ATP than glycogen stores can provide. After about 30-60 minutes of exercise they begin to rely increasingly on fat stores, and use fatty acids as their primary fuel—through aerobic metabolism.

Table 11-1: Two types of Energy-Releasing Reactions.

	Anaerobic	Aerobic
Uses oxygen?	No	Yes
Primary fuel	Glucose	Fatty acids
Type of exercise	Strength/power	Endurance
Cell-type with most capacity	Fast-twitch	Slow-twitch

Even the leanest endurance athlete has more than enough body fat to fuel an event like a marathon.

In contrast, strength-and-power athletes—such as weightlifters, shot putters, gymnasts, and sprinters—use ATP generated mainly from the anaerobic metabolism of glucose (glycolysis) to fuel their event. Oxygen isn't a limiting factor for these athletes. Because their event is short, they can rely on glycolysis, which doesn't require oxygen.

The main advantage of glycolysis over aerobic metabolism for strength-and-power athletes is that the reactions of glycolysis are much faster. In other words, ATP can be made much faster (for "bursts of energy") by anaerobic than by aerobic metabolism.

It follows that those athletes having a greater capacity for glycolysis will be more successful in athletic events that call for a short and intense burst of energy. Muscle cells differ in their capacity to use the anaerobic and aerobic energy-releasing reactions.

Muscle cells can be roughly divided into two types—*fast-twitch* and *slow-twitch.* Fast-twitch muscle cells have a high capacity for glycolysis (they have greater amounts of the enzymes needed for glycolysis), allowing them to contract (twitch) rapidly.

> Quarter horses and greyhounds are bred for speed; muscle cells in their legs are about 95% fast-twitch.

Slow-twitch muscle cells are geared toward the slower, aerobic energy production. They have more fat and mitochondria (the site of aerobic metabolism) than fast-twitch muscle cells. Slow-twitch cells are also rich in myoglobin, which is similar to the hemoglobin in red blood cells. Like hemoglobin, myoglobin carries oxygen.

Most people have fast-twitch and slow-twitch muscle cells in about equal proportion. Studies looking at cell types in the relevant muscles of top athletes, however, show that strength-and-power athletes, like sprinters, have a greater proportion of fast-twitch cells (>70%), whereas endurance athletes, like long-distance runners, have a greater proportion of slow-twitch cells (>70%).

The relative proportion of fast-twitch and slow-twitch cells in a muscle seems to be genetically determined. For athletes intending to break world records, heredity could well be destiny. Training, however, can markedly enhance the aerobic (and possibly the anaerobic) capacity of both types of muscle cells to produce energy.

Storing Excess Calories

What happens when we take in more energy-providing nutrients than we need? In other words, what happens to those excess calories when we eat too much? This was discussed in Chapter 2, but we all know from personal experience that the excess is stored as body fat.

The body does this by using some of the same chemical reactions that break down carbohydrates, protein, and fat. But as can be seen by comparing Figures 11-3 and 11-5, acetyl CoA and fatty acids are diverted from the aerobic core of energy production to energy storage (formation of triglycerides). It's clear from Figure 11-5 that we can become fat from excess calories, whether the excess calories come from carbohydrate, protein, or fat.

Starvation and Low-Carbohydrate Diets

The body constantly needs a certain amount of glucose for energy production. Brain cells, for example, need a lot of energy as ATP, but under normal circumstances can use only glucose as fuel. Where does the glucose come from during starvation or when on a low-carbohydrate diet?

When a person isn't consuming carbohydrate, for whatever reason, glycogen stores are soon depleted. The body must then make the glucose it needs from certain amino acids. *The body can't make glucose from fatty acids.*

Figure 11-5: Excess energy-providing nutrients are stored as body fat.

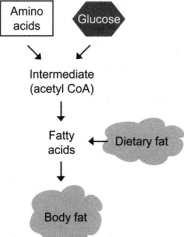

Glucose can be made from pyruvate, but not from acetyl CoA. The conversion of pyruvate to acetyl CoA (see Fig. 11-3) is a crucial reaction in that it's irreversible. Glucose can't be made from fatty acids because fatty acids are broken down to acetyl CoA rather than pyruvate (see Fig. 11-3). However, the amino acids that can be converted to pyruvate can be made into glucose.

The amino acids come from protein. During starvation, the body first breaks down the proteins least essential for survival (e.g., some proteins in the liver and skeletal muscles) to provide the necessary amino acids. As a last resort, the body starts breaking down such proteins as those in the heart muscle.

Starvation would be rapidly fatal if the body had to incessantly break down its protein to provide the brain with glucose. The body in its wisdom produces an alternative fuel *(ketones)* for the brain during starvation. It does this by using the lack of carbohydrate as a signal of starvation.

When carbohydrate is lacking, acetyl CoA doesn't readily proceed to aerobic metabolism. As a result, acetyl CoA accumulates. This unusual accumulation of acetyl CoA causes acetic acid (from acetyl CoA) to combine with each other to form ketones (see Fig. 11-6).

The brain uses the ketones as fuel in increasing amounts during starvation. This lessens its need for glucose, thereby slowing the breakdown of body protein. Of course, once the body's fat stores are used up, body protein is used unremittingly as fuel, and death is imminent.

Figure 11-6: Glucose and ketones are made when carbohydrate is scarce.

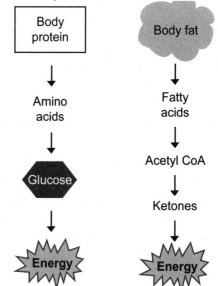

Ketones are acidic, and excessive amounts can cause a condition called ketosis or acidosis, a condition that can be life-threatening. About 50 grams (200 calories worth) of carbohydrate ("carb") a day will prevent ketosis.

A low-carb diet in one form or another shows up regularly in the steady stream of popular weight-loss diets. One reason why this diet is so popular is that it promotes rapid weight loss because body protein (and glycogen) is broken down to maintain glucose in the blood.

The early weight loss is mainly from water loss. Recall that protein and carbohydrate (which includes glycogen) hold about three times their weight in water, whereas fat doesn't hold any (see Chap. 8). (Longer-term weight loss is typically from simply eating a lot fewer calories. Cutting out carbs—candy, desserts, sugared drinks, bread, pasta, rice—cuts out a lot of calories!)

Another reason why low-carb reducing diets are popular is because the production of ketones causes a loss of appetite (sometimes in the form of nausea). Also, some of the ketones are excreted in the urine and breath.

Ketones have caloric value, and this "easy loss of calories" is touted in popular books promoting these diets. But, typically, this loss is less than 60 calories a day. Also, keep in mind that ketone production is basically a response to starvation, an assumed desperate situation in which the benefits of the response outweigh the risks.

Summary

Vitamin research started by looking for microbes, because the results of deficiencies look very much like disease. Through various experiments, scientists discovered that certain elements in the diet prevented these "diseases." But it was uncertain for some time just what role these vitamins played in the body.

The chemical reactions that occur in the body are collectively called metabolism. Metabolism includes the chemical reactions that release energy in the process of breaking down the energy-providing nutrients (carbohydrates, fat, protein) to carbon dioxide and water. Metabolism also includes the energy-requiring reactions in which larger molecules are made from smaller ones (e.g., proteins are made from amino acids).

Many complicated reactions are required for these processes, and B vitamins act as coenzymes in many of these reactions. This is why metabolism is impaired when any of these B vitamins is lacking in the diet.

Carbohydrate is made by plants, and is taken in by our cells as glucose when we eat it. The breakdown of glucose to provide energy is called glycolysis and produces pyruvate. Glycolysis includes many chemical reactions, each requiring its own enzymes and coenzymes. One of these steps requires a coenzyme that contains the B vitamin niacin.

The reactions of glycolysis take place in the cytoplasm, and don't need oxygen—the process is thus called anaerobic metabolism. Glycolysis can produce energy quickly, but only for a limited time. When the need for lots of energy is prolonged (as in sustained, strenuous exercise), the pyruvate forms lactic acid, which can build up and play a role in muscle fatigue.

The usual route for pyruvate is through the aerobic cycle, which takes place in the mitochondria. Pyruvate undergoes a series of chemical reactions (involving coenzymes that contain the B-vitamins thiamin, niacin, and riboflavin) to form acetic acid. Acetic acid attaches to Coenzyme A (which contains the B vitamin pantothenic acid) to form acetyl CoA.

Acetyl CoA combines with oxygen to produce carbon dioxide, water, and lots of ATP. In effect, the original process, in which plants gathered energy from the sun and through photosynthesis used carbon dioxide and water to build the molecules we call food, has been reversed, returning to carbon dioxide and water and releasing the stored energy.

The energy released from fat (i.e., fatty acids) comes exclusively from the breakdown of acetyl CoA. In other words, fat can't release any of its energy without oxygen—fatty acids don't take part in glycolysis.

Protein (i.e., amino acids) must have their amino groups removed before they can be broken down for energy. (The amino groups are removed as urea in urine.) This leaves a carbon skeleton, which enters the energy-producing reactions as pyruvate or acetyl CoA.

Athletes can be roughly divided into two groups: (1) endurance athletes, who rely mainly on fatty acids and aerobic metabolism for energy and (2) power athletes, who rely mainly on glucose and anaerobic metabolism (glycolysis). They tend to have a predominance of muscle cells best suited for their event: Fast-twitch cells depend mainly on glycolysis, and slow-twitch cells depend mainly on aerobic metabolism. Which cell type predominates is genetically determined.

When not needed for energy production, acetyl CoA and fatty acids are converted to triglycerides and stored as body fat. Since all the energy-providing nutrients go through acetyl CoA in their energy-releasing breakdown, excess calories—whether from carbohydrate, fat, or protein—can be made into body fat.

The body continually needs some glucose for energy. If the body doesn't get enough carbohydrate, it makes glucose from amino acids. (The body can't use fatty acids to make glucose.) During starvation, a relentless conversion of amino acids to glucose would hasten the loss of protein from both muscle and vital organs. So when carbohydrate is lacking (because of starvation or a low-carb diet), the body uses the acetyl CoA made from fatty acids to produce ketones for use as an energy alternative to glucose.

Chapter 12

Water—The Body's Inner Sea

We tend to take water for granted. We're never far from a spigot in our everyday lives and thirst is our usual gauge for water need. We might have felt differently if we had lived just a short distance back in history, or if we lived in one of the arid areas of the earth. When people have to haul their water in from the well or up from the river, or have to live with the constant menace of not enough water to sustain life, they don't take it for granted.

But even when water is hard to come by, we seldom think about its importance for bodily function and health. As is so often the case, we only become aware when there's a problem— extraordinary sensations of parched heat and/or thirst—and don't think of dehydration when the clues aren't obvious (as with jet lag or 'instant weight loss diets').

In fact, we are largely made of water, and water plays a crucial role in all of our bodily processes. We need a constant supply, and can quickly compromise our health (and a sense of physical well being) when we don't get enough.

As well as science can determine, it was in some quiet backwater of the sea that life began on earth. Indeed, life as we know it could hardly have begun anywhere else but in water.

In this chapter, we begin by looking at the role of water in life chemistry and how that role extends to water's various functions in the body, particularly its bodily role in circulation, cooling, and waste disposal. Then the variation in our water needs and the meeting of those needs through our food and drink are discussed.

Life Chemistry and the Primitive Sea

The first making of life's chemicals seems to have required few ingredients. In that time—the Precambrian Era—it's thought that the planet's atmosphere was rich in such gases as methane, ammonia, and carbon dioxide. These gases dissolve in water, allowing them to react with one another.

The reactions that combine these gases require intense energy. In that era, the seas would have been exposed to the energy from such sources as lightning and cosmic rays, which were then much more powerful than they are today. So it's thought that such a combination of water, primitive gases, and intense energy brought forth the first of life's chemicals.

Decades ago, scientists began to test this hypothesis of life's origins. They reproduced what was thought to be the ancient chemical soup of life. Into water, they dissolved the simple gases methane (CH_4), ammonia (NH_3), and carbon dioxide (CO_2).

These gases, along with water (H_2O), hold the key atomic elements of life—carbon, hydrogen, oxygen, and nitrogen. From the simplest plant to the complex brain, living substances are composed mainly of these four elements.

The scientists then exposed this chemical soup to a steady bombardment of electrical energy. And day by day, new chemicals emerged. First, the solution began to yield such new molecules as acetic acid (vinegar) and formaldehyde. Then, as the bombardment continued, these chemicals became

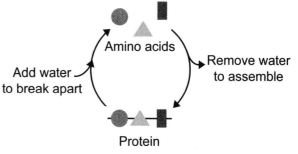

Figure 12-1: Water plays a key role in assembling and breaking apart proteins and other molecules.

richer in the solution, and the simplest amino acid appeared. Gradually, other more complex amino acids formed. And finally, these amino acids began to link together to make protein—one of life's most complex structures.

The Dual Role of Water

What part did water play in these formative reactions? First, there was the obvious role of solvent—dissolving. Once dissolved in water, the gases had a greater potential for combination. The components of the gases—such as the carbon and the oxygen of carbon dioxide—were then ready to separate and recombine.

We see many household examples of this common fact of chemistry, that many chemicals must dissolve before they can react. Consider the baking of a cake. None of the chemistry of cake-making occurs as long as the dry and liquid ingredients are kept separate. If this weren't so, cake mixes wouldn't keep on the supermarket shelf.

The liquids of a cake recipe—whether milk, applesauce, eggs, or any other fluid substance except oil—are mainly water. When these fluids are combined with the dry flour, baking powder, sugar, etc., the reactions begin. Dough is made, and it goes into action. Gases, mainly carbon dioxide, begin to form, and the dough rises. The relatively inert solids have suddenly become active. They change; they interact.

There's a message for us here. It's that the chemicals of life, like the chemical ingredients of a cake, change once they are dissolved. Water makes their reactions possible.

But water is far more than a holding place and meeting ground for the chemicals of life. It's far more than a transporter of chemicals through the body—whether in blood or cellular fluid. Water itself is an active participant in life chemistry.

In many biochemical reactions, a molecule of water is added or subtracted. We see this in the formation of protein, starch, and triglycerides, and in their digestion: A molecule of water is removed when an amino acid is joined to another in making protein (see Fig.12-1). The same is true when a glucose molecule is joined to another in making starch, or when a fatty acid is joined to glycerol in forming a triglyceride. The reverse happens as well: water molecules are added back in the digestive reactions that release amino acids from proteins, glucose from starch, and fatty acids from triglycerides.

To make the role of water as a participant in life's chemical reactions even clearer, recall that it's by combining carbon dioxide and water that plants are able to make carbohydrates and store the energy of the sun. Recall further, that as animal life uses these plant sources of carbohydrates for energy, the metabolic reactions yield carbon dioxide and water.

Clearly, water is central to the chemistry of life.

We are Mainly Water

Whereas many of us can survive months without food, none of us—fat or thin—can survive more than a few days without water. A lack of water is felt immediately. In extreme circumstances, as in a summer desert, the absence of water can mean death in as few as 12 hours.

Body water is often categorized as either *intracellular water* (water within cells, representing about 60% of total body water) or *extracellular water* (water outside of cells, representing about 40% of total body water) (see Fig. 12-2). But this categorization can be misleading when envisioned as two separate and distinct compartments of water. Rather, there's a constant exchange of extracellular and intracellular water. This exchange is the means by which nutrients are carried into our cells and the cells' products are carried out.

The sugar glucose, for example, needs to be dissolved in the water of digestive fluids

Figure 12-2: Body's fluid compartments.
About two-thirds of the adult body is water (60% intracellular, 40% extracellular).

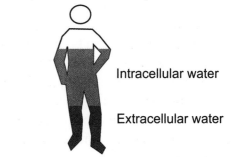

Intracellular water

Extracellular water

(extracellular fluid) before it enters the intestinal cell to become a part of its intracellular fluid. This glucose coming from food is then passed by way of blood plasma (an extracellular fluid) to the intracellular fluid of cells throughout the body.

We see an example outside of our bodies by looking at the one-celled animals of ponds and tide pools. This same flow of nutrients between extracellular and intracellular fluid takes place. These one-celled creatures are separate from, yet a continuous part of, the sea in which they live. Our own cells are much the same.

Although the percentage of our body weight that's water varies from person to person and diminishes from birth to death, water is always the major component of the body. The newborn infant has the most water, averaging about 75% of total body weight. The elderly person may be only slightly more than 50% water.

In between these extremes of age, the average adult body is about 60 to 70% water. How much water the adult body normally holds is mainly determined by the amount of body fat. Recall that fat doesn't hold water. It follows that the fatter you are, the smaller the proportion of water in your body.

Indeed, the fact that body water has little to do with fat suggests why it's futile to tamper with the water balance of the body when trying to lose body fat. There's no value in trying to restrict water intake or to promote water loss. Similarly, there's no point in devices and exercises which are intended mainly to cause water loss through sweating. While such water losses temporarily lower body weight, they don't reduce the true problem of fatness.

The Water Game in Quick Weight-Loss Schemes

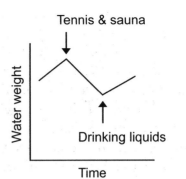

There really is a pill that will make you lose weight. Just as quick-loss diet programs advertise, you really can see your weight fall two, four, six pounds, even more, within a couple of days. It's a gratifying experience for the frustrated dieter.

Unfortunately, this "magic pill" is a *diuretic*. It works by stimulating the kidneys to take water out of the body and excrete it as urine. So the diuretic pill has shed pounds all right, but it has nothing to do with fat.

Our body water does have its ups and downs. For example, body water can vary by several pounds during a woman's menstrual cycle. Water retention generally peaks as the menstrual period begins, and can make the woman feel fat.

The amount of sodium in a day's food can raise and lower the body's water content, by a matter of pounds. Alcohol and caffeine tend to be dehydrating. We tend to be the lightest before breakfast—our stomachs are empty; we have lost some water through evaporation during sleep; and we usually urinate upon getting out of bed.

The ups and downs of body water create the impression that fat can come and go with incredible speed, and can easily deceive the reducer who relies only on the scale.

Take Sue, who says, "I sure wish I could control my appetite. I played grueling tennis last Sunday for 3 hours in that sun. Afterwards, I skipped lunch, and sat in the sauna instead. Sure enough, I'd lost 5 pounds. But then, you know what? At Ed's dinner party that night, I went crazy over the prime rib and had some daiquiris with a lot of appetizers. When I got on the scale before I went to bed, I couldn't believe it. All that work to lose 5 pounds, and then at that one dinner I ate it all back on!"

Such things happen all the time. The *weight* loss and gain are real. But there's an illusion that the food and drink really made the person 5 pounds fatter. Let's see what the body is actually doing.

To gain a pound of body fat, one must eat 3,500 calories more than one expends. For Sue to have eaten her way to a 5-pound gain in body fat would mean an extra 17,500 calories. Ten pounds of prime rib, 10 daiquiris, and 2 trays of appetizers? Probably not.

Sue may have spent 800 calories in 3 hours of vigorous tennis. (Though actually, she didn't spend the whole 3 hours playing tennis. She rested 10 minutes between each set and spent some 20 minutes changing courts and arguing scores.) And the sauna didn't use up much beyond basal metabolic need. But even at that, an 800 calorie expenditure represents less than a quarter pound of body fat.

But the sweat loss was considerable, and Sue neglected to drink water during the match. Between the tennis, the hot sun, and the sauna, 5 pints of perspiration were lost, actually representing the 5 pounds ("a pound a pint").

Weak after the sauna, Sue drank long at the water fountain. At home, while changing for dinner, she drank a couple of cans of diet soda. Famished, she had big helpings at the dinner party. Still thirsty, she had more water, a couple of daiquiris, and a few more cans of diet soda poured over a lot of ice. Her body water came back up.

Calorie-wise, her tennis, skipping lunch, and all that extra food at dinner balanced out to about zero. As usual, need and appetite stayed pretty close together. But the dip and then rise of body water had made her experience seem much more dramatic.

Water and the Body's Cooling System

Although as a whole, the body can survive in a very wide range of temperatures, most of our cells cannot. Instead, our cells are more like the single-celled animals of the seas and lakes, most of which can function only within a very limited temperature range. Our body's chemical reactions work best at our typical human body temperature, between about 98 and 99°F. Temperatures somewhat higher or lower can impair our body chemistry.

Moreover, many of life's chemical reactions are heat-producing. Because these reactions may be more intense in some cells than in others—for example, in muscle cells during exercise—water becomes important to keep body heat rather evenly distributed. Otherwise, our bodies would continually develop "hot spots," and cells in those areas might become inefficient or even be seriously damaged.

Because body cells can't survive when temperatures rise more than a few degrees, the removal of added heat must be prompt and dependable. Water not only carries the heat away from the cells that produce the heat, but water is also a key factor in disposing of the heat.

The Cooling Breeze

Evaporation of water is a key mechanism for heat disposal. Although we think first of the cooling evaporation of water in sweat, the evaporation of watery secretions in the lungs and mouth also contributes to cooling. Dogs provide a good example, since they can't sweat like we can. Dogs must rely on evaporation from their lungs, their throat, and their long and extendible tongues. That we humans don't respond to heat by extending wet tongues, panting, and drooling, isn't due to innately better manners; it's because we can sweat.

For humans, sweating—an obviously watery operation—is the most important means of heat loss. We sweat almost constantly, though we may not be aware of the fact. Indeed, about half of human sweat is called *insensible perspiration,* because it's so slow and subtle. Under normal conditions of comfort, with relatively little activity, water loss through evaporation accounts for more than 40% of the water lost by the body.

It follows that conditions that increase—or hamper—the evaporation of water substantially affect heat disposal. A hot day is particularly uncomfortable if the air is humid and still and we are covered with a heavy layer of clothing—conditions which minimize the evaporation of water. That hot day wouldn't feel so hot if the air were dry and breezy. What we call a cool breeze is usually, in fact, a cooling breeze. "Heat stroke" or "heat collapse" usually has its beginnings in dehydration: the body seeks to cool itself and doesn't have enough water to do the job.

Some sense of the urgency of water replacement in terms of body heat can be seen by how fast the water we drink can be put to work by the body when we're very dry. When water is drunk in such a state, its absorption and use is almost instantaneous. You may have experienced the phenomenon: You're hot and dry and begin to drink. Almost at once, sweat seems to burst out on your face.

Water and the Body's Wastes

Except for the breathing out of carbon dioxide, most of the waste products of body chemistry are discarded through urine and feces. Urine is clearly a watery instrument of waste disposal. The kidneys use rather large amounts of water to carry off waste products which they have removed from the blood.

The amount of water needed—and thus the volume of urine—becomes larger when a lot of waste must be disposed of through the urine. For example, excess salt intake increases the amount of urine. When we eat a lot of salty foods (table salt = sodium chloride), more water is needed to get rid of the excess sodium. Beer joints don't lose money on free bowls of salty peanuts, pretzels, or tortilla chips. We feel thirsty, drink more, and urinate more.

Sea water has so much salt that the kidneys need additional plain water just to dispose of it. So, ironically, when castaways drink sea water because of desperate thirst, they actually cause their bodies to become dehydrated faster.

Feces, the "solid" wastes of the body, also carry a fair amount of water. In fact, we might recall that dietary fiber does much of its work in speeding up "transit time" in the colon by holding water, making the stool softer and bulkier. The more fiber in our food, the more water carried by the feces.

But we should keep in mind that when the colon moves its contents through too fast, the colon doesn't have time to absorb all the water it should, and the result is diarrhea. Diarrhea can cause rapid loss of body water. The water loss from some diarrheal diseases can be life-threatening.

Dehydration resulting from severe diarrhea is a leading cause of infant death in developing countries. In these countries, infant diarrhea is commonly due to ingestion of disease-producing bacteria, often from fecal contamination of drinking water. As one might expect, an acute response to ingesting toxins, including disease-causing bacteria, is vomiting and diarrhea.

In developing countries, a mother's use of clean water with a bit of added sugar and salt to feed her infant (*oral rehydration therapy*) has rescued many an infant from fatal dehydration from severe diarrhea. The sugar and salt speed the absorption of water and provide a little nutrition.

In the extreme situation of cholera, for example, there's severe diarrhea. The cholera bacteria make a toxin that causes water to actually be drawn out of the tissues into the intestine. In addition, there's vomiting, which causes more loss of water and electrolytes. In the most severe cases, several quarts of body water are lost within a few hours. Treatment calls for the immediate administration of intravenous fluids. Untreated, the fatality rate from severe cholera is over 50%.

Ridding the Body of "Toxic Wastes"

Many popular diet-and-health books promote regimens for "ridding the body of toxins and toxic wastes." But these books define "toxins" and "toxic" rather vaguely. For good reason. The line between toxins and non-toxins isn't always sharp. Even essential nutrients or plain carbon dioxide can be toxic in excess, and toxins in small amounts can be harmless. The body has its own regimens for ridding itself of toxins—regimens far more sophisticated than those devised by such dietary manipulations.

Vomiting and diarrhea are, of course, the body's most violent response to toxins in our food and drink. But what of bodily "toxins"?

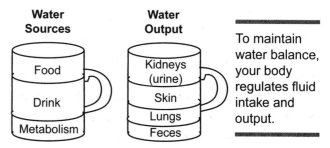

Water Sources: Food, Drink, Metabolism

Water Output: Kidneys (urine), Skin, Lungs, Feces

To maintain water balance, your body regulates fluid intake and output.

The body routinely gets rid of the "toxins" it produces. If this weren't so, we'd all soon be poisoned to death. Think of those whose kidneys don't function as they should in ridding the body of "toxic wastes." Modern medicine keeps them alive by "detoxifying" their blood through dialysis.

Water Balance

Water balance (amount taken in = amount lost) is carefully regulated by the kidneys and the thirst center in the brain. When water intake is less than we need, we become thirsty and our urine becomes more concentrated. Conversely, when our water intake is more than we need, we don't feel thirsty, and our urine becomes more dilute. Under normal, everyday circumstances, the body automatically regulates our water balance, and we don't have to be concerned with it.

But the thirst mechanism doesn't work as well in the elderly, so they need to make a point of drinking water, even when they aren't thirsty. Also, when extraordinarily large amounts of water are lost—as in severe diarrhea, vomiting, fever, or heavy sweating—the body's control mechanisms may not work well enough or fast enough to prevent dehydration (e.g., thirst isn't a reliable gauge of needed water replacement for the active athlete). Because so many bodily functions depend on water, the balance between loss and intake must be maintained within reasonable limits. There's only so much forgiveness (see Fig. 12-3).

As dehydration develops, the body has its priorities. As we've seen before, the body tends to protect first those organs and functions which are most necessary to survival. Foremost, the body needs to maintain its blood volume for adequate circulation. For this reason, the body will permit only so much water to be used for perspiration when we're hot and dry.

Figure 12-3: **Effects of Dehydration.**

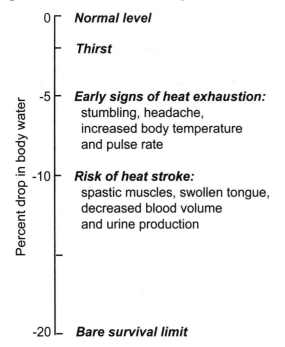

tioning that there's a psychological disturbance called compulsive water drinking—a compulsion to drink enormous amounts of water to the point where the kidneys can't get rid of the overload fast enough. It results in a potentially lethal condition called *water intoxication.* Tissues swell, making the brain particularly vulnerable because it's encased in the skull.

Early symptoms include headache and vomiting. (Recall that headache can also be a symptom of dehydration. Headaches often serve as a subtle—or not so subtle—indication that something is out of kilter.) Tragically, fraternity pledges have died from water intoxication from being forced to drink huge amounts of water during hazing.

Alcohol and Dehydration

Alcohol increases urination and can thus be dehydrating, and dehydration causes some of the misery of a hangover. So drinking plenty of water during or after cocktail parties can spare one from some of the discomforts of the morning after.

In hot weather, the body may have less water available to deal with alcohol. So a beer, with its higher water-to-alcohol ratio, is a better choice in hot weather than a cocktail.

Combine the hot weather with heavy exercise or a high altitude (where the drier air and reduced atmospheric pressure hastens evaporation from the skin and lungs), and alcohol can carry a lot more kick. For one thing, the effect of alcohol increases as it becomes a larger percentage of the blood.

When we're low on water, the volume of blood circulating in our bodies is less. So every ounce of alcohol we drink is a bigger percentage of the blood; it takes less alcohol to make us a lot more fuzzy.

So after a tennis match in the sun, have a drink of water before (or, better yet, instead of) one with alcohol. And on a passenger jet, you might want to take the same precautions. Dehydration can make a substantial contribution to jet lag. Despite pressurization, the air is thin and dry—like that of high altitude on land. Limit alcohol intake, and drink plenty of non-alcoholic beverages.

But this adjustment can work only so long. It's a kind of bodily stalling tactic, which has some strict time limits. As water ordinarily expended in sweat is held back when we're hot, the body temperature begins to rise, and it can't rise more than 6 or 7 degrees before collapse becomes imminent.

The first President Bush, at age 82, was hospitalized briefly after becoming dehydrated and dizzy while golfing in Palm Springs, California.

With just a 5% drop in body water, a person may begin to show early signs of heat exhaustion, such as weakness, headache, and a weak and fast pulse. When body water drops 10%, a person is at risk of *heat stroke,* which can be fatal if not treated promptly.

Even if heat isn't a problem, continued dehydration will cause a fall in blood volume. This can cause a fall in blood pressure and a weak pulse—and a fast pulse, as the heart beats faster in trying to maintain circulation. The fall in blood volume and circulation can lead to its own set of potentially fatal complications, such as an inability to produce urine.

Lest one think that the problem of water intake is always one of not enough, it's worth men-

The Variables of Water Need

Considering the variations in weather, individual activity, alcohol intake, etc., it should be clear that the need for water is quite variable. At a minimum, it's estimated that adults need about 2 quarts of water each day to replace normal losses. About a quart is lost as urine, and the rest is lost in perspiration, expired air, and feces.

A common rule of thumb is that adults need about a quart of water for each 1,000 calories consumed. Infants need more water—about a quart and a half per 1,000 calories. (As will be discussed soon, we meet our water need not only through drink, but also through the substantial amount of water in "solid" food.)

This amount doesn't take into account such stresses as a hot or dry climate or strenuous activity. Because the loss of water by evaporation from the skin and lungs is a primary way of cooling the body, a combination of heat and exertion can markedly increase water usage. Soldiers working in desert heat can lose up to a quart of water an hour.

Water and the Athlete

As with other nutrients, there are misconceptions about water and athletic performance. Even today, some parent coaches tell their young players to limit the amount of water they drink even during a vigorous soccer game on a hot day. In reality, unless one gulps enormous amounts of water, there's little or no risk of "cramps" or other problems.

To the contrary, the risk is one of substandard performance—or a serious health problem—if play continues when the players need water. Thirst isn't a discomfort to be endured. It's a warning sign of bodily need in almost all cases. (But an absence of thirst isn't necessarily a signal that the body doesn't need water.)

Strenuous athletic events in hot weather offer particular dehydration problems. As stated earlier, water loss may be so fast that athletes cannot depend on thirst, and often cannot even drink and absorb water fast enough to keep pace with their water need. For this reason, athletes should drink a lot of water before, during, and after athletic

events that last more than a half-hour, even if they aren't thirsty. Cold water may be preferable because it's absorbed a little faster, and is itself cooling. But unchilled water will do quite well.

Activity is partially taken into account by the tie-in of water need to calorie need—more physical activity requires more calories. All activity is heat-generating, but strenuous activity is all the more so.

Athletes can monitor their dehydration by weighing themselves before and after an athletic event or work-out. The aim is to minimize weight loss by drinking plenty of water, and to drink enough water afterwards. For every pound of weight loss, two 8-oz. glasses of water are needed for rehydration ("a pint a pound").

In most circumstances, "sports drinks" don't provide any performance advantage over plain water (except perhaps the psychological advantage of believing performance will be enhanced). But in endurance events lasting more than 90 minutes, consuming drinks containing about 6 to 8% carbohydrate (glucose, sucrose, or glucose polymer) beginning about 30 minutes before fatigue sets in, does seem to enhance performance. (Most sports drinks are 5-8% carbohydrate.)

One-third cup of table sugar (sucrose) per quart of water makes a "sports drink" of 7% carbohydrate. Add a bit of unsweetened Kool-Aid for flavor and color. Adding a bit of sodium also can help by speeding the absorption of the sugar and water. Adding 1/8 teaspoon of table salt (sodium chloride) per quart, provides about 70 mg sodium per cup.

Taking sodium or other electrolytes isn't generally necessary, and doesn't enhance performance. The one exception is the need for sodium in the drinking water during endurance events lasting more than 4 hours. In such situations, sweat losses are extraordinarily large and prolonged.

The sodium and other minerals lost in sweat is quite minimal and doesn't compromise performance except in the most extreme circumstances. Furthermore, the body adapts to regular, heavy sweating; the sweat of a trained athlete has less sodium and other electrolytes than that of an untrained person. Following the event, the lost minerals are readily replenished by a normal diet.

Other nutrients, such as amino acids and vitamins, taken immediately before or during an event are of no help, and can even be detrimental to performance if taken in large amounts. Such excesses means more waste products to excrete through the urine, and increased urine production hastens dehydration.

To sum up, it's very important for an athlete to drink plenty of water to keep from becoming dehydrated. For athletic endeavors lasting less than 90 minutes, plain water is all that's needed for optimal performance. For endurance events of more than 90 minutes, carbohydrate-containing drinks can enhance performance when taken during the event, starting about 30 minutes before the expected time of fatigue. For endurance events of 4 hours or more, sodium-containing drinks should be taken during the event.

For events lasting less than 90 minutes, plain water is a good "sports drink."

For all the emphasis placed on preventing dehydration, there's a caveat—don't over-do it. In many marathons, runners load up on water before the race, and then are offered water and sports drinks at every mile along the route.

A study of several hundred runners in the 2002 Boston Marathon found excessive fluid consumption in 22% of the women and 8% of the men, as measured by abnormally low levels of sodium in the blood (from water overload), regardless of whether they drank water or sports drinks.[1] Most of those with excessive fluid intake gained weight during the race—an indication of water overload ("a pint a pound"), just as weight lost during a race is a measure of dehydration. A 28-year-old woman who ran that race (but wasn't in the study) died soon afterwards from severe water overload.

Water in Food and Drink

Even if we knew exactly how much water we needed on a given day, it would be hard to know how much water we actually took in. This is because, for most of us, drinks can play a relatively small part in meeting our water needs—"solid" food is a big source.

Roughly half of the food we eat is water. If this sounds incredible, think of how much water you add to uncooked rice, and how the water "disappears" into the rice when cooked. Or how the thin package of dry spaghetti becomes a potful when cooked. Or how raw mushrooms shrink and seep as we sauté them in a bit of butter. Even when we eat low-moisture foods, we typically have something watery at the same time, whether we drink beer with our pretzels, pour milk over our cornflakes, or sip a soft drink between mouthfuls of movie popcorn.

We have a clear notion of which foods are solid and which are liquid. For example, we think of milk as a liquid, and of oranges or apples as solid. But the chemical truth is that milk, oranges, and apples all have about the same relative amount of water—about 85%.

Even solid-seeming meat is usually more than half water. And many vegetables, such as lettuce and asparagus, which appear to be more solid than milk, are actually less so, being about 95% water. Why would such "solid" foods have so much water?

Water and the Structure of Food

Whether vegetable, animal, or fungal, the processes of life hinge on water-based chemistry and must take place in a watery medium. This suggests that the solid structures of life, even though they serve important purposes, could, in large amounts, hinder life's chemistry. So nature keeps "real solids" to a minimum in living systems.

Since our foods are taken from one life form or another (either "animal" or "vegetable"), they follow this same rule of minimal solid matter. For example, the structural framework of plants, with the roots that hold them in the soil and the stems that lift their leaves to the sun, are very fibrous. To maximize structural integrity with a minimum of solid material, the fibrous structures of plants (and the bony structures of animals) are built in a honeycomb-like way—a lattice-work of supporting solid matter. It's this construction that deceives us into seeing as solid even the most watery of foods.

Figure 12-4: Percent Water in Various Foods.

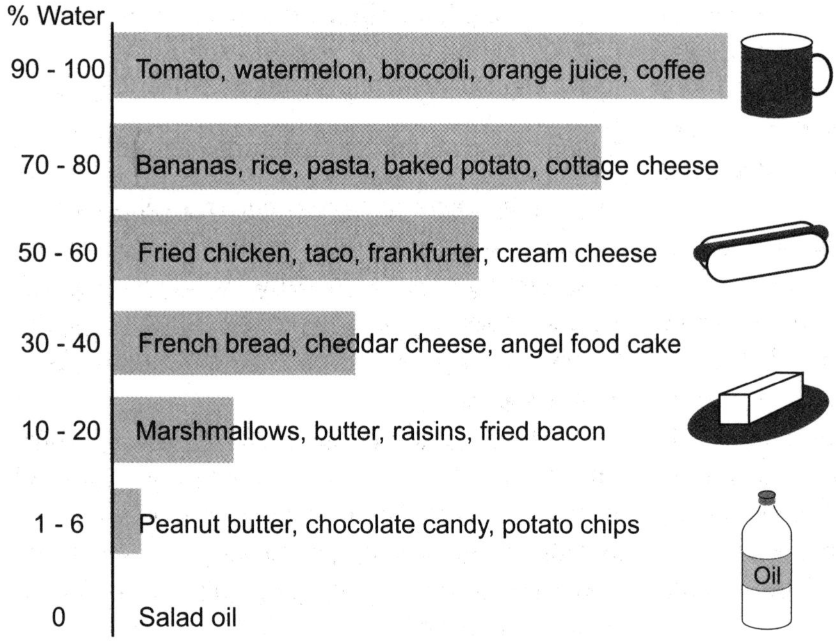

% Water	
90 - 100	Tomato, watermelon, broccoli, orange juice, coffee
70 - 80	Bananas, rice, pasta, baked potato, cottage cheese
50 - 60	Fried chicken, taco, frankfurter, cream cheese
30 - 40	French bread, cheddar cheese, angel food cake
10 - 20	Marshmallows, butter, raisins, fried bacon
1 - 6	Peanut butter, chocolate candy, potato chips
0	Salad oil

Watch raw spinach cook. When raw, the spinach fills the pot. Within a minute or two of cooking, the fibrous structure goes limp, and the spinach shrinks to a thin layer at the bottom of the pot. Yet even with this loss in structural integrity, the water content of the spinach changes little. So even in its seemingly condensed form, cooked spinach, like the raw spinach leaves, is still more than 90% water.

To get a more graphic image of the water-to-solid ratio of a "solid" food such as asparagus or lettuce, imagine a cup of water with about 2 spoonfuls of sugar dissolved into it. The relative amounts of water and sugar represents the water-to-solid ratio of these vegetables.

In other words, if it weren't for the cleverness of nature's structural arrangements, we could very well say that we live on "liquid" diets.

"Juicy" Fat and Sugar

Even if we took all our food as liquids, we can still be deceived as to how watery they are. Foods that are high in fat or sugar are particularly deceptive. The moisture illusion created by fat is easy to understand, as when we "moisten" our baked potato, rice, pasta, vegetables, bread, or popcorn with butter.

The moisture illusion of high-sugar foods is caused by their stimulation of saliva. So most people find hard candies (including cough drops) quite moist. But they aren't. This illusion can be counterproductive for athletic competitors like runners or cyclists who are dehydrating and suck on candies for an illusion of quenching thirst.

When the candy contains fat as well, this compounds the illusion. For example, most forms of chocolate are only 1-2% water, being mostly sugar and fat. It's not surprising that eating much moist-seeming candy is often followed by thirst.

Water and Deception in Food Choices

Comparisons of foods, whether for pricing or nutrient evaluation, can be distorted by water content. In pricing, a clear example is when companies inject broth into the carcass of the Thanksgiving turkey for a "juicier" turkey. Since we pay for turkey by the pound, we pay turkey prices for the added water. Different amounts of water in different brands of the same product make it hard to make cost comparisons.

In trying to compare the fat content of foods, water can distort the comparison. To repeat the example given in Chapter 9, milk is mainly water, so its fat content, by weight, appears deceivingly low.

By weight, whole milk is only about 3.5% fat, low-fat milks 1-2% fat, and non-fat milk is almost fat-free. These are very low percentages. But about 50% of the calories in whole milk comes from fat, while 35% of the calories in low-fat (2%) milk, 15% of the calories in "extra light" (1% fat) milk, and 5% of the calories in non-fat milk comes from fat. By expressing fat content in terms of calories from fat, as opposed to percentages of total food weight, comparisons of the fat content become realistic—the comparisons aren't distorted by water content.

Categorizing foods as liquids or solids can also be deceptive, especially for the dieter. For example, the perception is that a glass of clear apple juice has fewer calories than an apple. True, the apple is more filling and takes longer to eat. But it's the apple's non-caloric fiber that makes it so. A cup of apple juice is about 115 calories, whereas a medium sized apple is about 80 calories. So in many ways, the dieter is better off eating whole fruits rather than drinking their juices.

In thinking of meeting our water needs, we also tend to categorize foods as liquids or solids. But as we have seen, "solid" foods often have as much water as liquids. Even "real solids" can provide some water. Recall that the complete metabolism of the energy-providing nutrients provides water as a breakdown product. We can meet our water needs with a wide variety of beverages and foods. Plain tap water is, however, calorie-free and the least expensive.

Water–Plain and Bottled

Plain drinking water from the tap isn't so plain. As we have seen, water is a superb solvent, so depending on where it's been, substances of all kinds dissolve in it. Even rain water falling through clear air collects various gases before it hits the ground. The dissolved substances are what give various waters their distinctive tastes—and sometimes odors and colors—and are what determine whether or not the water is safe to drink.

Although our senses separate the good-tasting from the bad, they don't necessarily tell us which water is safe and which isn't. For example, drinking water rich in iron tastes and smells bad, but iron is safe to drink. But lead in the drinking water, even at toxic levels, is tasteless and odorless.

For the nation as a whole, *lead is* the pollutant of most concern in the drinking water. The developing nervous system is particularly vulnerable to the toxic effects of lead. Thus, lead exposure is most worrisome among pregnant women and young children—population groups that also tend to be low in iron and calcium. Diets rich in iron and calcium can lessen the amount of lead absorbed.

Progress is being made in reducing this source of lead. The amount of lead allowable in drinking water has been lowered, and water suppliers are required to notify customers of any lead in the water. Also, current safety regulations ban lead pipes in new plumbing to be used for drinking water. Homes more than 90 years old might still have lead pipes, which should be replaced.

Lead solder on pipes is less serious (but more widespread), especially if the solder is more than 5 years old (lead solder dissolves more easily during the first 5 years). If your household plumbing is suspect, the water can be tested, and local water departments usually offer advice and help.

Lead can come from various sources. In slum areas, for example, children often ingest the flakes or dust from old peeling lead-based paint (either directly or through contamination of other things they put in their mouth).

Despite the variations in tap water throughout the country, most drinking water from the tap is safe, especially when the water comes from large municipal water systems. Any lead contamination generally comes from the lead in plumbing. Other hazardous contaminants tend to be localized (e.g., water from wells in certain areas).

Another aspect of drinking water to consider is its *fluoride content* and whether the water is "hard" or "soft." Fluoride is found naturally in water and hardens the enamel of developing teeth, making the teeth highly resistant to tooth decay. (Fluoride in the drinking water also may possibly strengthen bones, offering some protection against osteoporosis.)

The optimum level of fluoride is about 1 ppm (1 part fluoride per million parts of water), a level which protects against tooth decay but isn't enough to produce [harmless] mottled tooth enamel. Some water supplies naturally have more than 1 ppm fluoride; other water supplies need added fluoride to reach this level.

Whether water is "hard" or "soft" depends on its content of calcium, magnesium, and sodium. Hard water is relatively high in calcium and magnesium, and low in sodium, whereas soft water is relatively high in sodium and low in calcium and magnesium. Unlike soft water, hard water leaves behind a hard [mineral] "scum" or deposit in the automatic coffee maker, bathtub, etc., and interferes with the action of various soaps. Soap doesn't "suds up" as well in the shower or dishpan, and hard water "grays" the white laundry.

So, many households prefer soft water. Some households install a water-softening apparatus to convert hard water into soft water (the apparatus exchanges the calcium and magnesium in the hard water for sodium). But because soft water is relatively high in sodium, this can be a concern for those on sodium-restricted diets. Also, soft water is slightly acidic, making it somewhat corrosive. (If there's lead in the plumbing more of it will dissolve in soft water than in hard water.) A compromise is to soften only the hot water supply, and use only the cold (hard) water for drinking and cooking.

Bottled water has become exceedingly popular. The supermarket shelves offer a large variety of bottled waters—flavored or unflavored, with or without minerals, carbonated or not. Although many people drink bottled water simply because they like the taste, many drink it because they perceive it as more healthful than tap water. This perception is certainly valid if the tap water is harmfully contaminated, but this isn't usually the case.

If your tap water doesn't meet the standards of the Environmental Protection Agency (EPA), the water company is required both to notify you and to clean it up. The standards set for bottled water aren't necessarily higher than for tap water, and most of the bottled water sold in the United States is in fact processed tap water. An argument against bottled water is environmental, e.g., energy and pollution costs of bottling and transporting the bottles.

Bottled water sometimes can be less healthful than tap water. Some, for example, are comparatively high in sodium. The various types and brands of bottled water can be confusing to the consumer. Although the brands vary and the types overlap, a few generalizations can be made:

Distilled water: Water is evaporated to steam, and the steam is condensed to make distilled water. Thus, the solid, mineral matter (including sodium) is left behind. (The distillation process doesn't, however, remove all organic chemicals.)

Since minerals give water their taste, distilled water tastes flat.

Mineral water: Water that contains minerals—which includes virtually all water except distilled water. Most bottled mineral water is, however, taken from a spring, and afterwards the mineral content of the water may or may not have been altered. When it's called "natural mineral water," its mineral content hasn't been altered.

Spring water: Simply water that comes from a spring. It may or may not have been processed and, as ground water, it may or may not be contaminated. "Natural spring water," means that it hasn't been processed before bottling.

Sparkling water: Water that's naturally or artificially carbonated. It tends to be relatively high in sodium.

Seltzer: Usually tap water that has been filtered and carbonated. Often, flavors are added, and sometimes sugar is added as well.

Club soda: Like seltzer, usually tap water that's been filtered and carbonated. But unlike seltzer, minerals (usually including sodium) are added.

Summary

Water is an important nutrient that's often overlooked in discussions of diet and nutrition. Yet our bodies are more than 50% water, and unlike the other nutrients, we can't survive more than a few days without it. Water works by acting as a solvent, allowing chemical reactions to take place, and also takes part in many of our biochemical reactions.

Our bodily water is both intracellular and extracellular, constantly moving, along with other dissolved substances, in and out of our cells. The amount of water in an adult body is inversely related to the amount of body fat, and decreases with age. Some of this body water can be lost or gained relatively quickly, from things like water intake, hormones, sodium, diuretics, exercise, and diet. Much of the quick weight loss that occurs within a few days of starting a diet or after exercising is really from water loss.

Figure 12-5: Functions of Water

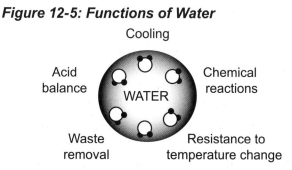

Water is critical for maintaining body temperature and also for removing body wastes and extraneous substances. Evaporation of perspiration cools our bodies, and this is occurring almost constantly. Removal of wastes and extraneous substances occurs through urine (waste products are dissolved and excreted in urine using relatively large amounts of water) and feces, which contain water. Diarrhea can cause enough water loss to endanger life.

Body water is regulated by the kidneys and our brain's thirst center. Urine will become concentrated if water intake is too low, and dilute when we get more than we need. When intake is too low, we become dehydrated, which can lead to heat exhaustion and eventually heat stroke, as the body loses its ability to regulate temperature. This can be fatal, and emphasizes the importance of drinking enough liquids, particularly in hot weather and during heavy exercise.

Because many variables can alter water balance, there's no specific daily requirement for water.

But in general, about a quart of water is needed for each 1,000 calories consumed. In addition, to drinks, the water in "solid" foods counts, as does the water produced when energy-providing nutrients are metabolized.

Athletes can have special water needs, especially in hot weather, and thirst isn't a reliable gauge of need. Any advantage conferred by "sports drinks" will generally be due to their carbohydrate content, and will be limited to endurance events lasting more than 90 minutes. While drinking enough water is important, it's also important to not drink too much.

Much of the water we consume is in food, which is roughly 50% water. Even solid-appearing foods have a lot of water, as their fibrous structures hide the liquid inside. Because water represents so much of food, it must be considered when measuring calorie content or food value.

Most of our drinking water is safe. Hazardous contaminants tend to be localized, as in water from wells in certain areas.

Fluoride in water helps protect against tooth decay, whereas minerals such as calcium and magnesium make the water "hard." Bottled water, in general, is processed tap water, or spring water, and some may have added carbonation and relatively high levels of sodium. Tap water and bottled water must meet the same Environmental Protection Agency standards.

Guest Lecturer: *Robert S. Swenson, MD*

Notes of a Nephrologist

A physician trained in the medical management of kidney disease is called a nephrologist. Surgery of the kidney, ureters, bladder, prostate, etc. is performed by urologists, whereas vascular surgeons and transplant surgeons provide the techniques used to manage kidney disease and kidney failure.

The kidneys are paired organs located at the back of the abdomen. In size and shape they resemble small adult fists, averaging 4 inches in length. Each kidney contains 1 million nephrons (the Greek *nephros* means *kidney*). Each nephron consists of a blood filter followed by a long, com-

plex tubule in which water and substances dissolved in it (*solutes*) are absorbed and/or secreted. The nephrons empty into the part of the kidney that leads to the ureter, the tube that carries the urine from each kidney to the bladder.

Two normal kidneys can filter 100 milliliters of water from the blood per minute—144 quarts per day. Fortunately, the amount of urine we excrete is less than 1% of this filtered volume. More than 99% of filtered water and solutes are reabsorbed within the tubule of the nephron back into the bloodstream. The amount of materials being filtered is breathtaking: the 144 quarts— one day's filtrate—contains about 900 grams of sodium chloride (almost 2 pounds of table salt) and about 320 grams of sodium bicarbonate (the content of a box of baking soda)! Most of these sodium salts are reabsorbed back into the bloodstream, leaving only 10-30 grams of sodium salts being excreted daily in the urine. Very importantly, our kidneys also filter out substances that would be toxic if retained.

When kidneys are severely diseased, the person suffers signs and symptoms of uremic toxicity, which are nonspecific (e.g., nausea, easy fatigue, itching, easy bruising, edema) and occur even when urine output is normal.

It follows that our kidneys provide a large degree of flexibility even when both kidneys are diseased. People born with only one kidney can lead normal lives, which is the reason why kidney transplantation works for both the donor and the recipient.

The kidney has many functions (e.g. synthesis of vitamin D precursors, and breakdown of blood-filtered compounds, such as insulin), but its most obvious function is to produce a pale yellow, slightly aromatic liquid called urine. The volume of urine excreted in health varies as a function of the water (food and drink) ingested.

Normal daily urine output ranges from a pint to several quarts, generally reflecting the water in your food and drink.

In health, 75-90% of an acute water load is excreted as urine within four hours. Taking in a lot of salt, however, can delay the excretion of an acute water load by hours to days. One result of kidney failure is a loss of the ability to concentrate and/or dilute urine. As such, urine volume doesn't respond as easily to your intake of water or salt.

People who are in kidney, liver, or heart failure may retain sodium, resulting in salt-water retention (edema) and weight gain. If they retain urea in their blood, the diagnosis is uremia, indicating acute or chronic kidney failure.

The normal pigment of urine is urochrome, a normal breakdown product of hemoglobin. Large urine volumes obviously dilute urochrome, and therefore produce a paler yellow urine. Urinary urochrome may be overwhelmed by other pigments. Eating a lot of carrots may result in an orange hue (carotemia). Similarly, eating a lot of beets can produce a red urine (beeturia).

Changes in urine color are as likely to be from drug-induced causes as from food pigments. An orange color can result from taking Pyridium (a urinary antiseptic), rifampin (an antibiotic), or large amounts of oral vitamins. Red urine can follow administration of Ex-Lax, or phenothiazines. Blue urine follows ingestion of methylene blue, once considered a college prank. A brown or black hue may also reflect Ex-Lax or dietary intake of rhubarb or fava beans. These new colors may alarm, but are rarely clinically significant.

A common complaint is a change in the smell of one's own or one's partner's urine. This may be due to changes in diet, or taking in less water, resulting in a smaller volume of more concentrated urine. It is commonly thought that a smelly urine is a sign of urinary tract infection. However, most urinary tract infections are not associated with a change in urine's smell.

A really smelly urine can follow eating asparagus, the whiff of which is thought to be due to the excretion of mercaptan (a sulfur compound, akin to the smell of rotten eggs). "Asparagus urine" has three components: 1) intake of asparagus even in small quantities, 2) an autosomal dominant inheritance of urinary excretion of the smelly substance, and 3) most interestingly an inherited ability to smell it. This means that some individuals (*who me?*) may be unaware that they are excreting a vile-smelling urine.

Garlic also is smelly, and some believe its odor on eating may permeate urine. However, it's more likely that the garlic permeates exhaled breath, and body perspiration. Dinner parties heavy in asparagus and garlic may have predictable results that affect hosts and guests alike.

Dr. Swenson, as faculty in the Nephrology Division of Stanford Medical School, taught clinical renal disease and urinalysis to medical students and postgraduate fellows for more than 20 years. His clinical activities included renal transplantation and acute and chronic dialysis. He was later Chief of Staff of Livermore's VA Medical Center, a teaching hospital of Stanford.

Part 6

The Micronutrients

Chapter 13

Some Practical Realities of Vitamins

Part of the art of selling is, of course, convincing people that they need whatever it is you have to offer. Clothiers prosper by implanting the idea that we need the latest fashions, even if we've hardly worn what we bought last year.

When it comes to health, enthusiastic sellers often find a willing audience—health is nothing to fool with. But the amazing thing is how badly people want to believe, and how little interest they have in the credentials and self-interest of the people doing the selling.

There are probably a lot of sincere people in the multibillion-dollar dietary supplement industry who feel they are providing products that will help people lead healthier, more vigorous lives. They are only giving people what they want, and passing on the heart-felt testimonials of all who have believed and benefited. It's only sensible to charge more for the "natural" supplements that people believe in. If "vitamin B-15" hasn't been shown essential for human health, perhaps the researchers are dragging their feet.

Much of the result is just wasted money. But sometimes there is bodily harm—or a failure to get the real help that is needed.

From the first, popular perception of the vitamins has been distorted, leading to much confusion of fact, error of nutritional choice, and quackery. Sadly, in many ways, the passage of time has only imprinted such misconceptions more deeply in the public mind.

The basic mistakes about vitamins probably are rooted in the most ancient ideas of the magical powers of foods. And the first discoveries of how vitamin-containing extracts of food could snatch people from such horrible diseases as scurvy, beriberi, and pellagra seemed only to confirm such magical belief, giving it scientific substance. It was as though science had finally identified the healing essences attributed to food.

The popular view was that vitamins were some new kinds of medicine, wonder drugs. It was as if the "goodness" in food had been extracted in the same manner that drugs were derived from plants—like morphine from the poppy, or digitalis (the heart stimulant) from foxglove. But how realistic is this popular view?

Before discussing individual vitamins in the chapters that follow, we'd do well first to examine more closely some myths and realities of the vitamins in general. We begin by looking at some basic truths about vitamins, and then matching these truths against some popular myths. We end this chapter by discussing how vitamin needs are measured, how we meet those needs, the question of dietary supplements, and again matching some basic truths against some popular myths. Much of what's said here about vitamins also applies to minerals and other dietary supplements.

Some Basic Vitamin Facts to Keep in Mind

In trying to separate fact from fiction, it helps to keep several truths in mind. First, we should keep before us the basic definition of a vitamin. Remember that it's a substance which, in very small amounts, is essential in our diet; each and every vitamin is essential to our health and survival. It's misleading to speak of an "essential" or "important" vitamin. Many advertisements use such language. If it's a vitamin, it's by definition essential and extremely important—a matter of health or sickness, life or death.

Second, we shouldn't forget that a vitamin can't be made by the body. So a vitamin must always come from an outside source. This is true even of the "outside" sources which are actually inside us—such as bacteria that make vitamins in our intestines. Remember, there are other substances which are necessary to human chemistry in very small amounts, but which the body can make. These can't be defined as vitamins.

An exception to the rule that vitamins can't be made by the body is vitamin D, which can be made in the skin upon exposure to sunlight. If sun exposure is inadequate, vitamin D is required in the diet.

Third, although in chapter 11 we saw vitamins at work as coenzymes, not all vitamins play such roles in taking food substances apart or putting them together as life chemicals. As we shall see, vitamins have a variety of functions. One function of vitamin A, for example, is as a structural part of a molecule that plays a key role in vision.

Fourth, we need to have some idea of how much of a vitamin is needed. There's a limit to the amounts our bodies can use. Beyond this limit, increased amounts of vitamins are pointless and may be harmful.

When vitamin intakes fall below a certain level, certain bodily chemical processes are inhibited. Body chemistry is either hampered, or is changed in injurious ways. The result is that symptoms of the deficiency begin to appear.

Fortunately, there are ways of detecting nutrient deficiencies before they occur. One is to measure a person's stores of a vitamin or mineral—low stores indicating a vulnerability to deficiency (see Fig. 13-1). More commonly, a person's dietary intake of nutrients is assessed and compared to recommended levels.

Dietary intake below the recommended amount is a measure of risk rather than an actual bodily deficiency. But it's a realistic measure in that it indicates an increased possibility of a deficiency, and calls for a closer look at the person involved.

As will be discussed in Chapter 18, the recommended amounts are called Recommended

Figure 13-1: Stages of Nutrient Deficiencies.

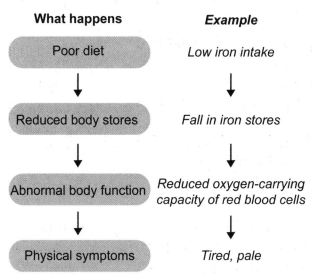

Dietary Allowances (RDAs) and are decided upon by the expert committee of the Food and Nutrition Board. The RDAs include safety margins which go beyond the true requirements of most people. Thus, many people can fall short of such amounts with no physical trouble at all. The recommended amounts aren't minimum requirements.

The Difference Between Vitamins and Medicines

The confusion between the roles of vitamins and medicines is an understandable one. Vitamins were discovered through studying and trying to relieve true deficiency diseases. When the early reports of vitamins appeared, scientists really didn't understand how they served in body processes. They only knew they made people well. Decades were to pass before questions of their precise functions could be answered—before, for example, anyone knew how B-vitamins did their work as coenzymes.

Yet even the early vitamin researchers realized what the modern public rarely seems to comprehend—that, with few exceptions, *vitamins can work their curative magic only when vitamins have been missing from the diet.*

Medicines, on the other hand, usually function by causing body changes of their own, changes which are somehow helpful to patients in a disease state. Aspirin and antibiotics are examples.

Aspirin can, for example, reduce the inflammatory reactions of arthritis. Antibiotics serve by killing disease-causing bacteria. In doing so, medicines act very differently from vitamins.

Where Medicines and Vitamins Overlap

The confusion between vitamins and medicines is made worse by the overlap in ways certain medicines and large doses of certain vitamins are used. Some medicines are given for the same reason that vitamins are given for a vitamin deficiency. That is, they are used to correct a deficient supply of a normal body chemical. Thyroid hormone is given when the thyroid gland can't make enough, and insulin is given to diabetics whose pancreatic production of insulin is inadequate.

But note that, like vitamins, such drugs only cure when there's a deficiency. And when these drugs are used to replace body chemicals, the physician takes care to prescribe only what's needed. Excesses—as well as deficiencies—of these body chemicals can be hazardous. The same can be said of vitamins.

Vitamins are sometimes prescribed for reasons other than correcting a vitamin deficiency. In these cases, huge doses of water-soluble vitamins are used—water-soluble so that the excess can be excreted in the urine, and a dose that far exceeds the amount the body can use or store as a vitamin.

It's crucial to keep in mind that, except when used to relieve a true deficiency, the huge dose isn't being given for its vitamin effect, but rather for a pharmaceutical effect. In other words, most drug-like applications of vitamins have nothing to do with nutritional problems.

There are two forms of niacin—nicotinic acid and nicotinamide. Both forms function the same as a vitamin, but huge doses of nicotinic acid (1,000 to 9,000 mg/day) lower blood cholesterol, whereas huge doses of nicotinamide do not. (The adult RDA for niacin is 14 to 16 mg/day.)

As an example, a particular form of niacin is used in huge doses to lower blood cholesterol in the treatment of people with high levels. Its role here is as a drug rather than a vitamin.

Let's look a little more at this failure to understand that vitamins taken in large doses function as medicines rather than vitamins. Vitamin C is useful as an example since it's taken so commonly in large doses.

Herbal supplements add to the food-medicine confusion because, for regulatory purposes, they are classified as food rather than drugs, yet are commonly used as medicine.

Vitamin C plays an important role in the immune system, but there's no good evidence that extra C enhances immunity. Controlled studies have failed to show that large doses of vitamin C are helpful in treating cancer or in reducing the frequency of the common cold.

Some Hazards of Using Vitamins as Medicines

Drugs have side effects, and vitamins used as drugs are no exception. Consider large doses of vitamin B-6. The ease with which excesses are excreted in the urine offers much protection against toxicity, but huge doses—particularly doses of 2000 milligrams or more—can cause permanent nerve damage.

As another example of the possible dangers, the large doses of niacin used to treat high blood cholesterol can cause liver damage. When physicians use this treatment, they check and monitor their patients' liver function.

The special danger of vitamins used as medicine is that vitamins can be purchased freely without prescription. So there's nothing to keep people from diagnosing and treating themselves—and they do.

For example, people sometimes get confused as to which form of niacin is the one that works in high doses against high blood cholesterol, and take the wrong form. Also, many of them fail to understand that in taking large doses they are really taking a drug, rather than a "harmless vitamin." In taking large doses of niacin, some of them have indeed suffered from serious liver damage, as well as milder side effects like flushing of the skin.

Table 13-1: Examples of Tolerable Upper Intake Levels (UL*)

Vitamin	Adult RDA	Adult UL
Vitamin A	0.7-0.9 mg	2.8-3.0 mg
Vitamin D	5-15 µg	50 µg
Vitamin B-6	1.3-1.7 mg	80-100 mg
Vitamin C	75-90 mg	1800-2000 mg

*UL is the maximum daily intake that is not likely to have adverse effects.
1000 µg (microgram) = 1 mg (milligram);
1000 mg = 1 gm (gram)

As with drugs, some of the side effects of large doses of vitamins are identified only when their use becomes widespread. If only a few people take a vitamin in large doses, their experience doesn't provide enough of a statistical base to establish that the vitamin supplement is, for example, causing a side effect of a headache, tremor, rash, or kidney stones. It's only as large doses of a particular dietary supplement become popular that previously unknown side effects are uncovered. Most of the side effects of large doses of vitamin B-6 became apparent only as its use became widespread.

Classifying dietary supplements as drugs would mean that, like drugs (e.g., aspirin), they'd have to meet certain standards of purity, safety, etc., and consumers would be warned of side effects.

Nutrition scientists have long advocated that dietary supplements be classified as drugs. But their voices are drowned out by the loud voices of those that sell supplements and those that buy them—billions of dollars worth.

The attitude was fostered that "vitamins are good for you." And from this, the belief spread that if a little of a vitamin would prevent disease, more would make a person extra healthy. Moreover, it began to be accepted thinking that everyone ought to play it safe by taking vitamins. Those selling dietary supplements have carefully reinforced this view.

What was the harm in such thinking? First, because dietary supplements were thought of as "good" and "harmless," they became stock-in-trade for promotion by shopkeepers, salespeople, and others who weren't licensed to prescribe drugs.

Such uses of supplements quickly built up a store of testimonials. It's well known that many ailments tend to take care themselves, without medical treatment. Thus, in most cases, when a person recovered after taking a dietary supplement, the supplement got the credit, whether or not any credit was due.

Second, believing that supplements might be the answer to ailments, many people delayed in getting proper diagnosis and treatment. It's much easier to accept the idea that one has a vitamin shortage or a problem that a supplement might "cure," than to face the threatening reality of disease. Of course such false reassurance and delay in treatment can be dangerous if medical attention is really needed.

Finally, the popular belief in some or all of these ideas has led people to waste astonishing amounts of money. Using vitamins in the search for health is usually pointless. Yet such thinking is now entrenched in our culture: "I've been feeling run-down lately; maybe I need some vitamins," is a lamentably common idea.

Look in some popular magazines, and you'll find vitamin relief suggested for an astonishing array of physical problems—from arthritis to anxiety, from baldness to itches. Yet many of these disorders have only the vaguest relationship, if any at all, to vitamin chemistry.

How "Deficiency Symptoms" Can Deceive

If we look at the long lists of deficiency symptoms, and look without real understanding of what they are and what they mean, it's easy to be misled. And, indeed, many are fooled.

One source of deception lies in the trickiness of identifying the symptoms themselves. For they may easily be confused with other bodily signs.

As one example, *cheilosis* is characteristic of a deficiency of riboflavin (a B-vitamin). Look up cheilosis in a medical dictionary, and you see that it is a swelling and cracking of the lips, especially at the corners of the mouth. Unless one is medically sophisticated, one can easily be led to believe that any case of chapped lips is in fact cheilosis.

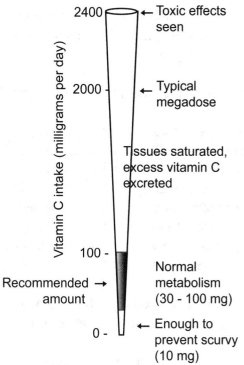

Figure 13-2: Consuming the right amount of a nutrient, using Vitamin C as an example.

Such swelling and cracking isn't uncommon for people who have plenty of riboflavin in their diets. Taking riboflavin won't protect the lips of the skier or the summer lifeguard.

Another common source of confusion stems from the assumption that deficiency symptoms appear in an isolated way. Knowing that sore and bleeding gums are among the signs of scurvy (vitamin C deficiency), many people assume that any gum disease, especially where there's bleeding, shows a need for more vitamin C. The mistake is an important one, for gum disease is the leading cause of tooth loss in America.

Gum disease resulting from poor dental hygiene is the usual and most common cause of bleeding gums.

But bleeding gums are merely one sign of the general tendency toward hemorrhage which develops with scurvy. Wounds don't heal well; hemorrhages under the skin and in the nose are common—often painful—scurvy signs; and there's muscle weakness, tenderness of the extremities, susceptibility to infection, and so forth. So bleeding gums alone aren't a sign of scurvy. And if scurvy isn't really present, it's irrational to believe that taking vitamin C will help one's gums.

Sensible Tests of Deficiencies

Before a reasonable diagnosis of vitamin deficiency can be made, there are a number of factors to take into account.

Is there only a single sign of deficiency?

If there is, it may be a situation where it's all too easy to generalize and assume, for instance, that all gum-bleeding signifies a vitamin C deficiency. On the other hand, you don't want to dismiss individual symptoms as unimportant; some early signs of vitamin deficiency may appear in a seemingly isolated way, as with the peculiar rash of pellagra. So we must ask another question.

Is the symptom really a deficiency sign, or is it merely something similar?

The rash of pellagra is distinctive. It isn't quite like other rashes. And telling the difference takes the eye of an expert—hard to find in the United States because the niacin deficiency which causes pellagra is now so rare here. But few of us are experts about disease symptoms. Before taking niacin for your "distinctive-looking" rashes, consider applying some other easy tests.

Do your dietary habits suggest that your vitamin intake is inadequate?

In considering your bodily needs, you look to the Recommended Dietary Allowances (RDAs). But you must remember that there are safety margins built into these recommendations. Your intake can fall below the recommendations without your having an actual nutritional deficiency. Small departures from the RDAs are unlikely to cause trouble. But the further you fall below your RDAs, the more likely you are to be deficient.

What of the idea that some people have some special high needs for vitamins? Contrary to the fear-talk of vitamin enthusiasts, these special needs are largely taken into account in setting the RDAs. The RDAs aren't minimal; they go beyond actual requirements in attempting to assure ample nutrition for all but a very few. The Food and Nutrition Board attempts to cover 97.5% (2 standard deviations above the average) of the U.S. population with its recommended amounts and even to anticipate the need for protection against life's stresses.

Let's go back to the example of the bleeding gums. What do you eat that would supply your needs for vitamin C? Perhaps you detest citrus fruits and their juices, often cited as the important common sources of vitamin C. What have we learned? Very little. Some C is included in most plant-source foods, especially in potatoes, strawberries, and green leafy vegetables. And vitamin C is added to many foods, from fruit-flavored drinks to breakfast cereal. So unless your diet is quite bizarre, a vitamin C deficiency is unlikely.

Do special stresses or other exceptional requirements spell deficiency?

Not likely, except in rare cases. For example, there's a common misconception that a smoker needs extremely large doses of vitamin C. But the fact is that while smoking can increase vitamin C needs, it's only by 20 to 40%. And this increased need is accounted for by a special vitamin C RDA for smokers (an additional 35 mg), making it 110 mg for women, and 125 mg for men.

How long have the symptoms persisted, and how fast are symptoms triggered?

True deficiencies are slow to develop and even slower to produce overt symptoms. It's true that the RDAs are daily allowances. But, in reality, the recommended amounts are for averages per day, since diets vary day to day. And the amounts allow enough to maintain reserves in the body—reserves even for the water-soluble vitamins, which the body can store to some extent.

Stores of water-soluble vitamins don't accumulate beyond a certain limit, so it's a common misconception that they need to be consumed daily to prevent a deficiency. Practically speaking, it's generally advised that nutrient intakes will be adequate if, over a period of a several days, they average the recommended amounts. But even failure here doesn't necessarily mean disease.

The fact is that vitamin levels in the blood are not so quickly exhausted. Typically, a month or more of complete deprivation of a water-soluble vitamin is needed before the blood supply is exhausted. And several months more of deprivation is usually needed before symptoms appear. In the extreme—as is the case with vitamin B-12—the body can store enough for several years.

It should be noted that the RDAs are for healthy people. Certain diseases and conditions can warrant a physician's prescribing larger doses.

Similarly, vitamin deficiencies are not relieved as quickly as many believe. For example, much popular belief about alcohol and B-vitamins is unrealistic. It's true that alcohol intake can require some extra B-vitamins. And it's true that alcoholics tend to take in too few B-vitamins when they replace many of their food calories with alcohol calories. (And it's also true that some alcoholics suffer from severe thiamin deficiencies that can result in psychosis.)

But it's not true that taking vitamins the morning after will counter the effects of the night before. A hangover isn't a vitamin-deficiency symptom—a true vitamin deficiency can't possibly occur so fast. So despite fake claims and fond hopes, vitamins won't cure a hangover.

While some organ systems do tend to be more vulnerable to vitamin deficiencies than others, a deficiency is a total body problem. Though clear symptoms may develop earlier in some organs or parts of organs than they do in others, there's a general chemical shortage, which chemical testing can confirm. The significant status is that of the body as a whole, even though some organs may show problems sooner than others.

To put it simply, if one has a deficiency of a vitamin, all the chemical systems which depend on that vitamin are affected, not just one.

But in times of vitamin shortage, the body often protects the most vital organs and functions, shorting the least essential organs first. This is thought to be why the first signs of deficiency are often shown in the skin and the last in vital internal organs. This is certainly the case with niacin deficiency, in which rashes and other skin problems appear first, and effects on the brain and nerves are experienced only in the final phases.

How Vitamin Needs are Measured

How certain can we be that our judgments of the need for vitamins are sound? Are nutrition scientists really confident that some of us don't need extraordinary amounts of vitamins— huge doses of niacin to prevent mental illness, or massive intakes of vitamin C to keep from catching cold? Let's look at a few of the principles applied in determining vitamin needs and judging when they're met in optimum ways.

Originally, the only measure of vitamin deficiency or adequacy was symptomatic deficiency. This served practical purposes, but it wasn't a satisfactory measure. We can see why from the vitamin realities we've observed. Deficiencies don't cause symptoms until they are severe and have persisted for some time. One wouldn't want to wait until signs of beriberi developed before getting more thiamin.

But as science began to understand how vitamins play their chemical roles, it became possible to set more and more precise standards for vitamin adequacy, and to assess the stores in a given person's body in terms of those standards.

In principle, the system isn't very different from the baking of a cake. If we know the chemistry of cooking, we can both predict how much of each ingredient is needed, and we can study the resulting cake to determine whether there wasn't enough or too much of something— or whether the ingredients were optimal for the best cake possible.

Suppose we used buttermilk to make a cake. Along with the buttermilk, we add a certain amount of baking soda. The object is to cause a reaction between the acid buttermilk and the alkaline baking soda, the product of which is carbon dioxide. The carbon dioxide forms bubbles, which are caught in the protein substance of the flour. And in baking, the gas bubbles form little balloons, surrounded by flour components, to make the cake rise, and to make it light and fluffy. One can roughly calculate the amount of buttermilk and baking soda needed to produce the desired reaction.

If we add too little baking soda, we don't get the full potential of the reaction with the buttermilk. Not only will the cake taste acid because of the excess buttermilk, there won't be enough gas bubbles, and the cake won't rise well. It will be dense and heavy, and the compliments will be strained at best.

But going the other way and adding too much baking soda, beyond the chemical requirements for reacting with the buttermilk, would be just as bad. There's just so much buttermilk to help yield carbon dioxide. The extra soda won't only be wasted, it will be tasted, giving the cake the characteristic bitterness of alkalinity. Any compliments will come through pursed lips.

In a similar way, if we don't get enough vitamins, our bodies' chemical processes won't take place as they should. The chemical reactions won't be completed as they need to be for good health. And in the same way, an excess of vitamins will simply be a burden, perhaps needing to be cleaned away by excretion, or perhaps causing chemical problems.

So it is that by understanding the exact role of each vitamin in chemical reactions that we can predict, say, how much thiamin is needed in metabolism. And by looking at body wastes and products of reactions in the blood, we can tell whether the chemical processes have gone forward adequately, or whether they have been hampered by the lack of a vitamin (and whether body stores of the vitamin are adequate).

Obviously, the problem of such assays is more difficult than it is with a cake, since so many more factors are involved. Body chemistry is infinitely more complex.

But the principles remain. And paramount among them is the concept that vitamin adequacy or inadequacy is measurable—not a matter of guesswork, faith, or subjective feeling.

As was pointed out earlier, the recommended vitamin intakes are amounts intended to assure that the body chemistry has what it needs, both immediately and for storage. Just as the bakery must continually make sure it always has ample supplies on hand, the body's storage of ingredients is important. The baker checks the cupboards. The biochemist takes measures of bodily stores and circulating levels of vitamins.

But there's no point in going beyond full. There will be no additional helpful reactions. There will be nothing but needless expense and the burden of excess.

Human needs can vary, just as cakes and their ingredients vary. But the variation isn't so great as is popularly believed. Gross distortions of vitamin intakes are no more valuable, and no less risky, than gross distortions of your favorite cake recipe.

Synthetic vs. "Natural" Vitamins

Because the role of vitamins is a chemical one, it's the success or failure of the chemistry which matters. So just as we're able to judge the amounts of vitamins needed, so also can we evaluate sources of vitamins for potency.

We can easily answer the old questions about whether the vitamins in foods are different from those made in a laboratory. We can apply simple tests, seeking simple answers to the simple question: Do the vitamins made in the laboratory enable the needed chemical reactions to take place as well as the "natural" vitamins do?

The purpose of vitamins is for body chemistry, so the absolute test of vitamin potency rests with chemical assays of pertinent biological reactions.

The results of such assays can be seen on any number of pill bottles and food packages, where the vitamin values are set forth in terms of effective amounts of the vitamins contained in each measure—a pill or a serving. And such labels are closely regulated by Federal law and monitoring.

The bottom line is vitamin potency. Vitamins don't function at different levels. They either function or they don't. Although there can be more than one natural form of a vitamin, whatever form is synthesized in the laboratory has the identical function as the natural model found in food. It's not just similar. It's the same. Vitamin C is vitamin C, whether synthesized in a laboratory flask or in an orange.

Vitamin C supplements that "contain natural C from rose hips" contain mostly laboratory-produced vitamin C. Adding a bit of vitamin C from rose hips adds to its allure—and price.

Wishful thinking and language confusion have muddled these clear-cut truths. Especially, the word *synthetic* has been corrupted by popular usage. To *synthesize* means to combine parts to make something. When that something is a vitamin, the end-product of the synthesis must be the vitamin.

The language problem may have begun with commercial use of the term synthetic rubber during World War II and after. It was really imitation rubber because, while it had some of the characteristics of natural rubber, it wasn't the same. Synthetic vitamins aren't imitation vitamins. They are the vitamins—nothing else.

The making of a vitamin is no less exact a task than the making of a key for a very sophisticated lock. If the key doesn't fit precisely, the lock won't open. So must the synthesized vitamin fit a precisely required chemical pattern. If the molecule isn't just right, it can't carry out its role.

We thus have two clear-cut tests for insuring successful vitamin synthesis, both similar to the tests for a well-made copy of a key. First, the vitamin molecule, like a good key, must exactly reproduce the original. Secondly, the synthesized vitamin must work. Just as the key must open the lock, so must the molecule enable the chemical reaction to take place.

All the forms—regardless of the brand, expensive or not—must be similarly usable, or they wouldn't be vitamins, merely related chemicals. Whatever the form, what matters is that the working part of the vitamin, the part of the molecule that must fit other molecules to function, is the same. Variations in another part of the molecule are no more important in this respect than are variations in the decorative handles of keys. The key works or doesn't work, whether the handle is gold or brass.

What really counts is whether the key moves the tumblers in the lock. It makes no difference if the key is a fancy one stamped Rolls Royce, or is a generic spare made at the local hardware store.

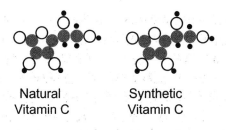

Figure 13-3: Natural and synthetic vitamins have the same chemical structure.

Natural Vitamin C   Synthetic Vitamin C

The Sources of Vitamins

A corollary to unscientific concerns about vitamins being "natural" or synthesized is a large body of myth about vitamins and their special sources. These myths are of three principal kinds.

• *Myth #1: Differences in the source make for different kinds of vitamins.*

The misconception here is distorted, but perhaps derives from a basic truth. In the case of vitamin A, some sources don't contain the vitamin itself, but instead hold provitamins. These are molecules which the body can easily convert to the vitamins, but which aren't actually the vitamins themselves. For example, there's no actual vitamin A in vegetables, such as carrots. But in practical terms, the provitamins in plant foods (e.g., beta-carotene in carrots) can serve the body just as well, because they can be converted to the vitamin by the body.

• *Myth #2: Differences in the source make for a different "quality" of vitamin.*

The basis of this misunderstanding is probably the fact that some foods are richer sources of vitamins than others. Consider the popular fantasy that "natural vitamin C from rose hips" has some special superiority. It doesn't. Despite the fact that rose hips, the seed pods of the rose, are an extraordinarily rich source of the vitamin, the vitamin C extracted from them is no different from any other. Each milligram of vitamin C taken from rose hips is identical to a milligram of the vitamin derived from oranges, cabbage, or broccoli—or assembled in a pharmaceutical factory.

• *Myth #3: Differences in the source mean that "extras" will accompany the vitamin.*

When vitamin values are shown on a label for vitamin pills, the source from which they are taken has no additional meaning. To believe otherwise is the same as believing that aluminum differs according to whether it's been extracted from the bauxite ores of Jamaica or taken out of old cans. The successful chemical objective is to purify the aluminum—or the vitamin.

Yet commercial promotion has tried to popularize the idea that the source determines the quality of the end product, as in "vitamin C from the sunshine tree." Such ideas are pathetically popular.

We see similar examples daily with other products. For example, some are convinced that sucrose (table sugar) differs somehow according to whether it comes from sugar cane, or from a sugar beet, or whether it's grown on the mainland or in Hawaii. But the sucrose which is refined from either cane or beet, no matter where it's grown, is still sucrose, a precisely defined molecule.

The only real difference between these two sugars, since they're chemically the same, is the price and the image, which the commercials for Hawaiian sugar relate to dancing Hawaiian maidens and virile Hawaiian men on surfboards.

Foods do differ from one another, of course. If we get vitamin C from Tang (the orange-flavored drink powder), it holds only the nutrients assembled by the manufacturer. If we get the vitamin C by eating a potato or an orange, we get the other nutrients which nature has included in the food. This is, in fact, one reason why nutritionists generally recommend that nutrients come from food rather than dietary supplements.

What About Vitamin and Mineral Supplements?

Even if we don't take vitamin and mineral supplements in pill form, virtually all of us in the United States eat foods that are supplemented with vitamins and minerals. As examples, milk is fortified with vitamin D; margarine is fortified with vitamin A and beta-carotene (a provitamin A); white flour—and the white bread, pasta, and pastries made from them—is enriched with iron and some B-vitamins; vitamin C is usually added to fruit-flavored sugar drinks; and even the most sugar-coated cereal typically adds a generous dose of vitamins.

Yet, as mentioned earlier, we're confronted with a multitude of advertisements that would have us believe that we're suffering from vitamin deficiencies of one kind or another. These advertisements are, of course, selling the very vitamins that they tell us we need. Indeed, most of us—even when doubting what the ads suggest—worry that we possibly might be deficient. And when in doubt, the general response is to take vitamins "just to be sure."

Vitamin Supplement "Rules of Thumb"

• Take single-vitamin supplements only when prescribed.
• Multivitamins should contain no more than 100% the Daily Value (100%DV).
• "Organic" vitamins have no advantage.

Let's look again at one popular refrain—that tobacco-smoking creates unusually high needs for vitamin C. In principle, this is true. The fact is made much of by some pharmaceutical firms. For example, there's a supplement called *Stresstabs 600.* The name apparently derives from the fact that the product has 600 mg of vitamin C—five times the amount recommended for smokers. Smoking is one of the "stresses" envisioned to create extreme vitamin requirements—and thus to justify buying quantities of a vitamin for which true nutritional deficiencies are virtually unknown in America.

But even if one looks at the supporting data issued by makers of such vitamin tablets, one finds only what was mentioned earlier—that smoking can push C recommendations up by about 35 mg—an extra amount easily covered by a normal diet. The advertisers' proposition thus appears to have little scientific substance.

What about those who, for example, "swear by large doses of vitamin C" in preventing their colds? Not to be forgotten is the placebo effect—the power of believing. In one study, for example, it was found that the subjects given either vitamin

C or placebo capsules had tried to guess what was in their capsules. There was no difference in the number of colds between the vitamin C and control groups, but those in the placebo group who *thought* they were taking vitamin C had fewer colds than those in the vitamin C group who *thought* they were taking a placebo.

We've already discussed the perils of self-prescribing and treating oneself with large doses of vitamins. But what about smaller doses?

There are, in fact, situations where supplements at RDA levels are recommended. When one is on a very low calorie diet, for example, it can be hard to meet one's nutritional requirements from the food itself, so a multivitamin pill makes sense. In another example (discussed in the next chapter), vitamin pills or fortified foods are recommended for certain people as a source of vitamin B-12 and folate.

Foods as the Best Sources of Nutrients

Studies of vitamin and mineral supplementation are often misunderstood by the public. If a study shows a benefit, people often are misled into thinking that the supplements themselves must be taken for such a benefit.

In the early days of nutrition research, scientists had only whole foods or crude extracts of foods to test, and when benefits were found, the public rushed to get those foods or extracts. Scientists now have available pure, single components of food. And testing only one pure component at a time provides more precise answers than testing all at once the hodgepodge of substances found in whole foods and crude extracts.

When nutrients come from foods, there's little danger of a harmful excess. This is important to keep in mind as scientists continue to isolate and investigate various components of food.

Just because scientists may test dietary substances in a pure, isolated form, we shouldn't be misled into thinking that we need to take them that way as well. But today, when a benefit is found in these tests of pure substances, all too often the public rushes out to buy them in pills, encouraged by the companies that make them.

There's more to good nutrition than meeting the RDAs. There are other substances in food that aren't essential, per se, but can be beneficial to health. Fiber and its benefit in reducing risk of diverticulosis and constipation is one example. Certain non-nutritive substances in cabbage-family vegetables that may be helpful in preventing cancer is another.

A varied diet that includes the recommended amounts of nutrients (preferably, for example, in orange juice rather than orange-flavored sugar drinks with added vitamin C) provides the nutritional components for health—without having to count individual nutrients to make sure recommended levels are supplied. Broccoli, for example, is not only rich in vitamin C, but is also a source of several B-vitamins, fiber, beta-carotene (provitamin A), potassium, and indoles (a non-nutritive substance that may be helpful in preventing cancer).

With this in mind, let's now consider the individual vitamins.

Summary

Throughout history, food has often been described as having magical powers. Then, when vitamin extracts were thought to have cured diseases, it led people to believe that vitamins were the answer to many health problems.

Vitamins are substances which are essential to our diet in very small amounts, can't be made by our bodies, and have a variety of functions. The Recommended Dietary Allowances (RDAs) are calculated to provide the amounts needed by over 95% of the population, and take into account variations found among healthy people.

The public often thinks of vitamins as a "natural" type of medicine but, in reality, vitamins can only "heal" by curing a pre-existing vitamin deficiency. When huge doses of vitamins are given, vitamins work as drugs, not as nutrients. Like drugs, vitamins given in huge doses have side effects, which can be unhealthy, even dangerous. Also, self-medication can delay getting a true diagnosis.

It's easy to be misled into thinking we have a nutrient deficiency. First, most symptoms are very general and easily confused. Second, we may latch onto one particular symptom, when in reality, a true nutrient deficiency has an array of symptoms.

What are reasonable tests of a diagnosis of deficiency? If there's but one symptom, it's important to consider whether it's due to something other than a vitamin deficiency. Checking to see whether one's diet is supplying less than the RDA for that nutrient is also helpful. But it must be remembered that the RDAs include safety margins, and take into account normal life stresses.

Real deficiencies take a long time to develop—months, not days. The deficiency will affect the whole body, not just one specific area, though signs usually appear in some areas earlier than others, as the body tries to protect vital organs at the expense of "lesser" organs like the skin.

To be labeled as a vitamin, the ultimate test is whether a substance functions as a vitamin in the body. Synthetic vitamins function just like "natural" vitamins, and thus have the same bodily functions. In reality, the working form of the vitamin is the same no matter what the source. In fact, the best way to get "extras" and the "most natural" vitamins is to eat a variety of healthful foods, rather than take supplements.

Many foods in the U.S. have nutrient supplements added to them. Many of us are convinced by advertising that we should take dietary supplements to be sure we are getting enough. Getting a vitamins from fortified foods or a vitamin pill are advised for certain people (e.g., folate for women of child-bearing age, B-12 for people over age 50). But, still, for all of us, the overall aim is to get our nutrients from a variety of healthful foods.

Chapter 14

Water-Soluble Vitamins

Pity the poor dietitian (most real nutritionists are dietitians), who so often finds that the best advice is "to eat a balanced diet." How undramatic! How unromantic! How uninteresting!

It's a hard sell competing against a theory of a single magic bullet—a shot of vitamin B-12, or a handful of 'C's'—with a story of the single dramatic curative effect to be anticipated. It's confusing trying to learn about intricate interactions between different nutrients, and no fun learning that some are useless without others, so that a deficiency of one nutrient can alter the requirement for another.

It's far easier to learn about single deficiency symptoms for a given vitamin, and to load up on that vitamin to turn that deficiency symptom into an extraordinary health asset. A shortage of thiamin makes you weak—a megadose will surely provide super strength.

In fact, bodily mechanisms are astonishingly complex. Nutrients generally play a variety of roles, and are often interdependent in their effectiveness. Learning something of these mechanisms and interrelationships adds a lot of credibility and personal relevance to eating a balanced diet.

The most obvious characteristic of the water-soluble vitamins—vitamin C and the eight B-vitamins—is that they dissolve in water. This means that, in contrast to the fat-soluble vitamins (the subject of the next chapter), excesses can be excreted in the urine, and they are less likely to be toxic in large amounts. This isn't to say that the water-soluble vitamins must be taken each and every day—body stores can hold some in reserve.

In this chapter, the water-soluble vitamins are discussed one by one. Their more interesting and instructive aspects are discussed selectively.

An underlying objective is to encourage a deeper understanding of the vitamins. There are reminders throughout that all the B-vitamins do their work as part of coenzymes, that vitamin deficiencies tend to occur together, that vitamins have broad functions (and broad symptoms), and that the functions (and the symptoms of deficiency) of one vitamin often overlap and intertwine with those of other nutrients.

To minimize tedious discussion, basic information about each vitamin is summarized in Table 14-1, and references to earlier discussions of some aspects of certain vitamins are noted. The Daily Reference Intakes, which includes RDAs, for each vitamin can be found in Appendix A.

Vitamin C

Chemically, vitamin C (ascorbic acid) is the simplest of vitamins. In fact, it's a close chemical relative of the simple sugar glucose. Not only do pharmaceutical companies make their vitamin C from glucose, so also do most animals, birds, and insects. Humans are among the very few in the animal kingdom that can't make vitamin C, but must take it from food. Others that can't make this vitamin include monkeys, guinea pigs, a few fish, and an obscure Indian fruit-eating bat.

It's been speculated that it was because the regular diets of the vitamin-C-requiring species included enough of the vitamin, that their cells surrendered vitamin-C-making as a needless function. This makes a nice evolutionary theory, but it's open to question. First, we don't know that humans ever had the ability to make vitamin C. Second, some species that make their own vita-

min C also seem to get plenty in their usual food.

The vitamin-C-deficiency disease, scurvy, was described as long ago as 1500 B.C. Most of us know that scurvy was once the bane of seafaring men on long voyages, and that the disease was attributable to the lack of C-rich fruits and vegetables. But many of us don't realize just how devastating scurvy was. It was so devastating that it seems amazing—or else tells something of living conditions in those times—that anyone would volunteer for a long sea voyage, knowing full well that so many wouldn't make it back alive.

General characteristics of water-soluble vitamins
• excreted in urine
• limited body stores
• less toxic than fat-soluble vitamins

Consider Richard Walter's account of the round-the-world voyage of the British ship Centurion in the early 1740s[1]:

...the scurvy began to make its appearance amongst us...at the latter end of April there were but few on board who were not in some degree afflicted with it...and in that month no less than forty-three died of it...In the month of May we lost nearly double that number...The mortality went on increasing...so prodigiously that after the loss of above two hundred men, we could not at last muster more than six foremast men in a watch capable of duty.

This isn't to say that no one knew of ways to combat the disease. Long before this time, there had been knowledge of anti-scurvy substances. The Chinese had found that while neither beans nor grains had an anti-scurvy effect, the sprouts that formed as they germinated did. The sea captains of England had found that the sprouting barley that went into beer could offer some protection against scurvy, and they sought passengers who could make the brew.

We can't expect to find vitamin C in today's beer—a far different brew. The beer of the ships was a kind of fresh brew made from a mash of the sprouting barley, briefly fermented, low in alcohol, and served without aging, heating, or filtering. Like an uncooked soup, it carried some of the nutrients leached from the green sprouts. It probably was just enough to delay the symptoms of

Table 14-1: Water-Soluble Vitamins.

Vitamin	Function	Source	Deficiency	Adverse effects of high dose
Vitamin C (ascorbic acid, ascorbate)	Antioxidant, synthesis of connective tissue	Citrus fruits, berries, potatoes, red/green peppers, broccoli, brussels sprouts	Scurvy, loose teeth, bleeding gums	Diarrhea
Thiamin (vitamin B-1, aneurin)	Coenzyme in carbohydrate metabolism	Pork, legumes, whole and enriched grains, liver, nuts, squash	Beriberi, impaired nervous system	None reported
Riboflavin (vitamin B-2)	Coenzyme in energy and protein metabolism	Liver, meat, dairy products, enriched grains, eggs, mushrooms, greens	Sore, red tongue, inflamed skin, eye disorders	None reported
Niacin (nicotinic acid, nicotinamide)	Coenzyme in energy metabolism	Liver, meat, fish, whole and enriched grains, legumes, mushrooms	Pellagra (diarrhea, inflamed skin, dementia)	Flushing of face and hands, liver damage
Vitamin B-6 (pyridoxine)	Coenzyme in amino acid metabolism	Liver, meat, fortified foods, enriched grains, legumes, potatoes	Inflamed skin, convulsions in infants	Weak and numb muscles, nerve damage
Folate (folic acid, folacin)	Coenzyme in cell division	Legumes, green leafy vegetables, whole grains	Anemia	None reported
Vitamin B-12 (cobalamin)	Coenzyme in amino acid/fatty acid metabolism, cell division	Animal products (meats, eggs, milk)	Anemia, nerve damage	None reported
Biotin	Coenzyme in carbohydrate and fat metabolism	Liver, yeast, whole grains, egg yolk, fish, nuts, legumes	Dermatitis, depression	None reported
Pantothenic Acid	Coenzyme in metabolism	Liver, yeast, eggs, whole grains, legumes	Fatigue, headache, nausea	None reported

scurvy before arrival at land.

We're reminded again that in looking at the nutrient value of any food, if the quantity consumed is large enough, even foods with low values can be protective. From all accounts, the seafarers had lusty thirsts.

The fact that scurvy continued to ravage so many, in the face of all the reports of successful means of a cure, is rather surprising. Part of the problem was that objective evidence was lacking. Looking back with today's knowledge, we can see why certain regimens worked. But at the time, there were only theories and anecdotal evidence.

Seafarers were often cured of scurvy upon arrival at land, but they weren't sure why. Was scurvy caused by the crowded conditions on board (an infection perhaps), or was it "sea air," or was it something missing in the diet, or was it something contaminating the diet?

Captain James Lind of the British Royal Navy is recognized as one of the first to provide objective evidence. In 1747, he performed the classic experiment in which he took 12 sailors with scurvy, divided them into 6 pairs, and gave each pair a different dietary supplement of either sea water, vinegar, sulfuric acid, hard apple cider, a medicinal paste, or oranges and lemons. Only the pair of sailors given oranges and lemons were cured of scurvy.

Fruits and vegetables had been found over and again to be effective. Yet even in the American Civil War, scurvy was still a problem for both sides. Scourges of scurvy persisted into the early 1900s. But until the discovery of vitamins in the early 1900s, it wasn't generally accepted that the lack of a substance in food could be the cause of a disease. The idea persisted that scurvy was a contagious disease.

Part of the problem also may have been that (as discussed in Chap. 6) plant foods were often disdained as the food of the poor. The famed explorer of the South Seas, Captain James Cook, kept his men from scurvy by stocking his ship with vegetables and fruits. But it wasn't so easy to get his men to eat them. He succeeded in doing so by insisting that his officers eat them with zest, in front of the men. As Captain Cook related in his journal, "…the moment they see their superiors place a value on it, it becomes the finest stuff in the world…"[2]

Albert Szent-Gyorgyi discovered that vitamin C was the substance which cured and prevented scurvy. For this, he received the Nobel Prize in 1937.

In 1796, daily supplements of lemon or lime juice became standard issue in the British navy, and the sailors were nicknamed limeys. Preventing scurvy with citrus juice and fresh fruits and vegetables is thought to have contributed to the superiority of the British navy at that time.

In 1932, vitamin C was identified as the substance which cured and prevented scurvy, and was named *ascorbic* (anti-scorbutic) *acid.*

Vitamin C and Body Chemistry

There's a huge body of research on vitamin C. The presence and influence of vitamin C are seen in a wide variety of bodily processes—including the formation of connective tissue and the matrix of bone, the body's use of calcium and iron, the integrity of the capillaries and the prevention of hemorrhage, the immune response, the making of key hormones and brain chemicals, and a host of other bodily work.

One of vitamin C's functions is to serve as an **antioxidant**, both in the food and in the body. The iron in plant foods, for example, is more readily absorbed from the intestine when the iron is in an unoxidized form. Vitamin C enhances iron absorption by keeping the iron in this form. For those with borderline iron intake or those whose primary source of iron is plant foods, this is good reason to include vitamin-C-rich foods in a meal.

We don't yet understand all the details of how vitamin C functions in some of its roles. This fact, together with the vitamin's broad range of func-

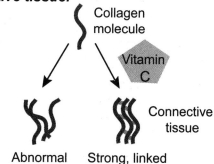

Figure 14-1: Vitamin C helps link collagen molecules together to form strong, stable connective tissue.

tions, leaves the door wide open to much guesswork and fanciful claims. But the basic functions of vitamin C are not, as some enthusiasts claim, open to anyone's guess.

Just because certain symptoms are associated with a vitamin deficiency, this doesn't mean that extra amounts of the vitamin will alleviate similar symptoms where there is no deficiency. People with scurvy are easily fatigued and more susceptible to stress. This has led to a popular idea that extra vitamin C will make one more energetic or better protected against stress. Studies indicate that when various stresses do induce a fall of vitamin C in the blood, that fall is brief and minor—too small to have an appreciable effect on anyone not at a scurvy level of vitamin deficiency.

Vitamin C Intake

The vitamin C content of the "typical American diet" far exceeds the RDA. Add to this the large numbers of people who eat or drink foods fortified with vitamin C, take vitamin supplements, and vitamin C deficiency is uncommon indeed. Most cases of vitamin C deficiency in this country are associated with poverty, alcoholism, and peculiar diets—such as a "tea and toast" diet or the brown-rice-based macrobiotic diet mentioned in the beginning chapter.

Those taking huge doses of C are at the other extreme. Excess vitamin C is readily excreted in the urine, but, as discussed in the previous chapter, massive amounts—particularly doses of 2 grams (2000 milligrams) or more—can be risky.

The adult RDA for vitamin C is 60-75 mg (see Appendix A), with an added 35 mg for smokers.

Thiamin

In Chapter 11, we had a peek at the thiamin-deficiency disease **beriberi** in discussing Eijkman's discoveries in Indonesia, and Funk's curative extract of rice polishings. But even before their discoveries, a Japanese Naval physician K. Takaki had shown he could cure beriberi by diet.

When Commodore Perry opened up Japan in 1854, one result was a new Japanese interest in both overseas commerce and sea-borne defense. Japan began to send ships to sea for long periods. This placed greater emphasis on the more easily preserved foods of their culture, with rice as the staple. Also, the overseas commerce of Japan led to the importation of finely milled rice. In short, the Japanese Navy began to travel longer and to depend more on highly polished grain for nutrition. And they came down with beriberi.

We get much of our thiamin from enriched grains and the products made from them (e.g., bread, tortillas, pastries) and fortified cereals. Compared to many other vitamins, there aren't many foods that naturally have much thiamin—pork is one of our richest sources.

As the work of Eijkman and Funk later indicated, the culprit was the polished rice—the thiamin lost in polishing had provided most of their dietary thiamin. The long time at sea magnified the problem, leading to beriberi.

In 1880, Japan had 4,956 sailors; 1,725 were lost to beriberi. In 1881, government annals show 4,641 naval personnel, with 1,165 lost to beriberi. In 1882, navy personnel totaled 4,769; beriberi losses were 1,929.

Navy physicians were instructed to look for a microbe, which it was felt must be causing the plague. There was a sense of urgency. Even among the survivors, as many as three-fourths of them were too sick to fulfill their duties.

Takaki noticed that British ships didn't have this problem. And he observed that one difference between the two navies was their diets. At first, his idea that food played a part was ridiculed and rejected. But, finally, a desperate naval command allowed Takaki to experiment.

Two ships were chosen. One was given the usual rations. The other—since Takaki had no idea just which food made the difference—was

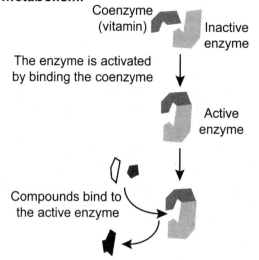

Figure 14-2: B vitamins function as coenzymes in metabolism.

Coenzyme (vitamin)

Inactive enzyme

The enzyme is activated by binding the coenzyme

Active enzyme

Compounds bind to the active enzyme

A chemical reaction occurs.

outfitted with a duplicate of British provisions, which included oatmeal, vegetables, meats, and condensed milk.

The ship with traditional stores returned with some two-thirds of its men either ill or dead of beriberi. The other ship had only four cases. And after intensive interviews, Takaki learned that these four men had not eaten the unusual and unappetizing British meals, but had secretly lived on their rice.

It wasn't easy to persuade Japanese sailors to eat Western meals. But word of the results spread fast, and the will to survive was persuasive. In 1884, the first year of Takaki's experiments, 718 out of 5,638 navy men were taken by beriberi. In 1885, the number of sailors grew to 6,918, with only 41 lost. In 1886, the number of deaths from beriberi fell to three, and reached zero in 1887.

In 1926, thiamin was isolated from rice polishings and pinpointed as the missing nutrient in beriberi.

Thiamin's Antivitamin

Some foods contain substances which actually destroy vitamins, or interfere with their use. These substances are known as **antivitamins.** And in some rare instances, these antivitamins can actually produce deficiencies. For this to happen, usually one must either take in very large quantities of the antivitamin, or very small quantities of the vitamin which it can destroy, or there must be some mixture of the two circumstances.

Thiaminase is thiamin's antivitamin, an enzyme that breaks apart thiamin. It's found in certain raw fishes, such as carp or herring, and also in a few shellfish, particularly clams and shrimp. The heat of cooking destroys thiaminase. So the fish must be eaten raw and, ordinarily, must be eaten in large quantity (comprising something like a fifth of the total diet) before thiaminase can do much damage.

One can't help but wonder if the predilection for raw seafood didn't have some effect upon the speed and severity with which beriberi took hold among the Japanese sailors. Adding to the force of this speculation is the fact that they apparently got beriberi but not scurvy.

We don't know what foods were consumed by the Japanese sailors, other than rice. But many foods with vitamin C also have thiamin. So why beriberi without scurvy? We can only speculate.

There was usually some fishing on 19th century naval ships. And fresh, raw fish does have some vitamin C, e.g., 3.5 ounces of Pacific herring has about 3 mg of vitamin C. Eaten in sufficient quantity, it could have been sufficient to prevent scurvy. Herring also contains thiaminase, and perhaps this provided part of the answer.

Teetering on a deficiency of both vitamin C and thiamin, eating enough raw fish may have spared the sailors scurvy but pushed them into beriberi.

The case can't be proven, but it's a useful exercise in applied nutrition. It shows that we must always consider the whole diet before making nutritional judgments. And in looking at nutrition in any culture, we must consider habits of food combination and preparation.

Thiamin and Body Chemistry

In our look at the metabolism of the energy-providing nutrients (Chap. 11), we saw that thiamin had a key role as a coenzyme. Without thiamin, our cells have a difficult time taking energy from food. No wonder that beriberi sufferers feel that they have no energy. It isn't surprising that beriberi means "I cannot."

Wernicke-Korsakoff Syndrome

Wernicke-Korsakoff syndrome is a degenerative disease of the brain caused by a severe thiamin deficiency. In this country, the most common cause is alcoholism. The body requires thiamin as a coenzyme to deal with alcohol metabolism. There's none in alcohol, so when alcohol supplies much of one's daily calories, the rest of the diet often can't furnish the needed thiamin.

The diets of many alcoholics are often severely deficient in thiamin as well as other nutrients, and chronic alcohol consumption impairs the ability to absorb, store, and use thiamin. Not all alcoholics with severe thiamin deficiency develop this disease, probably because of differences in genetic susceptibility.

The disease is characterized by severe mental confusion and memory loss. Also, many victims walk in an unstable and uncoordinated manner, and develop damage to nerves leading to the eyes—causing a tremor of the eyes or causing them to be fixed in a stare. If the disease is caught early enough, many of the symptoms can be reversed with immediate thiamin treatment.

Considering the cost of hospital treatment for these patients and the cost of nursing-home care for those permanently impaired by this disease, fortifying alcoholic beverages with thiamin as a means of prevention would be cost-effective.

Some Fanciful Claims for Thiamin

Reports of beriberi and its cure are perhaps the oldest sources of the popular idea that vitamins confer extra energy. Again, it must be said that a surplus of a nutrient won't provide extraordinary capacities for whatever is inhibited by the nutrient deficiency. In this case, extra thiamin won't provide extra energy. When one understands the role of thiamin coenzymes in energy metabolism, it's obvious why extra doses are pointless—just as extra sparkplugs won't make an automobile engine more powerful.

Thiamin is generously incorporated into "tonics" as "energy boosters." It's used in vain to better athletic performance. The fact that nerve and muscle impairments result from thiamin insufficiency leads to claims that extra thiamin will strengthen weak muscles for the jogger and relieve pains of rheumatism and migraine headaches. Unfortunately, there's no scientific basis for these beliefs.

Riboflavin

The history of riboflavin lacks the human drama of the stories of thiamin and vitamin C. And while the lack of riboflavin in the diet can certainly produce some appalling clinical effects—in some cases not unlike those of pellagra—the deficiency symptoms weren't even recognized for humans until after they'd been observed in rats. This doesn't mean that riboflavin deficiency wasn't occurring among humans. Rather, it was probably masked, or at least blurred, by the effects of other forms of malnutrition.

> Using purified diets, a rat's diet could be made deficient in just riboflavin. This identifies the specific effects of a riboflavin deficiency, confirmed by the relief from these effects when riboflavin is restored to the diet.

Severe riboflavin deficiency is generally seen only among severely malnourished populations. People in these populations suffer from so many deficiencies—such as niacin and protein deficiencies—that specific signs of riboflavin deficiency are hard to separate out. But specific effects of riboflavin deficiency have been established in human studies.

Riboflavin and Body Chemistry

Riboflavin is an essential part of coenzymes that are needed in the chemical reactions that extract energy from food. Like thiamin, and for much the same basic reasons, riboflavin needs are tied to energy needs.

There are some specific symptoms of riboflavin deficiency (see Table 14-1), but some of the symptoms are shared with those of niacin and vitamin B-6 deficiencies. This is because riboflavin-containing coenzymes play an important role in the functioning of these vitamins, and thus a riboflavin deficiency can cause symptoms of niacin and vitamin B-6 deficiencies as well.

Another reason for the overlap of vitamin-deficiency symptoms is that a dietary pattern that results in one deficiency also tends to result in others. We saw in Chapter 11 that those who suffered from the niacin-deficiency disease pellagra had diets that included very little milk or meat. Animal foods are a good source of protein, ribo-

flavin, and several other B-vitamins, so those with pellagra tended to be deficient in several nutrients in addition to niacin.

> A riboflavin-containing coenzyme is needed for the conversion of the amino acid tryptophan to niacin.

This fundamental lesson in nutrition—that signs of malnutrition don't usually occur singly—is one of surest commonsense defenses against faddism. Consider the claim of some promoters that riboflavin is an answer to baldness.

The idea seems to derive from some rat experiments in which animals deprived of riboflavin lost quite a lot of hair. But there's no evidence that hair loss is a sign of human riboflavin (or any other nutrient) deficiency. Moreover, if someone were to suffer from a vitamin deficiency as severe as that which causes hair loss in rats, one would expect to see also other symptoms of severe riboflavin deficiency (see Table 14-1).

Riboflavin Intake

Milk is a major source of riboflavin in the U.S. diet. Milk consumption has fallen, but it has been compensated for somewhat by increased consumption of other dairy foods such as cheese, yogurt, and ice cream. But when the dairy product is high in fat, as are cheese and ice cream, there's less riboflavin.

This is logical since riboflavin is a water-soluble, rather than a fat-soluble, vitamin. A cup of low-fat (1%) milk provides 105 calories and about a third of the adult RDA for riboflavin. But those 105 calories eaten as ice cream (~⅓ cup) or cheese (~1 oz) provide less than a tenth of the riboflavin RDA.

> Severe riboflavin deficiency in rats eventually leads to cataracts and partial blindness. In the long run, there's coma and death.

Riboflavin is destroyed by ultraviolet light. This posed a problem in the days when milk was commonly bottled in clear bottles and delivered on home doorsteps. When the milk bottles sat too long on the doorstep—exposing them too long to daylight—the riboflavin content fell. Direct sun could wipe out half the milk's riboflavin in a couple of hours. Today, of course, most of our milk comes in waxed cartons or opaque plastic containers and is purchased at grocery stores.

The liver, kidney, and heart of animals are very rich in riboflavin, but these aren't commonly eaten. Enrichment of bread and other grain products with riboflavin has boosted riboflavin intake in this country. Other good sources of riboflavin include meat, eggs, green leafy vegetables, and nuts such as almonds.

Niacin

As recounted in Chapter 11, Goldberger's medical detective work in relating pellagra to a dietary deficiency was a splendid clinical achievement—a feat of personal courage and determination. But in recalling the story, we must not lose sight of the fact that Goldberger made little headway in learning the actual nature of the "antipellagra factor" and how it serves in the normal processes of life.

Niacin in large doses is used as a drug; the form of niacin makes a difference. Massive doses of nicotinic acid—but not nicotinamide—are used to treat high blood cholesterol (see Chap. 9).

Niacin was isolated in the laboratory long before anyone understood that it had a role in life chemistry. In 1867, a German scientist made it by treating nicotine taken from tobacco (giving it its first scientific name, **nicotinic acid**). But, tragically, the cure for pellagra sat unrecognized on a shelf while tens of thousands died of the disease. It was 1937 before nicotinic acid was refined from food and clearly identified as a B vitamin.

Nutrition scientists were concerned that the name nicotinic acid would be confused by some with the nicotine found in tobacco, although the two compounds are very different. Nicotine has no vitamin activity. So niacin became the official name of the vitamin.

Niacin occurs in the form of nicotinic acid, and there's also nicotinamide. Both forms are called niacin and, in practical terms, are considered to have equal vitamin significance. Like thiamin and riboflavin, niacin is mainly used in body chemistry as an indispensable part of coenzymes needed to extract energy from nutrients and is needed by every cell in the body.

Niacin—and Tryptophan—Intake

The body can convert the amino acid tryptophan into niacin, so it's a bit tricky to assess the niacin adequacy of a diet. In stating the niacin values of foods, niacin equivalents are often used, to include the niacin which tryptophan can ultimately provide. Essentially, one niacin equivalent is the equal of one milligram of niacin.

This doesn't mean that all of our tryptophan is used to make niacin. Only part is used this way. Niacin conversion doesn't deplete the body of the tryptophan needed for protein synthesis and other functions. What's meant is that one doesn't necessarily have to eat niacin-containing foods to meet one's niacin requirement. In fact, the typical American diet provides enough excess tryptophan to meet niacin needs.

The way in which nursing infants get their niacin is strong testimony to the effectiveness with which tryptophan can serve as a source of niacin. Mother's milk has less than half of the daily need. The rest comes from the ample tryptophan content of the milk.

Generally, niacin is most plentiful in those foods which are good sources of protein. So in eating foods rich in tryptophan, we usually are also eating foods rich in niacin. Add to this the fact that niacin is added to a lot of foods, such as bread and cereals, and there's little need for concern about niacin in the typical American diet.

Niacin deficiency mainly concerns nations where the protein supply is very limited, especially if much of the protein comes from corn (low in tryptophan). In these nations, multiple nutritional deficiencies are common, and, again, attention must be paid to the whole diet.

If animal foods (meat, milk, eggs) are a regular part of the diet, one consumes not only a good bit of protein but also a good bit of both niacin and "potential niacin" as tryptophan. These foods are also good sources of thiamin and riboflavin. In

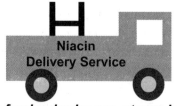

Niacin ferries hydrogen atoms between chemical reactions

cultures that prohibit meat, the well-to-do usually avoid nutritional deficiencies by consuming varied plant foods in ample amounts—not just corn, let's say, but wheat, peas, beans, millet, and a variety of vegetables.

There might have been much less pellagra in the American Southeast had plant sources of protein other than corn been widely available—more wheat, peas, beans, nuts, soy products, and the like. In general, one can expect nutritional deficiencies of several kinds when the diet is narrowed to only a few foods.

Some cultures whose diet centered around corn didn't have as much pellagra. Coffee has niacin—was coffee a common beverage? Was the corn soaked in lime water (water with calcium hydroxide), used to make the masa harina in traditional corn tortillas?

Some of the niacin in corn isn't easily absorbed; soaking the corn in lime water increases the amount of niacin we can absorb from the corn. Where intake is marginal, seemingly small aspects of one's diet can make the difference between deficiency and adequacy.

Vitamin B-6

Early in the 1950s, disturbing reports began to come in to the Food and Drug Administration (FDA). Here and there across the country, infants were developing a curious, unremitting irritability, with no apparent cause. There were odd muscle contractions. Some of the babies went into convulsions. All were receiving the same brand of infant formula.

Puzzling over this outbreak, nutritionists noted one clue. The formula was sold in two forms—one a canned liquid, the other a dry powder to be made into liquid formula by the mother. Only the babies on the canned formula seemed to be in trouble, and they became well as soon as the formula was replaced with some other.

A similar situation occurred again in 1982, just as quality control procedures stemming from the 1980 Infant Formula Act (requiring formulas to meet nutrient standards) were being adopted by the FDA.

What was wrong? An FDA scientist, recalling a study in which some young rats developed

similar nerve and brain symptoms when fed diets very low in B-6, correctly suspected a severe deficiency of vitamin B-6 in the infant formula.

But why should this formula, based, like most, on cow's milk, be so low in B-6? It happened that the manufacturer had instituted what it believed to be a superior new way to sterilize the canned liquid formula. It used higher heat than usual, which destroyed the B-6 in the liquid formula—not entirely, but enough to put babies, who were receiving little or no food other than the formula, in danger.

Vitamin B-6 and Body Chemistry

Vitamin B-6 is really a group of closely related chemicals. They are incorporated into coenzymes that play a part in a wide range of body chemistry, particularly in amino acid metabolism.

Its involvement with amino acid metabolism gives B-6 a wide variety of jobs in body chemistry. It's important in protein synthesis, because B-6 coenzymes are used to make the "non-essential" amino acids by transferring the amino portion of one amino acid to the carbon skeleton of another. In fact, if it were not for this B-6 coenzyme, 20, not 9, amino acids would be required in our diet.

The adult RDA of 1.4-1.7 mg/day of B-6 takes into account our typically high protein intake.

The job of shuffling the amino portions of amino acids is also important when amino acids are used as fuel. Recall that for such use, the amino portions must be removed—a job calling for a B-6 coenzyme. B-6 coenzymes are also needed to convert the amino acid tryptophan into niacin, and to convert tryptophan into serotonin (a chemical messenger in the brain) (see Fig. 14-3).

The UL (Tolerable Upper Limit) for B-6 is 35 mg/day. Doses of 2,000 mg or more taken for months can cause nerve damage, ranging from

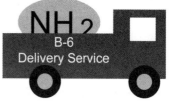

Vitamin B-6 shuttles the amino protions of amino acids.

Figure 14-3: Vitamin B-6 is important for amino acid metabolism. It's used as a coenzyme in the conversion of amino acids to glucose, and in the synthesis of niacin, serotonin, and non-essential amino acids.

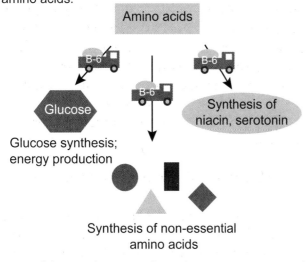

reversible numbness and weakness to severe and permanent damage.

Folate

Late in the 1920s, a puzzling epidemic occurred in Bombay, India that resulted in the death of many young women. The disease matched nothing in the textbooks. It had its own striking pattern, tragically occurring in pregnancy. It was an anemia, reminiscent of the pernicious anemia caused by vitamin B-12 deficiency, yet different. It was described as "pregnancy anemia."

Anemia represents a less-than-normal number of red blood cells, or a less-than-normal amount of hemoglobin in the red blood cells (hemoglobin is the red, iron-containing protein that carries oxygen). The common result is a reduced capacity of the blood to carry oxygen.

Anemia is often a sign of a nutritional deficiency, so it's important to know that there are different kinds of anemia, differing in cause and character. Otherwise, one can easily draw false conclusions from simple tests for anemia.

It's true that iron deficiency is the most common cause of anemia in this country, but it's not the only cause. Even when a test shows too little iron-containing hemoglobin, it doesn't necessarily indicate a deficiency of iron. Instead, there can be defects which keep the iron from being used, defects of the cells which make the hemoglobin protein, or deficiencies of other nutrients needed

Figure 14-4: Folate deficiency results in anemia. Developing red blood cells can't divide, leaving large immature cells (megaloblasts) and enlarged red blood cells (macrocytes).

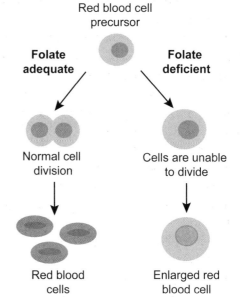

in the making of red blood cells or hemoglobin.

The young women in India with pregnancy anemia weren't well fed (their diets were mainly based on polished rice and bread), but their diets weren't deficient in any of the nutrients then linked to anemia. With no other treatment at hand, and aware that extracts of the "vitamin B complex" held substances that were still mysterious, the sick women were given extracts of yeast and liver. Dramatically, they began to get well.

To test for whether a vitamin was involved, monkeys were fed similar diets. They developed similar anemias, and were cured by yeast extracts. But a decade passed before researchers understood what was happening in even a general way.

Finally in 1941, researchers succeeded in making an impure extract of the missing vitamin from spinach leaves—giving it its first name, ***folic acid*** (from the Latin *folium*, meaning *leaf*). Its identity and structure were determined in 1946.

Folate Chemistry

Folate is found in many different forms. Folic acid is one form that's rarely found in food; it's chemically manufactured and used in vitamin pills and to fortify foods because it's so stable and easily absorbed. The vitamin value of various forms of folate are standardized as dietary folate equivalents.

The most dramatic functions of folate didn't become clear until the chemistry of heredity began to be understood. For folate is a part of coenzymes essential to the making of nucleic acids. We saw in Chapter 7 that the blueprint of life is found in the nucleic acids of DNA, and that protein synthesis is dependent on the nucleic acids of RNA.

Understanding that the folate coenzymes are necessary in this most fundamental body chemistry helps us to see why folate has a role to play in virtually every living cell.

The connection between folate and growth also becomes obvious. Cells can't reproduce and grow normally when their ability to make DNA and RNA is impaired. This leads to an understanding of why folate deficiency results in an anemia in which blood cells can't reproduce themselves properly.

Moreover, it isn't only through DNA and RNA that folate is important. The body needs folate coenzymes to make and use a number of amino acids.

As with some other B-vitamins, alcohol both hinders absorption of folate from the intestine and interferes with its use in metabolism. Again, as is true with some other B-vitamins, normal folate function can be upset by various drugs.

The drug—methotrexate—is a powerful drug used against the rapid cell division of cancer, precisely because it's so effective in interfering with folate's function in cell division. Methotrexate is a kind of chemical gamble. The cancer cells grow rapidly, in a disordered way. The gamble is that depriving the body of folate activity will kill the rapidly dividing cancer cells before it kills too many of the slower dividing normal cells.

After as many cancer cells as possible have been injured or killed, "rescue" doses of folate are given, hoping to save as many of the normal cells as possible. The heroic nature of this therapy is eloquent testimony to the urgency of folate needs.

Folate Intake

Folate is a difficult chemical to assay—it's hard to measure. This isn't only because of the various forms of folate itself, but because folate is usually bound to other substances that can affect both its

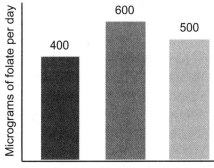

Figure 14-5: Folate requirements go up when pregnant or nursing.

chemical assay and its absorption from the intestine. This makes folate requirements and the folate content of food hard to measure.

As a rule of thumb, and as a matter of good sense, the less science is able to determine vitamin needs accurately, the more generous are the safety margins of intake it recommends. For folate, the margins are kept wide. But folate deficiency has been fairly common during pregnancy for women who have poor diets.

Pregnancy increases a woman's folate RDA, as does lactation (breastfeeding) (see Fig. 14-5). It's easy to see why pregnancy makes special demands for folate. A pregnant woman is supporting spectacular cell division, and a blood supply for two. The resulting increase of need is striking.

This brings us back to the 1920s mystery of the deadly "pregnancy anemia" among the young women of Bombay. Their diet of mainly polished rice and bread was markedly deficient in folate. Already deficient, the increased demands of pregnancy produced the fatal anemia.

A folate deficiency in the first month of pregnancy—before a woman may know she's pregnant—increases the risk of neural tube defects in the fetus. (The neural tube is an embryonic structure that develops into the brain and spinal cord). As of 1998, folate has been included with some other B-vitamins that are added, by law, to enrich staple grains like white flour. As a result, folate deficiency and related birth defects are now less common in the U.S.

Because folate is usually bound to other substances in food, the amount absorbed can be uncertain. Adequate folate is so important in early pregnancy that women of childbearing age are advised to get their RDA of 400 µg of folate in synthetic form (folic acid), as in fortified foods (such as fortified breakfast cereals) and vitamin pills. Many breakfast cereals are fortified with 100% DV of folate (400 µg), and one-a-day type of multivitamins also have this amount. Here, the recommendation is for the "synthetic" over the "natural" (as in food) form of folate.

Vitamin B-12

All during the 19th century, beginning in Scotland in 1822, there were reports of a strange and deadly anemia. So destructive was the ailment that by about 1850 it was called "the pernicious anemia." The name referred to its severe and insidious onslaught on life, progressing from an inflamed tongue to diarrhea and digestive misery, with nerve damage, brain damage, and finally, death. There was no effective treatment or cure.

Early clues suggested that pernicious anemia involved some inheritable tendency. The anemia seemed unrelated to malnutrition, since the victims usually seemed well fed.

In 1926, George Minot and William Murphy found a way to control this disease. The treatment was a dietary regimen that included about a half pound of liver a day. They didn't know then what caused pernicious anemia nor what in the dietary regimen cured it. For their discovery of an effective treatment for pernicious anemia—and the simultaneous discovery that the disease had something to do with nutrition—the two physicians were awarded the Nobel Prize in 1934.

A single atom of cobalt lies at the center of the very complex structure of B-12 (the most complex of all the vitamins), giving it its alternative name cobalamin.

In 1948, vitamin B-12 was isolated from liver. It was the last vitamin discovered. Then in 1955, Dorothy Hodgkins determined the complex structure of vitamin B-12, and received the Nobel Prize in 1964.

B-12 has much in common with the other water-soluble vitamins, but it stands out in special ways. For one, whereas plants can make all the other water-soluble vitamins, plants (except for certain fungi and algae) can't make B-12. For another, whereas the body has limited stores of the other water-soluble vitamins, it can store enough B-12 to last about 4 years.

Another feature—*cobalt* as part of B-12's structure—is worth a bit of digression because it gives some insight into the close relationship between our need for vitamins and our need for minerals.

In 1935 (before B-12's structure was known), an Australian scientist found that cobalt was an essential of life for sheep. For some years, when well-fed, healthy sheep were moved into certain pastures of Australia's Outback, they sickened and died. After painstaking analysis of the soils, the scientist found one difference between the soils that supported life and those that didn't. The healthful pastures had tiny measures of cobalt in their soil, which the unhealthful pastures lacked. This suggested that sheep required cobalt. Yet, if pure cobalt was given to the sick sheep, it was of no help.

It was years before this paradox was resolved. Finally, it was found that cobalt is used by microbes to make B-12. No higher animal can do this. So cobalt by itself is useless to higher animals until microorganisms have used it to make the complex molecule of vitamin B-12. Microbes in a cow's rumen (a chamber in a cow's stomach) make B-12, which the cow absorbs. We in turn get the B-12 from beef and milk.

Vitamin B-12 Absorption

A few years after Minot and Murphy's discovery that something in a liver-rich diet cured pernicious anemia, William Castle was able to outline the normal process by which this dietary factor is absorbed. He showed that:

- The stomach juices held some mysterious *"intrinsic factor"* (now known to be a protein-carbohydrate substance secreted by cells in the lining of the stomach).

- Animal protein had some *"extrinsic factor"* (now known to be B-12).

- The two factors combined to allow the absorption of an "anti-pernicious anemia principle" (see Fig. 14-6).

In his enlightening—and unappetizing—experiment, Dr. Castle ate a portion of beef, and then used a stomach tube to bring the meat-stomach-juice mixture back up. This mixture was then fed to patients with pernicious anemia and was found to be effective.

Present evidence indicates that pernicious anemia is an inherited autoimmune disease in which the body mistakenly "sees" as foreign its own stomach cells that make intrinsic factor. The body then makes antibodies against these cells, and destroys them as if they were foreign invaders. Thus, people with this disease must obtain B-12 by means other than diet, since their stomach cells can't make the intrinsic factor needed to absorb the vitamin in food.

The treatment usually involves injections of B-12. Lacking intrinsic factor, the object is to get past the intestinal barrier by putting the vitamin directly into the bloodstream. Once there, there's nothing to stop B-12's normal function in the body's chemistry.

So we must ask some questions about the first cures of pernicious anemia by a diet that included a lot of liver. Did the diet work because the liver provided so much of the vitamin that some managed to be taken up from the small intestine? Or could it have been that something else in the liver or the diet helped?

We don't know the answer for sure. But we do know that a small fraction of B-12 can be absorbed without intrinsic factor; liver has a lot of B-12; and a lot of liver was eaten. So the most likely answer is that "flooding" the intestine with B-12 was the key to the success of the diet.

Vitamin B-12 and Folate Connection

It's instructive to examine the alternate answer that there was "something else" helpful in the curative liver-rich diet. There's a close relationship between B-12 and folate. Liver is a superb source of folate, and the prescribed diet was also rich in folate-containing fresh fruits and vegetables.

Also, the anemia caused by a B-12 deficiency is indistinguishable from the anemia caused by a folate deficiency (see Fig. 14-7). But a crucial difference between the two deficiencies is that B-12 deficiency can cause permanent nerve damage whereas folate deficiency doesn't.

Nerve damage can occur because B-12 is needed in some reactions involving nerve tissue. This makes it very important to detect and treat

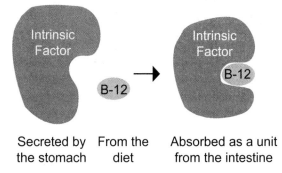

Figure 14-6: The Combination of Intrinsic Factor and Vitamin B-12 is Absorbed.

Secreted by   From the   Absorbed as a unit
the stomach   diet   from the intestine

the deficiency early to prevent permanent nerve damage. Often, the first sign of B-12 deficiency is the anemia.

The anemia of B-12 deficiency can be cured by large doses of folate. But the folate won't do anything about the damage to the nerve tissue from B-12 deficiency, and can, in fact, make the damage worse. In other words, large amounts of folate can mask the presence of B-12 deficiency by curing the anemia and thereby delaying the diagnosis of B-12 deficiency. This delay increases the risk of permanent nerve damage.

This effect of folate was taken into consideration in planning for the fortification of refined grains with folate in 1998.

Vitamin B-12 and Body Chemistry

Like the other B-vitamins, B-12 plays its roles as a part of coenzymes. B-12 coenzymes have a wide variety of uses in body chemistry, some so fundamental that B-12 is found in virtually every human cell.

Normal adult storage of B-12 is about 2 to 3 milligrams (2,000-3,000 micrograms). Yet, the adult RDA is only 2.4 micrograms (1/10,000,000 of an ounce)—the smallest RDA of all the nutrients. So, for the normal person, B-12 stores are not very quickly or easily exhausted (normal storage holds about a two-to-four-year supply). This means that an actual B-12 deficiency may not occur for several years after the loss of intrinsic-factor-secreting cells. The symptoms usually appear gradually, rarely before age 50.

When we look at some biochemical roles of B-12, we can see why it's universally required by the cells. Like folate, it's necessary to form the nucleic acids which hold the chemical blueprints

Figure 14-7: Both folate and B-12 are needed to synthesize nucleic acids and DNA. A deficiency of either causes anemia.

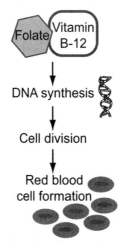

of heredity and control our synthesis of proteins.

Three body systems make the primary demands for B-12: the bone marrow (where blood cells are made), the nervous system, and the digestive tract. Failures of these processes—through an insufficient supply of the vitamin in food, insufficient absorption, or some combination of the two factors—suggest the origin of the leading deficiency symptoms. We can see why anemia, nervous-system defects, and diarrheas and other intestinal complaints are among the first signs of deficiency.

B-12 has a very low toxicity. Nevertheless, nutritionists are concerned about popular use of massive amounts of B-12. Such uses seem to be based on unscientific interpretations of how the vitamin plays its part in the blood, in forming nucleic acids, and in serving the needs of the nervous system.

Claims have been made for megadoses of B-12 for the prevention of a wide variety of problems, ranging from senility to emotional disorders. There's no known benefit to large doses of B-12, except in cases of deficiency. (That is, except to promoters, since it's cheap and large amounts can be given in a small pill or injection.)

Vitamin B-12 Intake

As a practical matter, B-12 deficiency is generally not a matter of concern for most people in the U.S. Animal foods are excellent sources of the vitamin, and most of us eat a lot of these. Most people with a B-12 deficiency then, are those who can't absorb the vitamin. As noted earlier, those who lack intrinsic factor can get B-12 by injection.

About 10-30% of people over age 50 don't absorb B-12 as well, partly because their stomach secretes less acid, which helps release food-bound B-12. For this reason, people over age 50 are advised to eat foods fortified with B-12, as in fortified breakfast cereals, or take a vitamin pill that includes B-12.

Strict vegetarians *(vegans)* are also a concern since they eat only plant foods that, for all useful purposes, are naturally devoid of the vitamin. But vegans can eat special vegetable proteins or other foods which are fortified with B-12, or can take B-12 supplements.

> Plant foods can be a source of B-12 when "contaminated" with the B-12 made by microbes or with the microbes themselves.

For adult vegans, vitamin B-12 deficiency generally develops only after a severe and long-term shortage. The body can store enough B-12 to last several years, and only a very tiny amount of the vitamin is needed. But, one concern is that vegans might have a delay in the diagnosis of a B-12 deficiency. A strictly vegetarian diet often has large amounts of folate, which, as mentioned earlier, can cure the tell-tale anemia of B-12 deficiency without protecting against potentially irreversible nerve damage.

Most vulnerable to B-12 deficiency are infants born of mothers who have been vegans with long-standing B-12 deficiency. These infants are born with low body stores, and, typically, are fed only breast milk during early infancy. As one would expect, the breast milk of a mother long deficient in B-12 has very little B-12. Some of the infants develop nerve damage. Also vulnerable are growing children on a vegan diet.

Pantothenic Acid

While one can scarcely overstate the importance of this vitamin in the chemistry of the human body, its story, in terms of human health and life, is devoid of drama. It's a vitamin for which no deficiency disease has ever been defined, except in very strictly controlled laboratory experiments.

The name ***pantothenic acid*** comes from Greek roots which suggest that it's "found everywhere." There's scarcely a food in nature which doesn't have some of this vitamin. It's easy to see why there's little or no concern among nutritionists about the intake of pantothenic acid. Getting enough seems unavoidable as long as there's food to eat.

This helps explain why there's so little drama about pantothenic acid—clear-cut deficiencies are not seen. If such deficiencies do occur—and they probably do—they're lost among other deficiencies which would be inevitable.

The deficiency can be produced readily in laboratory animals, but it took some 15 years of work with human volunteers to produce the deficiency in man. It not only took a specially synthesized diet, but also the use of a pantothenic acid antivitamin—a substance that interferes with pantothenic acid use—to make the deficiency worse.

The first signs of deficiency occurred in three to four weeks, with some vomiting, followed by a bewildering assortment of broad symptoms. The volunteers tired easily, suffered personality changes, and abdominal discomfort with diarrhea. Given inoculations against disease, they failed to produce antibodies normally. There were muscle cramps and other abnormalities of the nervous system, with sensations of tingling and pain, and a curious tenderness of the heels which some have called "the burning feet sign."

For ethical reasons, studies of human deficiencies were carried no further. But it was clear that pantothenic acid is a vitamin (and thus essential) for humans.

The best known role of pantothenic acid in life's chemical processes is as ***Coenzyme A***. We have seen this coenzyme at work in metabolism (Chap. 11) as one of the keys to the body's use of fuel. Coenzyme A is essential not only to the release of energy from carbohydrate, protein, and fat, but to the body's ability to synthesize them. It's involved in a variety of processes—from making hormones and cholesterol to the transmission of nerve impulses. It's easy to see why pantothenic acid is "found everywhere."

Biotin

Biotin is made by our intestinal bacteria. And the amounts they make seem to be generally greater than our requirements. Deficiencies have been seen only under the most unusual of conditions. So, as with pantothenic acid, there's little dietary concern about biotin.

In the 1930s, the substance was found to be a vitamin for yeast. So, in reference to the fact that the life of yeast requires it, the vitamin was christened *biotin* from the Greek *bios*, meaning *life*.

The essentiality of biotin for humans was determined with the help of raw egg white. In fact, for a brief time, biotin was known as "anti-egg-white-injury factor." The reason is that raw egg white contains a substance, called *avidin*, which binds biotin and prevents its absorption from the intestine.

The first studies produced biotin deficiencies by feeding subjects a low-biotin, 15 to 20% egg-white diet. This required the raw whites of about 24 eggs day for each volunteer. Cooking destroys the avidin (as a protein, avidin is denatured by cooking). For the anti-biotin effect, the egg white must be raw.

The symptoms found for biotin deficiency are good grist for the faddist mill. They include such vague and common signs as skin problems, lost appetite, depression, sleeplessness, and muscle aches—symptoms which also happen to be popular in the marketing of dietary supplements. But since biotin deficiencies are practically nonexistent unless deliberately created, it's a rare condition indeed that is relieved by biotin.

There are rare genetic defects in biotin metabolism that can be overcome by massive doses of biotin.

As with pantothenic acid, the virtual absence of naturally-occurring deficiency signs doesn't lessen the importance of biotin in body processes. Biotin coenzymes are used widely. They take part in the making of fatty acids, the breaking down of nutrients to yield energy, and in the producing of some amino acids. They are also necessary in some reactions which require Coenzyme A (the pantothenic-acid coenzyme).

The functions of biotin coenzymes seem to be closely related to those of vitamin B-6, folate, and vitamin B-12. In cases of severe malnutrition, it is possible that biotin deficiencies are hidden among the more evident signs of other deficiencies.

Summary

There are nine water-soluble vitamins—eight B-vitamins and vitamin C. The B-vitamins are components of various coenzymes important in metabolism.

Vitamin C is used by the body to form connective tissue, bone, and capillaries. It also facilitates the body's use of calcium and iron, helps immune function and hormone production, and serves as an antioxidant. A severe deficiency of vitamin C leads to scurvy, which in the early 1900s was thought to be a contagious disease. Most Americans get enough vitamin C in their diets.

Thiamin prevents the deficiency disease beriberi. It's part of a coenzyme used in energy production, but consuming extra thiamin won't make one more "energetic." Wernicke-Korsakoff Syndrome is a degenerative disease of the brain related to thiamin deficiency, and is most commonly seen in alcoholics.

Riboflavin is part of another coenzyme that aids energy production. Deficiencies are rare, and usually accompany severe malnutrition that includes deficiencies of other B vitamins (riboflavin also helps niacin and B-6 function). A deficiency of this one vitamin doesn't normally result in a single symptom (e.g., hair loss).

Niacin, like thiamin and riboflavin, is part of a coenzyme that aids energy production. Severe deficiency causes pellagra. The body can make niacin from the amino acid tryptophan, so the need for niacin is related to how much protein is in the diet.

Vitamin B-6 coenzymes are needed in amino acid metabolism, e.g., helping make "non-essential" amino acids, remove amino groups to allow amino acids to be used for energy, and convert tryptophan into niacin.

Folate is part of a coenzyme needed to make DNA and RNA, making it crucial in cell division. A deficiency symptom is anemia, but deficiencies are less common now that folate is added to enriched grains. Needs are higher during pregnancy; a deficiency in early pregnancy increases the risk of neural defects in the newborn. All women of child-bearing age are advised to get enough folate from fortified foods or vitamin pills.

B-12 is the only B vitamin not made by plants. It's also unique as a B-vitamin because the body can store up to about 4 years' worth. Intrinsic factor, secreted by the stomach, is needed for B-12 absorption. A lack of intrinsic factor thus prevents the absorption of B-12 from the diet, in which case B-12 is typically given by injection.

Vegans (and infants born of vegan mothers) are at risk for deficiency, since B-12 is found naturally only in animal foods. Vegans should make sure they get enough B-12, either as a supplement or by eating foods fortified with B-12.

A deficiency can also occur in those over age 50, due in part from less stomach acid. The acid helps release food-bound B-12. To over-ride this problem, those over age 50 are advised to get B-12 from fortified foods or vitamin pills.

Large amounts of folate given to those who are B-12 deficient will alleviate the B-12 deficiency anemia but won't do anything about the nerve damage that also can result from B-12 deficiency. This "masking" of the anemia caused by a B-12 deficiency can delay the diagnosis, risking permanent nerve damage.

Pantothenic acid is found in almost every food, so deficiencies are nearly impossible without severe malnutrition. Its role is as a part of Coenzyme A, which plays a crucial role in energy metabolism.

Biotin is provided by our intestinal bacteria, and deficiencies usually accompany only severe malnutrition. Biotin also has a role in producing energy, fatty acids and amino acids.

Chapter 15

Fat-Soluble Vitamins

In a world of instant news and a media system constantly on the look-out for eye-catching news, research findings have become a favorite source of copy. The more astonishing, the better.

That complicates life for the serious scientist. The accumulation of scientific knowledge is seldom a story of breakthroughs, and all findings must be subjected to a process of peer review and verification before they can legitimately join the body of acknowledged scientific fact. And even then, there must be care in defining exactly what has been learned.

Nutrition provides abundant examples. Animal studies are often the only practical form of much research, and the results may or may not apply to humans. And then there is always the popular tendency to believe (and the alert merchandiser to encourage the belief) that more will cure what inadequacy would have caused, even where there has been no inadequacy. If too little of vitamin X causes hair loss and diminished sexual desire, a surplus, even for the well nourished, will surely grow hair on the bald and enhance the libido of the most reluctant lover.

There are no better examples than the fat-soluble vitamins. They are wondrous indeed, but not in the way the supplement sellers often would like us to believe.

Like the water-soluble vitamins, the fat-soluble vitamins are chemical substances needed by the body in tiny amounts, which must be supplied from outside sources. But unlike the water-soluble vitamins, they can be stored in large amounts, especially in the liver. So dietary excesses—much smaller excesses than in the case of the water-soluble vitamins—can become toxic.

The vitamin overdoses stimulated by nutrition faddism become serious business when we look at the fat-soluble vitamins. Some can be dangerous at levels as low as five times the RDA, which—according to some vitamin supplement enthusiasts—is not excessive at all.

General characteristics of fat-soluble vitamins
• Absorbed with dietary fats
• Stored with body fat
• Not readily excreted
• More easily toxic (A and D)

The four fat-soluble vitamins—vitamins A, D, E, and K—play many diverse roles, roles which are quite different from the predominantly coenzyme roles of the water-soluble vitamins. Starting with vitamin A, we will see what these roles are.

As with the water-soluble vitamins, the more interesting and instructive aspects of the fat-soluble vitamins are selected for discussion. Also, to minimize tedious discussion, basic information about each vitamin is summarized in Table 15-1, and the RDAs are found in Appendix A.

Vitamin A

Many of the earliest insights into nutritional deficiency concerned the fat-soluble vitamins. Among the first recorded references to the relationship between vitamin A-rich foods and **night blindness** are found in writings which are some 3,500 years old. Eber's Papyrus, an Egyptian document from about 1500 B.C., defines the phenomenon of night blindness and suggests a cure of feeding patients the roasted livers of oxen or roosters. (The livers of virtually all animals are rich sources of vitamin A.)

Vision

Besides being one of the oldest accurate nutrition observations, the relationship between foods rich in vitamin A and vision is one of the best known. It is a rare child who has not been told to eat carrots in order to see better. Or who has not heard that a lack of vitamin A can result in night blindness

It is less well known that such night blindness is far more than an inconvenience. It is an extremely serious warning sign of a problem all too common among the world's poor.

Night Blindness, a Deadly Omen

The night blindness which results from a deficiency of vitamin A is characterized by a difficulty of adjusting, from seeing in bright light to seeing in poor light. All of us have experienced this adjustment, when the bright light was especially intense and the succeeding low light especially weak—as when we drive from brilliant sunshine into a dark tunnel, or after a flashbulb has fired. A chemical change is demanded of our vision system, and it takes a little time to occur even when our vision is healthy.

Keep in mind that a reduced ability to see in dim light doesn't necessarily mean a vitamin A deficiency. Eye changes related to aging, for example, can reduce one's ability to accommodate from bright to dim light, and one's ability to see in dim light. Again, if the problem isn't caused by a vitamin deficiency, taking the vitamin won't help.

The chemical involved in this change is **rhodopsin.** Vitamin A is the **photosensitive** part of the rhodopsin molecule, and this visual process begins when vitamin A is altered and released when light strikes it. This change sends an impulse from specialized cells at the back of the eyes, along the optic nerve to the brain (see Fig. 15-1).

This mechanism is perhaps the most basic phenomenon of seeing, for it enables us to tell the difference between more light or less. Thus do we see not only outlines but also the complex system of light and shadow that gives distinction to what

Table 15-1: Fat-Soluble Vitamins

Vitamin	Function	Source	Deficiency	Possible Toxicity
Vitamin A (retinol, retinoids, provitamin A carotenoids)	Vision, gene expression, maintain tissues, reproduction, immunity	Liver, carrots, spinach, winter squash, apricots, papaya, greens, tomatoes	Night blindness, xerophthalmia skin lesions	Fatigue, nausea, headache, hair loss, liver damage, birth defects
Vitamin D (calciferol)	Absorb calcium and phosphorus, mineralize bone	Fortified milk and breakfast cereals, fatty fish, sunshine on skin	Rickets, osteomalacia, osteoporosis	Fatigue, nausea, calcify soft tissue, kidney damage
Vitamin E (tocopherol)	Antioxidant	Vegetable oil, margarine, whole grains, egg yolk	Hemolytic anemia	Increased tendency to bleed.
Vitamin K	Blood clotting	Intestinal bacteria, liver, green leafy vegetables, milk, meat	Lessened ability of blood to clot	Jaundice in infants

we see—that enables us to distinguish the face of a friend from that of a stranger.

The vitamin A portion must then be replaced before rhodopsin can be used again. So for continuing good vision, our eyes must be able to restore rhodopsin quickly. Otherwise, a bright light will leave us with too little rhodopsin for vision in dim light.

In 1958, George Wald discovered the action of vitamin A in vision; he was awarded the Nobel Prize in 1967.

When an insufficient amount of vitamin A is available in the eye, restoration of rhodopsin takes place very slowly. And during that time, to some extent, one is blinded. In other words, a shortage of vitamin A means a limitation on our ability to see. Conversely, we have no difficulty maintaining rhodopsin if we have sufficient vitamin A.

What Night Blindness Means

Recall that when vitamin deficiencies exist, there are shortages throughout the body, not just in one body system. True, some systems are more acutely dependent on the vitamin and show shortages sooner. But we may be certain that the rest of the body is also threatened with deficiency.

Among fat-soluble vitamins, a deficiency means that the body's reserve has been exhausted. So when vitamin A shortage reaches a point at which the eyes can't function optimally, other threats to health also exist.

What kinds of threats? For one, the night blindness indicates a condition known as **xerophthalmia**. The word derives from the Greek words for *dry* and *eyes.*

Indeed, the eyes of the vitamin A-deficient person do look dry. The whites of the eyes are especially flat and dull. The effect is much more than cosmetic. It means that eye tissue is beginning to dry out and die. Small ulcers can occur and result in little scars on the lens of the eye. Like the cataracts common in older people, these scars block areas of vision and can lead to permanent blindness.

The familiar trade name Xerox derives from the fact that its copies are dry—unlike the common office copier of the 1950s, which produced copies that literally had to be "hung out to dry."

Another threat to health is that a vitamin-A deficiency impairs the immune system, leading to higher death rates in children with measles or severe diarrhea, for example.

How Common is Severe Vitamin A Deficiency?

Striking signs of vitamin A deficiency are rare in the U.S., but according to the World Health Organization (WHO) of the United Nations, about 254 million preschool children (half of them in Southeast Asia) are vitamin A deficient, based on clinical eye signs and/or very low vitamin A levels

Figure 15-1: Role of Vitamin A in Vision. When light strikes, vitamin A changes shape and is released. This sends an impulse to the brain. Vitamin A must be restored for rhodopsin to function in vision.

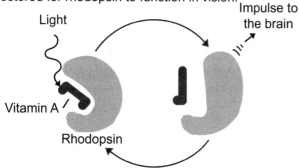

in the blood, and about 800,000 deaths worldwide can be attributed to vitamin A deficiency.[1]

An estimated 250,000 to 500,000 vitamin-A deficient children become blind every year, and about half of these children die within a year of becoming blind.[2]

For those of us in developed countries, it seems incredible that such a huge and tragic health problem exists when its cure/prevention is an inexpensive vitamin. In fact, huge strides have been made in combating vitamin A deficiency, including providing vitamin A capsules to young children and fortifying various foods with vitamin A (e.g., sugar in Guatemala).

What is Vitamin A?

Vitamin A itself is found only in animals, not in plants. But plants contain substances (***provitamin A***) that our bodies can convert to vitamin A. Thus, we get vitamin A from food by eating provitamin A—vitamin A precursors—in plant foods or by eating vitamin A itself in animal foods or foods to which vitamin A has been added (e.g., fortified breakfast cereal).

> The vitamin A that we get from animal foods originally came from carotenoids by conversion to vitamin A in an animal body.

The provitamin A in plants are among a group of pigments known collectively as ***carotenoids***. The carotenoids bring color to life. They are a group of several hundred bright yellow, orange, and red pigments that are made in plants. They are found in fruits, vegetables, flowers, and foliage, giving leaves their beautiful fall colors.

Some of these carotenoids can be converted into vitamin A in the body (***provitamin A carotenoids***). ***Beta carotene***, the most common and most potent of these, was first isolated from carrots in 1931, giving it its name.

> Many animals can make vitamin A from carotenoids but cats can't. So cats must get their vitamin A from meat or milk—a vegetarian diet doesn't work for cats!

Carotenoids are found in yellow-orange fruits and vegetables. They are also found in dark-green vegetables—the green color of chlorophyll masks the yellow-orange color.

Carotenoids are only made in plants, but can be found in animal tissues when animals eat plants rich in them. The yellow-orange color of egg yolk is from carotenoids (only some of which have vitamin A value). In fact, poultry and egg producers routinely add carotenoid concentrates (e.g., from alfalfa or corn) to poultry feed so that the egg yolk and chicken skin will be more attractive to the consumer. Carotenoids are also added to margarine (otherwise, it would be white).

> Although vitamin A itself isn't found naturally in plants, processed plant foods (e.g., breakfast cereals) often have vitamin A and/or beta carotene added to them ("fortified with vitamin A").

Like vitamin A, carotenoids are fat-soluble. Unlike vitamin A, however, they are fairly safe when consumed in large amounts. The body stores excesses, rather than converting the provitamin A carotenoids into toxic amounts of vitamin A.

The skin of people who eat a lot of carotenoids (e.g., drink carrot juice) looks yellow-orange because, as fat-soluble substances, carotenoids color the fat under the skin. Foods rich in carotenoids include sweet potato, mango, kale, pumpkin, carrots, cantaloupe, spinach, hot chili peppers, apricots, broccoli, and romaine lettuce.

Vitamin A and Body Chemistry

Vitamin A plays a crucial roles in many other body functions besides vision, but the chemistry of its action in these roles is not as well understood. Possibly, the broadest and most important function

Beta-carotene

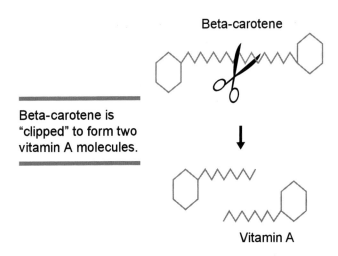

Beta-carotene is "clipped" to form two vitamin A molecules.

Vitamin A

of vitamin A is to maintain *epithelial tissues*—our skin, and skin-like structures (such as the tissues that line our respiratory and digestive tracts).

The word *epithelium* comes from the Greek, and it is instructive to look at its roots. The prefix *epi* is the same as in such words as epidemic or epicenter, meaning *on, upon,* or *over.* The *thelium* part refers to the nipple. Then why use it to describe the outer and inner protective tissues of the body? Because these tissues protect not only by covering but also by secreting important substances. When there is a vitamin A deficiency, the skin, intestinal lining, and other such tissues lose some of their integrity and their ability to secrete.

> Vitamin A values are standardized as micrograms (ug) of Retinol Activity Equivalents (RAE), e.g., 1 ug RAE = 12 ug beta-carotene or 3.3 International Units (IU) vitamin A.

When there is a shortage of vitamin A, the eyes take on a dry look because the tissues are, in fact, dry. These tissues are among the first to be affected when there is a vitamin A deficiency. Eventually, tissues of the respiratory system and digestive tract are also affected. The normal cleansing and protective mechanisms of the body don't work as well.

Infectious organisms which are normally swept away, remain, and infections are harder to combat. Infections of the eyes, nose, throat, lung, and digestive tract become much more common. Vitamin A deficiency also reduces the effectiveness of white blood cells that fight infection—compromising further the ability to overcome infection.

A vitamin A deficiency can mean the difference between life and death in fighting infection. Measles epidemics, for example, regularly take the lives of many of the world's vitamin-A-deficient children.

Vitamin A in Foods

Liver, the main storage organ for vitamin A, is the main high-density food source of vitamin A itself. Other organ meats, eggs, butterfat, and foods we fortify with vitamin A, such as milk and many breakfast cereals, are also key sources.

> The vitamin A used to fortify foods or used in dietary supplements is often listed as vitamin A palmitate, retinyl palmitate, vitamin A acetate, etc. Vitamin A is manufactured in these combinations to make it more stable.

We get the rest of our vitamin A indirectly through carotenoids, mainly from plants. As was mentioned earlier, color—particularly yellow-orange and dark green—provides a good clue as to the amount in plants. However, unlike vitamin A, which is readily absorbed and already in usable form, carotenoids vary a lot in how well they are absorbed, and in the extent to which they can be converted to vitamin A.

> How many carrots does it take for Carol to meet her RDA for vitamin A? The RDA for adult females is 700 ug RAE (see above). The carotenoids in a medium carrot provide about 1,400 ug RAE. Thus, Carol only needs a half a carrot to meet her RDA for vitamin A.

When diets are very low in fats—as they are in most of the poorer nations of the world—carotenoids are less readily absorbed. It then becomes important to pay particular attention to the quantity and quality of the available yellow-orange and dark green fruits and vegetables. Vitamin A deficiency can be a major concern when there are severe seasonal problems, as when cold weather cuts off the harvest of plant foods. Remember, most poorer nations cannot count as we do upon canned, frozen, and imported fruits and vegetables.

The possibilities of vitamin A shortage become great among such people. Their low fat consumption often means that there is also a shortage of vitamin A itself, compounding the deficiency problem. We saw such a case in tales of the fat shortages among the Athabascans of the far north. Winter had eliminated fresh fruits and vegetables, and forage conditions had been poor for the animals they hunted. Since the game consumed by the Athabascans were less well fed, they were not only less fat, but could be expected also to have provided less vitamin A and carotenoids.

Cooking increases the amount of carotenoids absorbed from food, as does fat in the meal.

In many parts of the world, vitamin A depletion occurs with appalling frequency. When vitamin A intake is reduced—as in the case of strict vegetarian diets or when animal foods are scarce—the carotenoid intake must be substantial to avoid depleting liver stores of the vitamin. The one saving aspect is the liver's ability to store the vitamin. It allows one to take advantage of any surpluses, and provides a challenge to the nutritionist to do whatever is possible to increase regular vitamin A intake, including enough to provide for liver storage so it can be drawn upon as needed.

Ironically, countries in which vitamin A deficiency is common often have plenty of cheap, leafy sources of carotene. But it's hard to change eating habits. And even if the parents understand and try to cooperate, it is hard to generate much affection for greens among small youngsters.

Golden Rice was produced as a way to provide vitamin A to deficient populations where rice provides as much as 80% of calories. Carotenoids aren't normally made in rice, so the necessary genes to do this (one of them from a daffodil!) were inserted. The resulting beta-carotene gives the rice its golden color.

We face the same challenge with eating habits in our own country, but our children are better protected. They have greater access to such popular vitamin A sources as milk, butter, cheese, eggs, ice cream, and the like, as well as many sweet, carotene-rich fruits and fruit juices.

Figure 15-2: Vitamin A toxicity and deficiency.

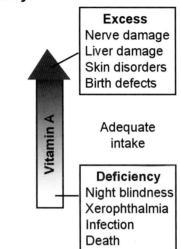

In addition, we have widespread vitamin A fortification, particularly in such foods as milk and ready-to-eat breakfast cereals.

The Toxicity of Excess

Large doses of vitamin A are dangerous, unless current intakes and liver stores are low. Toxic effects are most commonly the result of excess vitamin supplementation. Particularly vulnerable is the unborn child, susceptible to malformations when large doses of vitamin A supplements are taken during pregnancy.

Vitamin A poisoning brings on a wide variety of symptoms. They range from dry, itchy skin to swellings over the bones, and can include blurred vision, irritability, lost appetite, hair loss, headaches, diarrhea, nausea, liver damage, and neurological problems, including brain damage. Efforts to use vitamin A therapeutically, especially to correct skin and hair problems have generally proven futile. Indeed, much of what we know about vitamin A toxicity comes from misguided attempts to correct skin problems.

Vitamin A, Carotenoids, and Vitamin-A Analogs as Medicine

Vitamin A deficiency has been associated with an increased risk of lung cancer, leading some enthusiasts to interpret this as a call for vitamin A supplementation for cancer protection. Since vitamin A is needed to maintain the epithelial tissue that lines the lungs, it is logical to suppose that a vitamin A deficiency will make lung tissue more vulnerable to the assaults of cancer-causing substances, such as those found in tobacco smoke. Again, however, supplementation can help only where there is a deficiency.

Beta-carotene may have a protective effect against cancer that is separate from its role in providing vitamin A, e.g., it can act as an antioxidant (the role of antioxidants in possibly reducing cancer risk will be discussed in the section on vitamin E).

Observational studies have shown that smokers who ate more beta-carotene-containing food had less lung cancer, and it was plausible that beta-carotene was protective. However, randomized, double-blind studies (see Chapter 1) of smokers taking pills of either beta-carotene or a placebo had a shocking result—the beta-carotene group got more lung cancer than the placebo group! A randomized double-blind study of non-smokers, however, didn't show a harmful (or beneficial) effect of taking beta-carotene.

This reinforces the view that it's better to get our carotenoids from a normal diet that regularly includes yellow-orange and dark-green vegetables and fruit, i.e., food, rather than supplements. People who eat more foods containing certain carotenoids have been found to have lower risk of some diseases. So people take lutein supplements to prevent macular degeneration (an eye disease occurring mostly in people over age 65), and lycopene supplements to prevent prostate cancer. (Neither lutein nor lycopene have vitamin A value.) But the lesson of the smokers and beta-carotene pills is that eating carotenoid-rich foods is not the same as taking carotenoid supplements. (Spinach is a rich source of lutein; tomato products are a rich source of lycopene—put more catsup on those fries!)

Vitamin A analogs (laboratory-produced drugs that are similar in structure to vitamin A) have been produced as prescription drugs for specific medicinal roles. The vitamin A analog isotretinoin (Accutane), for example, has been used successfully in the treatment of severe acne and in preventing the recurrence of head and neck cancers. Unfortunately, isotretinoin has some toxic effects in common with vitamin A. Those being treated with this drug are carefully monitored for toxicity symptoms, including liver damage. Strict measures (not always successful) are taken to avoid pregnancy while being treated, because normal doses of the drug can cause birth defects.

Vitamin D

Like vitamin A, vitamin D has a long history. Rickets, the most striking sign of D deficiency, was recognized at least 2,500 years ago. And centuries ago the deficiency disease was understood to be curable or preventable by eating certain foods—which eventually were found to be potent sources of vitamin D.

Rickets and Osteomalacia

Rickets is a deceptive and pathetic disorder. Infant victims may not look as if they suffer from malnutrition. But, in fact, they can suffer from a hidden failure of development which may not be apparent until they start to walk.

The condition is technically a form of osteomalacia, literally a softening of the bone. It is the result of failure to absorb enough calcium—either because there isn't enough calcium in the diet, or because the body's absorption and use of calcium is limited by a shortage of vitamin D.

Such infants may be uncomfortably restless. The abdomen may be somewhat distended. The muscles are usually lacking in tone, and flabby. As the infants get older and begin walking, the weight of the body on the legs can cause the bones to become deformed, and the child is described as knock-kneed or bow-legged. The bones of the chest, spine, and pelvis may also become permanently deformed. The "sunken chest" of rickets can lead to lung problems, and a deformed pelvis can cause problems for women during childbirth.

In a sense, what happens in cases of rickets is akin to building the framework of a skyscraper with soft iron instead of steel. The framework may seem sound at first, but as more weight is placed upon it, the iron twists and bends. So also do the bones of children with rickets.

Although this pathetic disorder of development was long known, it became much more common with the coming of civilization, particularly in northern lands. The osteomalacia of adults also became more common, especially among poorer women in northern industrial cities, who regularly went through many pregnancies and long periods of breastfeeding.

By the 17th century in England, there was much speculation about the disorder and its causes. And by the latter portion of the 19th century, up to 75% of the children living in the poor areas of industrial cities had rickets.

By the early 1800s, some practical answers to the problem had been found, but with no real understanding of why they were effective. In 1807, an English physician name Bardsley tested the old Scandinavian idea of giving cod-liver oil (a vitamin D source) to babies and young children, and found that the oil cured osteomalacia.

We are reminded again of the interrelationships between nutrients. Osteomalacia can result from a lack of either calcium or vitamin D, or a combined deficiency.

But Bardsley's report went largely unrecognized. It was not until 1889 and 1890, that two sets of experiments caught medical and public attention. In one, lion cubs at the London zoo were cured of rickets when fed a mixture of crushed bone (a calcium source) and cod-liver oil. Another experiment showed that, in some cases, sunlight alone could cure rickets. During the next 30 years, more bits and pieces of the puzzle gradually emerged.

By 1920, it was speculated that there was a "calcium-depositing, fat-soluble vitamin." Vitamin D was finally isolated and synthesized in the 1930s, but it was learned even later that vitamin D must go through elaborate chemical pathways before it can take part in human chemistry. Some key parts of this work were accomplished as recently as the 1970s, and the story is not yet complete.

Today, rickets is a relatively uncommon problem in world nutrition, although milder vitamin D

Figure 15-3: The active form of vitamin D

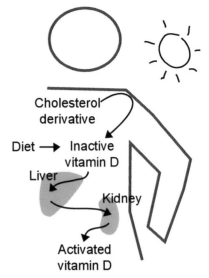

deficiency is still common.[1] In industrialized countries, it has been understood since early in this century that certain food sources provided protection; and there has been steady progress in finding cheap ways to assure ample sources of the vitamin in commonly consumed foods.

The Sunshine Vitamin

The active form of vitamin D is made in our body either from vitamin D in our diet, or from a derivative of cholesterol in our skin. When the cholesterol-derived precursor is struck by sunlight, there is a chemical change. It becomes vitamin D and is taken up into the circulating blood. Thus, when there's adequate exposure to the sun, vitamin D isn't required in the diet.

We can begin to understand why the widespread rickets of the 19th century has been called a disease of civilization, and even of the industrial revolution. In Europe, for example, the factory towns of the north received little sunlight, and the workers (many of whom were children) had little chance to be outdoors. Also, in cold climates, more clothing is needed and less skin is exposed to sunlight.

Women workers had few daylight hours outside the factories. They spent as few days as possible away from their machines during and after pregnancy. They drank little milk and could afford little butterfat in foods during either pregnancy or lactation. Birth control methods were limited.

Thus, in short, they had little of either sunlight or food sources of vitamin D, and poor reserves of either vitamin D or calcium. With repeated pregnancies and breastfeeding during young adulthood, their own bodies were rapidly depleted, and they became common victims of osteomalacia.

Another factor contributed as well. Much of milk was either watered or skimmed of some fat, thereby removing vitamin D. (Most of the low-fat and non-fat milk sold today in the United States is fortified with vitamin D.) Butterfat (the source of vitamin D in milk), was the most valued part of dairy products. Creams, cheeses, and other butterfat-rich products were not for the poor.

Vitamin D and Body Chemistry

Even after vitamin D has been consumed in food or made in the skin, further chemical changes are needed before the body can use it. First, the liver makes a chemical change. Then, the kidneys make a second change, and the vitamin D is now called activated vitamin D (see Fig. 15-3).

When either the liver or kidney is compromised by injury or disease, vitamin D activation is impaired. Chronic kidney disease can produce some of the signs of vitamin D deficiency, since the necessary modification of the vitamin does not occur at a normal rate.

Activated vitamin D is needed for the absorption of calcium and phosphorus. It also controls both calcium and phosphorus in the mineralization of bone. These two minerals are used together in about equal amounts to form bone and teeth.

Moreover, we know that calcium and phosphorus are chemically necessary to the nerve-muscle systems of the body, and are involved in muscular contraction and relaxation. And apparently, wherever these two minerals are used, vitamin D is used. The vitamin appears to signal various cells to produce special proteins needed to transport these minerals.

These more recent insights suggest why the symptoms of rickets (and other forms of osteomalacia) extend beyond weak and malformed bones. The involvement of vitamin D with the muscular and neurological systems explains why deficiencies can cause rickets-associated muscle spasms

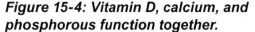

Figure 15-4: Vitamin D, calcium, and phosphorous function together.

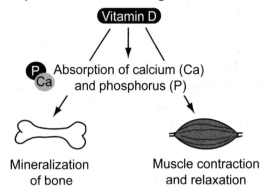

Absorption of calcium (Ca) and phosphorus (P)

Mineralization of bone

Muscle contraction and relaxation

and weakness, and such psychological effects as irritability and restlessness.

Vitamin D Requirements

It could be said that civilization made vitamin D a vitamin (in the sense that it was needed in the diet). Since vitamin D can be made as long as sunlight is allowed to fall on the skin, deficiencies apparently began when civilization took people out of the sun.

Sunlight production of vitamin D varies according to the intensity of the light, time of exposure, amount of skin exposed, color of one's skin, and the use of sunscreen. The lighter the skin, the more efficient the absorption of solar radiation. Conversely, the pigmentation of dark-skinned people can keep as much as 95% of solar radiation from reaching the deeper layers, where most of the vitamin production occurs.

Moderation and Balance: Not enough sun exposure means less vitamin D production, but too much increases the risk of skin cancer.

There have been studies that link living at higher latitudes, where people have less sun exposure, to higher rates of colon, breast, and prostate cancers. It is uncertain that the link is due to a vitamin D deficiency. But low blood-levels of D have also shown this link.[4] Intriguingly, African Americans have amongst the highest rates of prostate cancer in the world, and they get less vitamin D because of darker skin and more avoidance of [vitamin-D fortified] milk because of more prevalent lactose intolerance.

People of all races can get all the vitamin D they need with enough sun exposure, but many simply cannot or do not get enough sun exposure. For these people, vitamin D must be ingested. The Food and Nutrition Board has set an adequate intake to be 5 μg per day from birth to age 50, 10 μg/day for ages 51-70, and 15 μg/day for those over age 70. In the elderly, there is not only less sun exposure, but vitamin D production from sun exposure is less efficient.

Infant formula has enough vitamin D, but human milk doesn't. So infants fed only breast milk need more vitamin D from sun exposure or a supplement.

Vitamin D in Foods

Unless foods are fortified with vitamin D, few are very potent sources. Fish livers, certain fatty fish, and liver and fat from seals and polar bears are good sources of vitamin D, but many people do not eat much of these. The most common source of vitamin D in our diet is vitamin D fortified foods such as milk and many breakfast cereals. Cow's milk is a convenient vehicle for vitamin D fortification, especially with milk being an important source of calcium.

The Toxicity of Excess

Excesses are stored in the liver, and toxic amounts are typically from supplements. (Sun exposure does not result in toxic amounts.) Excess vitamin D can lead to weight loss, vomiting, irritability, and destructive deposits of excess calcium in soft tissues, like those of blood vessels, lung and kidney. The UL (Upper Limit) for vitamin D is 25 μg/day from birth to 12 months, and 50 μg/day for all other ages.

Vitamin E

For decades after its discovery, vitamin E presented an awkward and baffling problem to nutrition researchers. It has been called a vitamin in search of a disease.

The reason is simple: Even after the long years it took to discover, isolate, and synthesize vitamin E, decades passed before it could be shown that a deficient intake leads to any specific symptom or disease in humans.

There is a special irony in this problem. For even though scientists have labored to find specific health effects of vitamin E deficiency, the vitamin has been heralded by the public as a virtual cure-all. Such belief has little reality. It seems to stem from two misinterpretations: First, the general misinterpretation so often at the root of megadose supplementation theory— that if a little will clear up a deficiency symptom, a lot will bring superior protection against whatever problems the deficiency caused. Second, the mistaken extension of theories based on animal deficiency to humans.

On the basis of such misinterpretations, the public doses itself with E to achieve better athletic or sexual performance, to prevent or cure heart disease or stroke, to negate the effects of smoggy air, and to stave off ailments from muscular dystrophy to cancer. But science is still unaware of any major human disease which is caused by a lack of vitamin E. Nor is it known that vitamin E supplements prevent or relieve any illness or confer any special health benefit, although studies continue to explore this possibility. Let us contrast some popular ideas about this vitamin with some scientific realities of what it is and does.

Science Identifies Vitamin E

In 1922 it was reported that an unidentified fat-soluble substance from several common foods was important for rat reproduction. When female rats were fed diets deficient in this substance, the ovum could be fertilized, but pregnancy could not proceed. When they were fed wheat germ or lettuce within 7 days of conception, however, pregnancy went forward normally. (It may seem curious that so unfat a food as lettuce could provide a fat-soluble vitamin. But there are small amounts of oils in most vegetables, and only very small amounts of vitamin E are required.)

It is evidently because of its relationship to fertility that vitamin E has won its mythical link to sexuality. Some later research showed a relationship between reproduction capacity and E deficiency for male rats as well. But for neither male nor female was there evidence of change in sexual activity—only in its result. Vitamin E deficiency did not discourage rat romance—only the birth rate.

Fourteen years were to pass from the time of these animal studies, before vitamin E was isolated in 1936. It was isolated from the oil of wheat germ, and was named *tocopherol,* meaning *to bear young.*

In the ensuing years, there has been continuing confusion about vitamin E's human function. In the 1940s, for example, *Time* magazine reported claims that large doses of vitamin E protected against cardiovascular disease. Later experimental evidence consistently refuted the idea. But popular impressions die hard—and vitamin E remains a darling of supplement takers and supplement sellers.

What is Vitamin E?

Vitamin E is a tocopherol, as noted above. There are alpha, beta, gamma, and delta forms of tocopherol, but the alpha form is the "real vitamin," so the RDA for vitamin E is for alpha-tocopherol specifically.

The various forms of tocopherol lead to a bit of confusion because all of them can perform as vitamin E. Thus, they are often referred to as "different forms of vitamin E." However, there is only one known carrier of vitamin E in the body--a carrier for alpha-tocopherol, and it's only alpha-tocopherol that is maintained in the blood. The other tocopherols don't have specific carriers to transport them to the various tissues that need vitamin E, nor are their levels maintained in the blood. This indicates that they are not essential nutrients.

To convert the IUs of supplements to milligrams (mg), multiply IUs of "*dl-alpha-*" tocopherol, tocopheryl acetate, or tocopheryl succinate by 0.45; multiply the "*d-alpha-*" forms by 0.67: If the label says 300 IU *dl-alpha-*tocopherol, it has 135 mg (300 X 0.45) of the form specified in the RDA. Likewise, 300 IU of *d-alpha-*tocopherol = 200 mg (300 X 0.67). The adult RDA for vitamin E is 15 mg.

To further add to the confusion, the alpha-tocopherol in supplements come in various forms and are often given in International Units (IU).

Vitamin E Chemistry

The chemistry of vitamin E centers on its notable antioxidant effect. The natural presence of the vitamin in many foods protects against rancidity—the oxidation of fats. This is particularly the case with vegetable oils expressed from seeds of cotton, sesame, wheat, corn, and the like, and with oils of nuts, especially almonds. These oils are polyunsaturated (their fatty acids have many double bonds in their structure), and vitamin E guards against their oxidation (see Fig. 15-5). Indeed a fairly good rule of thumb is that vitamin E is likely to be found where there's highly unsaturated fat.

This is true, not only of our food, but of our body as well. Vitamin E is found in our cell membranes, where it confers antioxidant protection to the unsaturated fat found there (see Fig. 15-5). When there is vitamin E deficiency, the polyunsaturated fats are more easily oxidized, leading to cell damage.

Symptoms of Vitamin E deficiency have not been seen in healthy populations, even in those whose diets with little vitamin E. Deficiencies have only been seen in unusual circumstances. It can occur, for example, in cases of cystic fibrosis because of the fat malabsorption associated with the disease. Vitamin E supplements are routinely given to such at-risk groups.

Vitamin E and False Hopes

Vitamin E may well have raised more false hopes than any other micronutrient—hopes spurred both by dramatic animal experiments and by biochemical theory.

In animal experiments, vitamin E has offered promise for human difficulties ever since it solved rat infertility. E deficiency has not been shown to cause infertility for humans, nor have supplements of E been found to cure it.

In a similar way, it was seen early that vitamin E deficiencies in chicks and rabbits led to degen-

Figure 15-5: Vitamin E helps protect the unsaturated fatty acids in our bodies and in our diets.

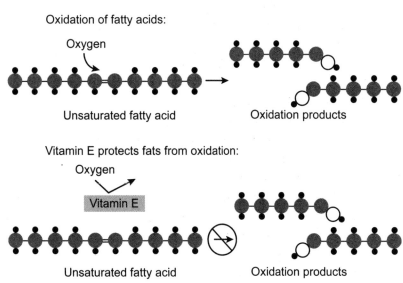

eration of the liver, and to muscular dystrophy. But vitamin E hasn't been proven to play such roles in human illness. A continuing belief that vitamin E can relieve human muscular dystrophy remains a cruel deception.

In calves, and in some other animals, a shortage of vitamin E can cause heart and blood-vessel damage, raising the hope that extra vitamin E might provide humans with extra protection against such ills. But not so, according to human studies.

In rabbits, low vitamin E intake can limit growth. Evidence that vitamin E may be involved in forming nucleic acids and in the respiration of cells has hinted that vitamin E may play some role in growth and aging. But in human tests, extra vitamin E has failed either to spur growth or to prolong cell life.

Inappropriate conclusions are still being drawn from vitamin E research. The animal studies tying vitamin E to cell growth and reproduction triggered claims for the healing of wounds and burns and the prevention of skin aging. Testimonials as to the effectiveness of vitamin E in burn healing may derive from the fact that putting fats on burns to soothe is common practice, and vitamin E ointments come in oily bases. The oil, not vitamin E, is probably what comforts.

There's certainly much to be learned still about vitamin E. But there's yet no reason to be concerned about the adequacy of the RDAs.

Many of the human studies of vitamin E supplements are in high-risk groups—people with diabetes, Alzheimer's disease, heart disease, etc. In these groups, risk is more acceptable if there's a clear benefit to their disease. The situation is far different for healthy people. When smokers, who have a higher risk of cancer and heart attacks, were given 50 mg vitamin E in one randomized study, they had 5% fewer deaths from heart attacks, but 50% more deaths from hemorrhagic stroke as compared to those not given vitamin E (and no difference in lung cancer).[3] In this light, it's not wise for even a disease-free smoker—much less a disease-free non-smoker—to take vitamin E supplements.

Vitamin E in Foods

Vitamin E is found naturally in the fatty parts of food. Vegetable oils are a particularly rich source because vitamin E is found along with polyunsaturated fats to protect them from oxidation/rancidity (see Fig. 15-5). The oils have different amounts of vitamin E, because all the tocopherols (alpha, beta, gamma, delta) protect the oil from oxidation, but only the alpha form fulfills our RDA for vitamin E.

Salad dressing is a major source of vegetable oil. Removing the oil, as in fat-free dressing, removes its vitamin E as well. But vitamin E is being added to more foods. There's even vitamin-E-fortified orange juice.

Vitamin E Toxicity

The UL for vitamin E is specifically for supplements because the popularity of massive and longterm, self-prescribed doses of vitamin E is still cause for concern. Excesses of vitamin E are relatively non-toxic, but can present problems in some cases. Large doses can, for example, interfere with vitamin K activity and thereby hamper blood-clotting. This can further increase the risk of bleeding in people who are taking medications to lessen blood-clotting, e.g., aspirin, Coumadin.

Vitamin K

In 1929, Danish biochemist Dr. Henrik Dam was studying chicks to learn how their bodies made cholesterol. A key factor in the study was a tightly controlled diet in which much of the fat was extracted from the food. Through this diet, Dam hoped to learn what raw materials the birds used to make cholesterol.

To the scientist's surprise, the chicks began to hemorrhage after they had been on the diet for as few as 10 days. And once the bleeding started, the clotting which should have stopped it was slow or almost absent.

Dam could not explain the clotting failure and suspected that it must have something to do with the narrow experimental diet—something must be missing. The characteristics of the three then-known fat-soluble vitamins (A, D, and E) did not provide an answer. Could there be a fourth fat-soluble vitamin?

In 1935, Dam reported his answer. He was certain that a fourth fat-soluble vitamin existed. He called it vitamin K, from the Danish word Koagulation. Eight years later, he shared the Nobel Prize for his discovery with American Edward Doisy, who had worked out the chemical structure of the vitamin.

Vitamin K can be made by bacteria living in the digestive tract. This protects us from deficiencies—unless the bacteria are somehow destroyed or disease interferes with the absorption of K into the blood.

Blood Clotting

To the untrained eye, blood clotting is deceptively simple. In truth, there is a chain of intricate reactions in which vitamin K and a dozen different protein factors take part.

It is fortunate that the process is complex because it is not only life-saving, but also can be life-threatening, and so requires some fail-safe controls. Obviously, the ability of the blood to form a seal and close a wound is invaluable. It is precisely the failure of this ability which can make the hereditary disorder hemophilia so deadly. Before the availability of outside sources of clotting factors, the hemophiliac faced death with every cut or bruise.

But if clotting takes place too quickly or too easily or when there is no wound to seal, clots can block a blood vessel. Such a block in a vessel leading to the brain can cause a stroke. In a vessel feeding the heart, the block can cause a classic heart attack. Or the clot can form in one vessel and travel through the circulatory system until it becomes lodged in a narrow place and does its damage.

Often the formation of such clots can be detected by physicians, along with narrowed portions of blood vessels in which clots are more likely to block the flow of blood. A common medical response when clots are discovered or considered imminent, is to give drugs which "thin" the blood (i.e., lessen its readiness to clot).

This way of dealing with unwanted clotting was discovered in 1922, when some Canadian cattle fed on spoiled clover began to hemorrhage. By 1931, it was found that the spoiled clover contained a chemical known as coumarin, which interferes with vitamin K action, thereby inhibiting the clotting process. Today, coumarin (Coumadin) is commonly used to treat patients whose blood needs "thinning." Conversely, vitamin K can serve as an antidote when there is an overdose of coumarin.

We are reminded that "the dose makes the poison" when we consider that a large dose of coumarin is used as a rat poison—the rats bleed to death.

What happens in the clotting process? Any child who has ever fallen and skinned a knee knows that very soon the blood coming from the scrape will stop flowing. It will form a red "scab," creating an illusion that it is the red stuff of blood which clots. Not so.

The substances used for clotting are in the plasma of the blood. This is a rather clear, yellowish liquid, about 90% water, which is both protein-rich and also holds slightly less than 1% of its weight in

Figure 15-6: Vitamin K and calcium are needed for blood clotting.

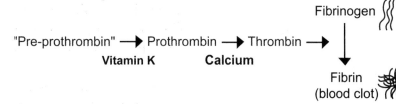

certain minerals, including calcium. The clotting agent in plasma is a dissolved protein called fibrinogen—meaning loosely, "fiber-making."

The usefulness of plasma for much more than just acting as a liquid carrier of blood cells is evident from the fact that plasma alone is sometimes used to replace blood lost in wounds, shock, and surgery.

What happens in clotting is that fibrinogen is converted to a substance called fibrin, which forms a tangled web of fiber-like molecules. The web traps blood cells and proteins, and creates the clot.

The mysteries of clotting and of vitamin K lie in how the conversion from fibrinogen to fibrin takes place. The process involves a complicated series of reactions. As shown in the diagram of one small segment of the clotting process (see Fig. 15-6), calcium and vitamin K are needed in the chemical reactions that form thrombin, the enzyme that catalyzes the crucial reaction in which the blood clot (fibrin) is formed.

Other roles of vitamin K have since been discovered. Indeed, we now know that vitamin K plays certain previously unsuspected roles in very basic life chemistry. For example, it's needed for the synthesis of the bone protein osteocalcin (see Fig. 15-7) and is essential to photosynthesis in plant cells.

Vitamin K Sources and Requirements

The fact that plant cells require vitamin K in using sunlight to store energy and make food suggests the fact that green leafy vegetables are good sources. In general, the greener the leaf, the more vitamin K. The outer, greener leaves of plants may have several times as much K as the inner, paler leaves. There are other vegetables which are

not so green that also have good amounts—among them cauliflower and cabbage.

Certain oils, especially that of soybeans, are sources. But most meats, legumes, grains, and fruits have little vitamin K. Liver is a good source, because animals store it there. Egg yolk is another good source.

There are RDAs for vitamin K, but intestinal bacteria produce amounts that can lessen or make unnecessary a dietary source. Since vitamin K deficiency is unusual, apparently the bacteria make sufficient amounts.

One dietary source of vitamin K is food which has begun to putrify through bacterial action.

The importance of the bacterial source is confirmed by the fact that deficiencies can occur when antibiotics kill intestinal bacteria or when there are none to begin with—as at birth. Newborns in the U.S. are, in fact, routinely given an injection of vitamin K for this very reason.

Overview of the Vitamins

Our review of the vitamins leads us to two broad and rather paradoxical conclusions. One is that we have a lot to learn about these nutrients. And the other is that we already know a lot.

It's important to understand both of these facts, because they help explain the false premises so often exploited by both the naive and the unscrupulous, and especially by those who market vitamins as medicine. In general, it's well to remember, vitamins relieve only those physical ills which are caused by shortages of vitamins.

Thus, the question of what constitutes vitamin adequacy, and what levels of intake may be considered inadequate (and thus causative of ill health) is central. When dealing with this question, our knowledge is imperfect, but it is also considerable.

It's worth noting that, overall, with each step toward greater knowledge, with each reconsidera-

Figure 15-7: Key Functions of Vitamins.

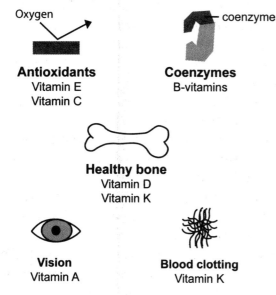

tion of the RDAs, the trend has been toward confidence in setting lower—not higher—intakes, as we refine our understanding of the biochemical functions of vitamins. And with each such refinement toward smaller and surer estimations of adequacy, the proofs grow steadily clearer that vitamins, in our society, are rarely the answer to diseases.

To say this is not at all to refute the importance of vitamins in life chemistry. It is not in any way to deny the appalling effects of narrow, limited diets, especially in the poorer nations.

But in our society, what we know about the limits to vitamin usefulness can spur healthy skepticism when it is implied that large doses of vitamins can prevent loss of hair, cancer, heart disease, or emotional disturbance. It reminds us that, unless vitamin shortages can be plainly and biochemically defined, magical claims for their benefits are illusions, not realities. And realities are the business of nutrition science.

Analogous in many ways to realities of the vitamins, are those of the second family of micronutrients, the minerals. Let us see how, and why.

Summary

There are four fat-soluble vitamins—vitamins A, D, E, and K. Vitamin A is found naturally only in animal foods. Plants provide carotenoids, some of which can be converted to vitamin A in the body (e.g., beta-carotene).

Vitamin A is critical for night vision. It's part of a chemical found in the eye called rhodopsin. When light strikes rhodopsin, vitamin A is released, causing an impulse to be sent along the optic nerve. Vitamin A must then be replaced in rhodopsin for the process to occur again. If there isn't enough available, the impulses slow down and vision is impaired.

Vitamin A also maintains epithelial tissues (e.g., the outermost layer of the skin and the lining of the nose, lungs, and digestive tract), allowing them to secrete substances. Without this ability, we are more susceptible to infection. The epithelium of the eye, for example, needs vitamin A, and when there is a deficiency, eye tissue begins to dry out, causing a condition called xeropthalmia. The eye is then susceptible to infection, which can lead to blindness.

Animal products such as liver are rich sources of vitamin A. Excesses of vitamin E, commonly the result of regular supplementation, can be toxic. Large doses are especially dangerous to the fetus, causing malformations.

Yellow-orange and dark green plants provide us with pro-vitamin-A carotenoids, which aren't toxic. The body doesn't convert them to vitamin A in excessive amounts. Carotenoids can also act as antioxidants, and foods rich in them may be protective against cancer. A normal diet can supply all the body can use. In some developing countries, however, vitamin A deficiency is a serious problem, causing blindness and many deaths from infections.

Some vitamin A analogs (laboratory-produced drugs that resemble vitamin A, but do not have vitamin activity) are used by physicians to treat conditions such as severe acne and to prevent the recurrence of head and neck cancers.

Vitamin D deficiency is associated with rickets, a form of osteomalacia, which results in bone softening and skeletal defects. We get vitamin D from our diet and from exposure to sun. A cholesterol precursor in the skin is changed by ultraviolet light to inactive vitamin D, and moves to the blood.

The inactive vitamin D from the skin (or the diet) must then be chemically changed both in the liver and the kidney, becoming "activated vitamin D." Activated vitamin D helps calcium and phosphorus to be absorbed in the intestine, and controls their use in bone and tooth formation.

Vitamin D requirements depend on sun exposure and skin pigment; many foods are fortified, and rickets and osteomalacia are rare for Americans. But it's relatively easy to overdo consumption of vitamin D to toxic levels. Toxicity is usually from supplements; toxic levels aren't reached by sun exposure alone.

Vitamin E works mainly as an antioxidant, preventing the oxidation of fats in various body tissues. It also prevents the oxidation of the fats in plants; therefore, plant oils are a good source of vitamin E. Vitamin E in large doses is relatively non-toxic. However, many people regularly take doses of vitamin E that far exceed the RDA and far exceed the amounts found naturally in food. The upper limit (UL) only applies to vitamin E supplements, and not the amounts found naturally in foods.

Vitamin K is provided in our diet, particularly by green leafy vegetables, but is also made by our own intestinal bacteria, and, thus, deficiency is rare. Vitamin K is critical for normal blood clotting. Clotting involves a series of chemical reactions, requiring both calcium and vitamin K.

With respect to all vitamins, it's important to stress that they aren't cures for diseases, unless the disease stems from a deficiency. It's also important to remember that results of animal studies don't necessarily apply to humans.

Chapter 16

The Major Minerals

For most of us, the word mineral *hardly brings to mind food. Minerals mean ore and mining, mineral-rich countries, metallic substances. We may have heard the word grouped in a dietetic-like way, as in getting lots of vitamins and minerals, but surely that's not the same thing as the minerals that miners mine and armies fight over.*

There's nothing very metallic about the human body. (Even the Tin Woodman had his parts added by a metalsmith—and there's no mention of the dietary fare in Oz.) In general we seem to get along quite well thinking very little about particular minerals in our diet. Can we run into trouble if we just ignore them? Are they really necessary?

As we shall see, some minerals are plentiful in a wide variety of foods, and deficiencies are rare. Others, however, are not so widely available, and shortages (and in some cases excesses) can be devastating for certain population groups

As used in human nutrition, the definition of the term *mineral* is a hangover from 19th century chemistry, when, on the burning of plant or animal materials, the residual ash was considered the mineral matter. It was first looked upon as a kind of single food factor—as *the* protein and *the* vitamins were once seen. In everyday terms, a mineral is anything which is not vegetable or animal; but in biological terms, a mineral is surely part of both.

A broad definition of a mineral as a nutrient would be: *An inorganic substance which is essential in small quantities for life processes.* (*Inorganic*, in chemistry, refers to matter which isn't constructed with a carbon skeleton.) What we are really discussing here are the needs for some special atoms for making essential life structures and chemicals.

Minerals and Vitamins Compared

Much of what's been said about vitamins may also be said about minerals. With a few rare exceptions, all the minerals needed by the body can be found in an ordinary, varied diet. In a similar way, they perform crucial bodily functions, and mineral excesses, carried far enough, can be toxic.

Carbohydrates, fat, protein, and vitamins are all organic—they all have a carbon-based chemical structure.

But minerals do differ from vitamins in some striking ways. For one, minerals aren't destroyed by burning. As has been noted, when food is burned, minerals form the ash left behind. The adult body contains several pounds of minerals— a fact confirmed by the ashes left after cremation (see Fig. 16-1).

Our mineral content, therefore, is measured in pounds, whereas our vitamin content is measured in ounces. As might be expected, some minerals are required in much larger amounts than any of the vitamins.

Calcium, phosphorus, magnesium (the three found mostly in bone), and the electrolytes sodium, potassium, and chloride are called the *major*

minerals, and are the subject of this chapter. The adult recommended intake for each of these minerals is more than 300 mg per day(see Appendix A).

The other minerals, called the *trace minerals,* will be discussed in the next chapter. The adult recommended intake for these minerals (except for the pregnancy recommendation of 27 mg iron) is less than 20 mg per day.

Calcium

Almost everyone knows that calcium—the most abundant body mineral—is a basic component of bones and teeth. (The dairy people hardly let us forget.) But most of us tend to liken the human skeleton to the steel framework of a building—solid, fixed, and constructed but once in the original building process. Actually, our bones are constantly changing and interacting with the rest of the body.

Bone is well supplied with blood, and minerals constantly move in and out of bone throughout the lifespan. Furthermore, certain bones contain red marrow, which makes red and white blood cells. Our skeleton is very much alive.

In addition to its functions of support, protection, movement, and blood-cell production, bone serves as a mineral reservoir—about 99% of the body's calcium, 85% of the body's phosphorus, and 60% of the body's magnesium are found in bone. These minerals are crucial to body chemistry. Without calcium, blood can't clot, muscles can't contract, and nerve cells can't send their messages. Phosphorus is a key component of ATP (the energy molecule), and magnesium is needed to regenerate ATP.

Calcium, phosphorus, and magnesium are needed in only tiny amounts for these purposes, but their presence is crucial, and the body is wisely constructed in a way that insures that it never runs out. Whenever there's a demand to fill the needs for body chemistry, bone minerals are readily mobilized to make up for any shortfall.

Calcium levels are kept quite constant in the blood. Whenever blood calcium rises, one hormone (calcitonin) takes calcium out of the blood

Figure 16-1: Minerals in a 130-Pound Adult: Major minerals and the most common trace minerals.

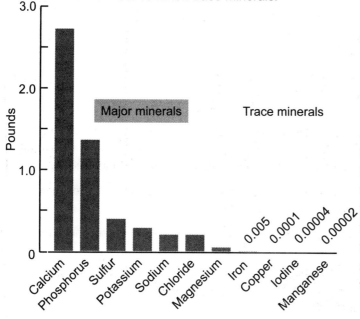

and deposits it in bone; whenever blood calcium falls, another hormone (parathormone) draws calcium out of bone (see Fig. 16-2).

Problems occur when the blood-calcium level gets outside of its narrow range. For example, nerve cells become more easily excitable with an abnormal drop in blood calcium. This can result in *tetany,* where there's such a rapid stimulation of muscle nerves that the muscle cramps or "freezes" in contraction.

Some popular health books falsely attribute tetany to a deficiency of calcium in the diet. We're easily convinced of this if we're under the illusion that 99% of body calcium is immutably locked in the skeleton. In fact, dietary calcium doesn't ordinarily alter blood-calcium levels.

Disturbances in blood calcium come from disturbances in the levels either of vitamin D, or of one of the hormones that regulate the movement of calcium in and out of bone. (We saw in the last chapter that calcium and vitamin D are closely intertwined, and that a deficiency of either can cause the bone diseases rickets and osteomalacia.)

Over the long run, we can't wisely continue to borrow from bone more calcium than we deposit. There will be an over-all loss of calcium, and eventually bone health will be compromised. The object of good nutrition is to provide enough calcium for strong bones, and of course to supply

proportionately larger amounts to children and adolescents, whose skeletons are growing. For similar reasons, pregnant or nursing mothers also have greater calcium needs.

Calcium in Foods

The main source of calcium in the American diet is milk and foods made with milk. Milk is a particularly good source— the vitamin D, protein, and lactose in the milk promote the absorption of calcium. In the U.S., calcium intake generally is related to the amount of milk or milk products in the diet. (Dark, leafy, green vegetables are a source of calcium in this country for those who don't drink much milk.)

Calcium-fortified foods (foods with calcium added) are an increasingly popular source of calcium, and include calcium-fortified orange juice and calcium-fortified soy milk.

Some foods eaten more commonly in other cultures contain a fair amount of calcium. Traditional Mexican corn tortillas are rich in calcium. Corn itself isn't rich in calcium, but the corn is soaked in lime water (a solution of calcium oxide) before being ground to make the tortillas. (This calcium-fortified cornmeal is called *masa harina.*)

The calcium-rich antlers of deer shed onto the forest floor provide dietary calcium for small animals.

Soybean curd (*tofu*) is also made rich in calcium by processing in a calcium-rich solution. Sesame seeds are rich in calcium, and a paste of ground sesame seeds is the main ingredient in *halvah,* a Turkish confection. Fish bones (as in canned sardines and salmon) and fish sauce *(bagoong)* also provide calcium.

When animals (including humans) need a lot of calcium but must subsist on foods that are low in calcium, they must eat tremendous amounts. Cows spend virtually all their waking hours munching on grass or hay.

The amount of dietary calcium absorbed from the intestine varies, depending on a number of factors. Spinach is rich in calcium, magnesium,

Table 16-1: Minerals

Mineral	Function	Source	Deficiency	Possible Toxicity
Calcium	Bone and teeth structure, muscle and nerve function	Milk, milk products, sardines, collard greens, calcium-set tofu, masa harina	Stunted growth, osteoporosis	Kidney stones
Phosphorus	Bone and teeth formation, energy production	Meat, fish, milk, eggs, legumes, cereals, nuts, soft drinks	Irritability, weakness, muscle ache	Poor bone mineralization if low calcium intake
Magnesium	Cofactor in metabolism	Green leafy veggies, whole grains, nuts, legumes, shrimp, broccoli, seeds, milk	Weakness, muscle pain, cramps, spasms	Diarrhea, nausea, abnormally slow heartbeat, weakened reflexes
Sodium	Water balance	Salt, soy sauce, fast foods, processed foods	Weakness, cramps	High blood pressure
Chloride	Fluid balance, stomach acid	Salt, soy sauce, processed foods	Rare; upset acid-base balance	High blood pressure
Potassium	Nerve function	Dried fruits, winter squash, legumes, potatoes, spinach, tomatoes, citrus fruits	Weakness, irregular heartbeat	Irregular heartbeat

and iron, but also contains a lot of oxalic acid, a substance that can bind to these minerals and hinder their absorption. In contrast, as discussed in the previous chapter, vitamin D promotes calcium absorption.

The rate of calcium absorption improves as the body adapts to a lower calcium diet over a long period, and also in times of higher need (e.g., during early childhood, pregnancy, and lactation). On the other hand, absorption is diminished in the elderly. This variability in calcium absorption is taken into consideration in setting the recommended intake.

It's important to get enough calcium, particularly during childhood, adolescence, and early adulthood when bone is growing and increasing in calcium content. The recommended intake for calcium is the same for both sexes, but males generally meet the recommendation, whereas females 11 years and older generally don't.

Girls and women drink less milk, and eat less food than males the same age. The more food we eat, the more nutrients we take in.

In population studies, adequate calcium intake is associated with a lower risk of colon cancer and high blood pressure.

Calcium Supplements

Different calcium supplements contain varying amounts of calcium. Calcium carbonate is the most concentrated form (40% calcium). Calcium citrate is 21% calcium; calcium lactate is 13%; calcium gluconate is 9%. Also, to be effective, the supplement must dissolves easily in the acid fluid of the stomach.

Some brands of supplements don't dissolve as they should in the stomach. Put a tablet into a half-glass of vinegar at room temperature, and stir vigorously every 5 minutes. If the tablet isn't completely dissolved in 30 minutes or less, try another brand.

Taking supplements of ground-up dolomite (a natural rock rich in calcium) or bone ("bone meal") isn't advised—they might be contaminated with lead or other toxic elements. Look for calcium supplements having a USP (United States Pharmacopeia) seal of approval.

Calcium supplements are better absorbed when taken with a meal, and in doses of 500 mg or less. Calcium supplements can increase total calcium intake far beyond recommended amounts. Excessive calcium can interfere with the absorption of other essential minerals.

Figure 16-2: *Calcium moves between blood and bone.* The amount of calcium in blood is kept steady by hormones (calcitonin and parathormone), which move calcium in and out of bone.

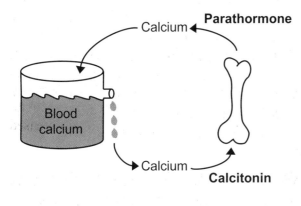

Osteoporosis

Osteoporosis literally means *porous bones.* The interior of bone is normally porous (styrofoam-like), but the size of the pores increase (become lace-like) as bone minerals—mainly calcium—are lost (see Fig. 16-3). Osteoporosis is the condition in which bones become so porous and brittle that they (especially the bones of the wrist, spine, and hip) are easily fractured. These fractures can lead to severe pain and disability. Osteoporosis is especially common in white, thin, elderly women.

After age 50, wrist fractures become more common, usually from extending the arm to break a fall. While wrist fractures aren't usually serious, they can indicate underlying osteoporosis. Fractures of the spinal vertebrae, which tend to occur after about 55, are often painless, though some people suffer severe pain and disability. The outward signs of these fractures are a loss of height and the stoop of old age—often called "dowager's hump" (see Fig. 16-4).

Fractures of the hip are the most serious and are most common among women over age 70. Many of these women either die from complications, or are so disabled that they can no longer live independently.

A key factor in the development of osteoporosis is the density (calcium content) of bone in early adulthood. The higher the *bone density* at its peak, the less likely that osteoporosis will occur later (see Fig. 16-5).

Figure 16-3: Dense vs. Porous Bone.

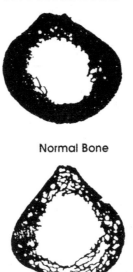

Normal Bone

Osteoporotic Bone

At comparable ages, osteoporosis is more common among women than men, and more common among whites than blacks. The increased susceptibility of women and whites can be explained by their lower peak bone density and increased longevity, compared to men and blacks. Women also have increased risk because of about 5 years of accelerated bone loss that begins at menopause. Estrogen has a protective effect on bone, and estrogen production by the ovaries falls after menopause.

Although osteoporosis can be detected to some extent by taking note of losses in a person's height, osteoporosis usually is brought to medical attention by a bone fracture. A puzzling aspect of osteoporosis is that the amount of bone loss doesn't necessarily correlate with the amount of pain or disability that a person suffers. One person may have compression fractures of the vertebrae and severe loss of bone density yet not suffer pain or disability, while another person may have much less bone loss and experience debilitating pain.

Osteoporosis has been a hard disease to study because most of the studies of changes in bone mass compare people of different ages within a population rather than following the same people as they age (which gives better information).

Another complicating factor is that bone is not lost evenly throughout the skeleton or even throughout a single bone. Certain bones are often studied because of convenience, cost, etc. The heel bone may be easier to study than the spine, but what one sees in the heel may not be indicative of what's happening in the bones of the spine or hip.

In other words, much of what is known about the development of osteoporosis is still rather tentative. Osteoporosis is a very active area of research, and more sophisticated methods of

Figure 16-4: Osteoporosis often results in a loss of height and a misshapen body.

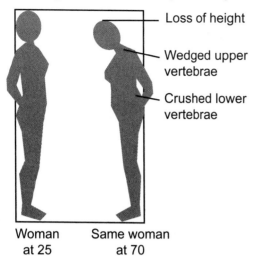

Loss of height

Wedged upper vertebrae

Crushed lower vertebrae

Woman   Same woman
at 25   at 70

measuring bone loss, e.g., CAT (computerized axial tomography) scans and DEXA (dual energy x-ray absorptiometry), are now providing better information. DEXA is also used as a screening test to identify people with or at high risk of osteoporosis.

Risk Factors

Looking at all the advertisements for calcium supplements, one would think that osteoporosis was simply caused by a deficiency of calcium in the diet. In fact, osteoporosis is a very complex disease brought about by an interplay of many factors (see Table 16-2). Some of these are:

Gender: As said earlier, women are at higher risk. They have smaller bones, their bones are less dense at their peak, their rate of bone loss accelerates at menopause, and they live longer than men. Both the male hormone *testosterone* and the female hormone *estrogen* help preserve bone mass. Whereas there's a rapid fall in estrogen for women at menopause, aging men have a small and gradual fall in testosterone. In addition, men's estrogen levels increase with advancing age. (These hormonal changes in men may contribute to their "mellowing" as they age.)

Family history: Having a close relative (e.g., parent, grandmother) with osteoporosis increases risk. Genes not only influence bone density but also bone size. Small-boned women have less

bone to lose. (Also, of course, families share food and exercise habits.)

Race: Osteoporosis is more common among whites, asians, and hispanics than among blacks, presumably because of racial differences in bone density. At comparable ages, blacks have higher bone density (even though their calcium intake is lower), and, as a result, black women have about half the number of hip fractures of white women. Women who have very light skin (e.g., those with naturally blond or red hair) have an increased risk.

Physical activity: Normal physical activity preserves bone mass, whereas prolonged bed rest results in marked bone loss. The importance of stress on bone is most dramatically demonstrated by astronauts' rapid bone loss during space travel, when they escape the pull of gravity.

The greatest effect of physical activity on bone mass occurs in the range of minimal to normal physical activity. In addition, moderate, stress-bearing exercise is helpful. As with muscles, the effects are very specific. Bone density is higher (and the muscles larger) in the playing arm of a tennis player than in the other arm.

Also, we sometimes need to be reminded that "getting exercise" doesn't necessarily mean we have to take up a sport or "work out." Such activities as vigorously scrubbing the bathroom or using a manual lawn mower also provide good exercise. A caveat: premenopausal women who engage in strenuous exercise to the point of *amenorrhea* (stoppage of menstruation) can lose bone mass. Amenorrhea has some of the same characteristics as menopause.

Body weight: Osteoporosis is less common among those who are overweight, perhaps because carrying extra weight puts more stress on bones (and extra body fat provides more cushioning for the bone in a fall). Also, because fat cells make some estrogen, they become an important source when ovary-produced estrogen falls after menopause. Among premenopausal women, extreme thinness to the point of amenorrhea (many ballerinas and women with anorexia nervosa have this problem) can result in losses of bone mass.

Smoking: Smoking appears to increase the risk of osteoporosis for both men and women. The reason for this isn't entirely clear, but women who smoke tend to have an earlier onset of menopause (by about 5 years). This results in accelerated bone loss at an earlier age. Also, smokers tend to weigh less than non-smokers. As noted earlier, a heavier body weight and more fat tissue can offer some protection against osteoporosis.

Alcohol: Osteoporosis is more common among alcoholics, presumably because they tend to have poor diets that are deficient in calcium and other nutrients, and because excessive alcohol can lessen the absorption of nutrients by damaging the intestinal lining. Also, excessive alcohol consumption increases the risk of falling, and consequently the risk of fractures.

Dietary calcium: Dietary calcium does play a role in osteoporosis, but its role isn't as large as advertisements for supplements would have you believe. It's important, of course, to meet your dietary requirement. The advertisements and magazine articles encouraging calcium intake are mostly directed at women, but young girls should be the focus.

Beginning at about age 11, girls' average intake of calcium falls below recommended levels—and persists for females at every age thereafter. Adequate calcium intake during childhood and young adulthood is crucial for obtaining a high peak bone mass. Of special concern are growing girls who are thin, small boned, sedentary, fair-skinned, continually dieting, and who consume very little milk or milk products.

Other nutrients: Various other nutrients can potentially affect risk of osteoporosis, mainly through their effect on calcium absorption and losses. We saw in the previous chapter, the important role of Vitamin D. High amounts of sodium and protein can increase the loss of calcium in the urine, but its effect on the risk of osteoporosis hasn't been established.

Prevention

As can be seen from the discussion of risk factors, the best that children, adolescents, and adults

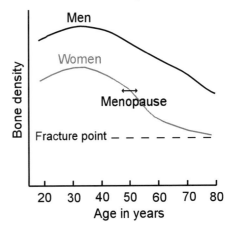

Figure 16-5: Peak bone density is a crucial factor in the risk of osteoporosis.

can do to prevent osteoporosis is to eat a good diet, get a moderate amount of stress-bearing exercise, and not smoke.

Preventive therapies to retard bone loss for post-menopausal women include estrogen-replacement therapy beginning at the start of menopause. Studies have shown that when estrogen therapy is begun at menopause, the number of hip and wrist fractures is about half that of comparable women who aren't given estrogen. Not all women are suitable for this therapy, including those who are many years past menopause and have already lost a lot of bone, women who have had breast cancer, and women with certain health problems such as liver disease or very high blood pressure.

As with all medications, there's concern about possible side-effects of estrogen-replacement therapy, a major concern being estrogen-related cancers. Estrogen used to be given alone, and this was found to increase the risk of cancer in the lining of the uterus (endometrial cancer). Now, estrogen is given together with another hormone (progestin) that greatly reduces—and possibly eliminates—the risk of this cancer.

In the Women's Health Initiative study, more than 16,000 postmenopausal women ages 50-79 were randomized into estrogen-progestin and placebo groups. In the 5.2-year average follow-up, the estrogen-progestin group had fewer bone fractures and fewer colon and rectal cancers, but more breast cancer, heart disease, and stroke.[1]

As a result of this study, many women on hormone replacement therapy stopped abruptly.

Table 16-2: Factors Associated with Bone Maintenance vs. Bone Loss.

Maintenance	Loss
Normal menses	Lack of menses
Estrogen replacement	Early menopause
Black race	Alcoholism
Physical activity	Cigarette smoking
Dietary calcium	Slender figure
Heavy body weight	Bed rest (months)
	Anorexia nervosa

Instead, many women are taking bisphosphonates (e.g., Fosamax) to prevent osteoporosis. Bisphosphonates retard bone loss, but like all medications, they have side-effects.[2,3]

Phosphorus

Phosphorus—the second most abundant body mineral—is found mainly in teeth and bones, and is closely associated with calcium in the building of these tough structures. About 85% of the body's phosphorus is in bone. The rest can be found throughout the body in phospholipids (recall that phospholipids make up cell membranes), and in such important molecules as DNA, RNA, and ATP (see Fig. 16-6).

The recommended intake for phosphorus is less than for calcium, but our diets tend to be much richer in phosphorus than calcium. Phosphorus is widespread in foods. Meat, milk, fish, grains, and nuts are rich sources.

A phosphorus deficiency is unlikely under ordinary circumstances. In a general way, almost every good source of calcium is also a good source of phosphorus. However, many calcium-poor foods are phosphorus-rich—for example, meat and cereal. Even diet soft drinks can contain a fair amount. As a component of many food additives, generous amounts of phosphorus can also be found in many processed foods.

Phosphorus deficiency has been found in premature infants fed only breast milk. Breast milk has enough phosphorus for a full-term infant, but not enough for a premature infant. Thus, supplemental phosphorus may be needed for

Figure 16-6: Phosphorus is found in bones, teeth, phospholipids, DNA, RNA and ATP.

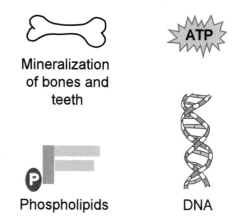

Mineralization of bones and teeth

ATP

Phospholipids

DNA

these infants to prevent inadequate mineralization of bone (rickets).

Phosphorus deficiencies have also resulted from the prolonged use of aluminum hydroxide as an antacid. Aluminum hydroxide can combine with dietary phosphorus and prevent its absorption from the intestine. A phosphorus deficiency can result in bone loss, weakness, and pain.

Phosphorus intakes can be high when people drink large amounts of phosphorus-containing soft drinks, like colas. Excessive amounts of phosphorus reduces calcium absorption from the diet. Of special concern are youngsters with diets that are both high in phosphorus and low in calcium. Studies with young animals show that such a diet promotes bone loss.

Magnesium

About 60% of body magnesium is found in bone. The rest has a wide involvement in body chemistry. Magnesium is needed in over 300 enzyme systems, and plays a vital role in such basic functions as maintenance of our nerve and muscle cells. Magnesium is crucial to plant life as well. It's a part of chlorophyll, the dark green pigment of photosynthesis.

Magnesium is easily available from a wide variety of foods. The richest sources are vegetables and whole grains. It's found in varied amounts in all unprocessed food.

Magnesium deficiency is uncommon, but can occur in cases of severe malnutrition or certain

Figure 16-7: Factors that affect mineral absorption from the intestine.

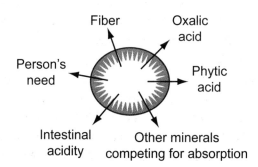

diseases (e.g., intestinal diseases that interfere with magnesium absorption). Deficiency symptoms include weakness, irritability, nausea, irregular heartbeats, and mental derangement.

A high intake of magnesium from food isn't thought to be harmful, except when kidney disease interferes with the excretion of the excess through the urine. Toxic levels of magnesium usually are brought on by magnesium-containing drugs rather than diet. Toxicity symptoms include nausea, an abnormally slow heartbeat, and weakened reflexes.

Electrolytes: Sodium, Chloride and Potassium

As we saw in Chapter 12, bodily fluids are mainly water, and substances change when dissolved in water. Sodium, potassium, and chloride are called *electrolytes* because when they dissolve in water, their salts separate into **charged particles (ions)** that can conduct an electrical current. For example, common table salt—sodium chloride—separates into positively charged sodium ions and negatively charged chloride ions.

The electrical charges of ions along the cell membrane serve as ways to transmit electrical impulses within the nervous system, and from nerves to muscles, to cause contraction and relaxation.

About 60% of body water is found inside our cells *(intracellular water)*. Here the water is rich in potassium. Outside and surrounding each cell is *extracellular water* (which includes blood plasma). Its main minerals are sodium and chloride (see Fig. 16-9).

Intracellular and extracellular waters are divided by the cell membrane. As the ions move across this membrane, they take the surrounding water along with them; or water will move toward a higher ion concentration inside or outside cells.

The ions serve to regulate the amount of water inside and outside of cells. We see how this works when we sprinkle salt (sodium chloride) on sliced cucumbers or cabbage to draw out water from the plant cells—or when we salt the garden slug and watch it "melt" as its water is drawn out.

Sodium

Most of our sodium comes as sodium chloride (ordinary table salt). We're warned so often of the hazard of excessive salt intake that we tend to forget that sodium is an essential nutrient.

Table salt is 40% sodium and 60% chloride. One teaspoonful has about 2,000 mg of sodium.

Our desire for salt and its importance to us are reflected in our everyday vocabulary—such words as *salary* [from the Latin *salarium*, meaning *money for salt* (given as a part of a Roman soldier's pay)], and descriptive phrases such as "above the salt" (*an honored position*), "salt of the earth" (*fine, noble*), and "worth one's salt" (*worth one's wages*).

In ancient times, people sought out salt deposits and settled near them. Inland from the salty sea, salt was a precious commodity.

Today, of course, salt is widely available and widely used. An Adequate Intake (AI) [see Dietary Reference Intake (DRI) in Chap. 18] is 1500 mg sodium (the amount in ¾ teaspoon of salt) for adults under age 50, 1300 mg for ages 50-70, and 1200 mg for those over age 70.[4]

These amounts are much higher than minimum requirements (less than 180 mg) because it would be hard to meet other nutrient requirements on a diet that low in sodium. Also, the Adequate Intake amounts are inadequate for people who sweat heavily, e.g., competitive athletes, manual laborers in hot weather.

The DRI gives 2300 mg as an upper limit[3]—the amount we should aim to stay below. The usual

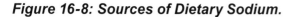

Figure 16-8: Sources of Dietary Sodium.

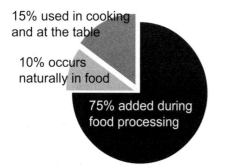

15% used in cooking and at the table

10% occurs naturally in food

75% added during food processing

daily intake in the U.S. ranges from about 2,000 to 6,000 mg, so the sodium in our diet is clearly excessive.

The main concern with excessive sodium intake is its relation to high blood pressure (as was discussed in Chap. 9). High blood pressure increases the risk of cardiovascular disease and kidney disease.

On average, blood pressure goes up as sodium intake goes up. But there's a lot of variation here. African-Americans, older people, and people with high blood pressure, diabetes, and kidney disease are more likely to be affected, and there's also a genetic component. Even among people with normal blood pressure, a lower sodium diet helps prevent the increases in blood pressure that occurs with aging.

As has been the case in discussing many nutrients, it's hard to evaluate the effects of excessive sodium in isolation. Excessive sodium doesn't affect blood pressure as much if the diet is low in fat and meets the recommended intake of calcium and potassium. Other factors like excess body weight raises blood pressure. To complicate the picture further, people who eat a lot of processed food and fast food tend to have diets high in sodium and fat, and low in calcium and potassium—and they tend to be overweight.

The bottom line is that we should all try to lower our salt intake (read food labels!) to below the upper limit of 2300 mg. Even if our blood pressure isn't salt-sensitive (most of us don't know whether it is or not), we probably cook for, or eat with, people whose blood pressure is affected.

Of course, this is easier said than done. Salt is tasty and cheap, helps preserve food, and is calorie-free. Also, high blood pressure itself doesn't normally make you feel bad.

Although foods in their natural state contain some sodium, most of the sodium in our diet comes from salt added during food processing (including food served at fast-food restaurants) (see Fig. 16-8). Salt added in processing was important when there were few ways to preserve food.

Today, with refrigerators and freezers in common use, there isn't the same need for processing meats with salts (as in ham, frankfurters, luncheon meats, etc.), storing vegetables in brine (as in pickles and kim chee), and making salty hard cheeses. But these foods are still popular for their taste and convenience.

Then there are the more obvious snack foods with added salt—chips, nuts, pretzels, crackers, and the like. Add to this the salted water often used to cook pasta or rice, the salt in most recipes, whether it be for ordinary bread, a casserole, or chocolate chip cookies, and the salt in such sauces as soy sauce, steak sauce, fish sauce, and mustard. It's no surprise that we get more than enough sodium in our diet. There are other sources of sodium—MSG (monosodium glutamate, the flavor enhancer), baking soda (sodium bicarbonate), etc.—but these are relatively minor sources, except for those on severely restricted sodium diets.

1 oz cheddar cheese: 174 mg sodium[5]
1 oz low-sodium cheddar cheese: 6 mg sodium
1 cup unsalted frozen or fresh peas: 7 mg sodium
Burger King Whopper® with Cheese: 1450 mg
BK Tendercrisp™ Chicken Garden Salad: 1080 mg

Sodium is readily absorbed from the digestive: tract. The amount of sodium kept in the body is controlled in the kidney; the urine carries little sodium when it's scarce, but excretes the excess when levels are high.

The role of the kidney in sodium balance is dramatized by patients with kidney diseases that interfere with the removal of excess sodium. Their faces, legs, and feet become swollen because the excess sodium in their tissues causes excess water to be retained (edema).

The main route of sodium loss is through urination. As was discussed in the chapter on water (Chap. 12), excess salt intake increases urine. When we eat a lot of salty foods, we feel thirsty, drink more, and urinate more.

Sodium is also lost in perspiration, the amount varying according to climate and physical activity. As was also discussed in Chapter 12, the amount of sodium and other minerals lost in perspiration is quite minimal under normal circumstances. Also, the body adapts to regular, heavy sweating. The sweat of a trained athlete contains less sodium and other electrolytes than that of an untrained person. But in the extreme situation of endurance events of 4 hours or more, athletes are advised to consume sodium-containing drinks during the event.

Sodium deficiency can occur as a result of heavy and prolonged sweating, prolonged vomiting or diarrhea, and as a result of certain kidney diseases. Sodium deficiency symptoms include muscle cramps, dizziness, and nausea. As is true of required nutrients generally, deficiencies can be fatal if severe enough.

Chloride

We hear much less of chloride, the companion to sodium in table salt. In addition to its bodily role in water regulation and nerve function, chloride is also a component of stomach acid (hydrochloric acid), which plays an important role in digestion and absorption (see Chap. 10),

As we might suppose, we get plenty of chloride in our diet, because our diet is so salty. The marriage of sodium and chloride as salt is functionally important. The chloride component intensifies the salty taste of sodium,[6] and is also thought to contribute to salt-sensitive high blood pressure. But chloride's separate effect on blood pressure is difficult to pinpoint—a diet high in chloride usually means one high in sodium as well.

A dietary deficiency of chloride has been found only in cases of infants fed exclusively a commercial infant formula deficient in chloride.

Sodium and chloride parallel each other in other ways. A chloride deficiency is uncommon. When it does occur, it's usually in conjunction with large losses of sodium—as in instances of heavy and prolonged sweating, prolonged vomiting or diarrhea, and certain kidney diseases. Since

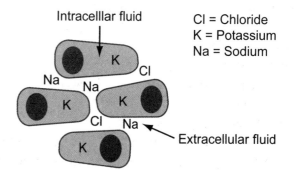

Figure 16-9: Electrolytes sodium and chloride are in fluids outside of cells; potassium is in fluids within cells.

sodium and chloride parallel each other in intake and loss, their deficiency symptoms are similar.

Potassium

Potassium shares many functions with sodium and chloride, except potassium predominates in intracellular fluid, whereas sodium and chloride predominate in extracellular fluid. Potassium thus regulates the amount of fluid within cells, and also participates in cell metabolism. Potassium is particularly noted for its role in conducting electrical impulses—especially in the heart. Either a deficiency or an excess of potassium can disturb the rhythm of the heart beat.

Potassium is an essential part of all living cells—both animal and plant. Since potassium is found in the intracellular water, more water in the cell (as when there's less fat in the cell) means more potassium. So it is that lean cuts of meat contain more potassium than fatty cuts—and fruits and vegetables are especially rich in potassium.

Although a high sodium intake is seen as the main culprit in salt-sensitive high blood pressure, a diet rich in potassium is thought to have a protective effect. It may be a matter of combination: a low potassium diet (one sparse in fruits and vegetables) is often a high-salt diet.

Like sodium and chloride, potassium is readily absorbed from the intestine, and its main route of excretion is the urine. Potassium deficiencies great enough to cause symptoms are unusual. Deficiency symptoms include loss of appetite, weakness, nervous disorders, and heartbeat irregularities.

The usual cause of a deficiency is excessive potassium losses, either through the digestive tract (as in cases of prolonged diarrhea or vomiting, or laxative abuse) or through the urine (due to the prolonged use of diuretics, or some kidney diseases). Those with bulimia, the eating disorder characterized by a continual cycle of binge eating followed by induced vomiting (discussed in Chap. 3), can be at particular risk when both laxatives and diuretics are abused.

As is the case with the other electrolytes, potassium toxicity is also uncommon under ordinary conditions, since excesses are readily excreted in the urine. Kidney diseases can, however, interfere with the process. One major concern with respect to potassium toxicity is that it can cause the heart to stop beating. A potassium-rich solution is, in fact, used in lethal injections for carrying out capital punishment.

Summary

Minerals are inorganic substances, some of which we require in small amounts. Those described as major minerals have an adult recommended intake of more than 300 mg per day, and include calcium, phosphorus, magnesium, sodium, potassium, and chloride.

Bones and teeth contain most of the body's calcium. Bone seems like a separate, structural part of our bodies, but calcium and other minerals move in and out of bone all the time. In fact, bone serves as a mineral reserve whenever dietary intake is low.

In the blood, calcium levels are kept constant by the hormones calcitonin and parathormone. A drop in blood calcium levels can cause tetany; levels are affected by these hormones, not by diet. Low levels of dietary calcium will result in calcium being taken from bone.

Low calcium content in the bone leads to osteoporosis—brittle, easily broken bone. Many factors affect the risk of osteoporosis, including gender, family history, race, and body weight. Smoking and alcohol, along with low dietary intake of calcium, increase risk of osteoporosis. Other nutrients such as phosphorus and vitamin D also have an effect. Stress-bearing exercise strengthens bones, and estrogen-replacement or bisphosphonate therapy can prevent or delay osteoporosis for postmenopausal women.

It's important to get enough calcium during growth, when bones are developing. Most of our calcium comes from milk products, but there are other foods that have significant amounts. It's best to get calcium from foods, since supplements may cause other health problems, and natural supplements (e.g., bone meal) can be contaminated with lead or other toxins.

Phosphorus is found in bones and teeth, but also in phospholipids and other molecules (e.g., DNA, RNA, ATP). A deficiency is unlikely under normal circumstances; it's been found in premature infants fed only breast milk, and after long use of aluminum hydroxide as an antacid.

Magnesium is required for many cell functions. It's hard to become deficient, and toxic amounts come from magnesium-containing medications rather than food.

Sodium, chloride, and potassium are called electrolytes because they dissolve into charged particles that conduct electrical current. Potassium is mostly found inside cells (intracellular), whereas sodium and chloride are mostly found outside cells (extracellular). Electrolytes help regulate water movement, and transmit electrical impulses in nerve and muscle cells.

The adult recommended intake of sodium is 1200-1500 mg per day, and the typical American diet contains more than this. The Upper Level is 2300 mg per day; excessive sodium can lead to high blood pressure. Sodium is excreted in urine, and to some extent in perspiration; sodium levels are regulated by the kidney. Deficiency can occur after heavy and prolonged sweating, or from certain diseases.

Chloride parallels sodium intake and is important in water regulation and nerve function and is a component of stomach acid (hydrochloric acid). Deficiency and toxicity are rare.

Potassium is important for electrical impulses in the heart, and also cell metabolism, and may be protective against high blood pressure. Deficiency can be caused by drugs, diarrhea or vomiting, or bulimia. Toxicity is rare, but can affect the heart.

Chapter 17

The Trace Minerals

Iron, zinc, copper, etc.—the "trace" minerals —could hardly sound less nourishing. They seem not a real part of food, but instead almost magical potions that line the supplement shelves and supply the fine print on the boxes of some "fortified" foods.

Perhaps it is the non-food aspect that creates the allure and makes it easier to associate them with abundant vigor, potency, and agelessness. They never were this much fun when associated with "eating your spinach." And it's not always politically or environmentally correct these days to encourage consumption of red meat.

There are appropriate times for supplements, of course. But the danger is usually on the side of the excesses to which supplements make us vulnerable. As we shall see, a nutrient essential for health can become a lethal poison at excessive levels. Learning about them is serious business.

Trace minerals are so named because they are needed and generally present in the body in extremely small amounts. Some are needed in such small amounts that scientists have had a hard time measuring them or proving they are essential to health. Iron, for example, wasn't even discovered in the blood until the 18th century. (Afterwards, the scientist delighted in demonstrating his discovery by using a magnet to lift out the iron from pulverized, dried blood.)[1]

In those days, minerals such as iron were barely measurable in food and tissues. Sometimes, when scientists wanted to create deficiencies of certain trace minerals in test animals, they had to filter the air to keep them from getting enough.

Many of the trace minerals were identified in body tissues quite early, but knowledge of their functions had to await a more sophisticated chemistry. Now, as scientists are able to look deep into molecules, they're beginning to understand how the placement of a single mineral atom can determine the proper function of giant, complex molecules.

The essential trace minerals—iron, zinc, iodine, selenium, copper, manganese, fluoride, chromium, and molybdenum—are the subjects of this chapter (see Table 17-1).

Iron

Iron is a key part of several important proteins, but hemoglobin contains the most iron. One of the many ancient folk sayings about food is, "Pale foods can't make red blood." This is generally true. The redness of blood depends on iron, and iron—like beta-carotene—is a food colorant. Among the best sources of iron are such dark foods as red meats (especially beef liver), dark whole grains, prunes, raisins, molasses, and all the dark green, leafy vegetables.

Because iron can be found in many foods, one might not expect iron shortages to be widespread. In fact, it's the most common nutritional deficiency in the world. Growth, menstruation, and childbearing make a big dent in body supplies of iron, making iron deficiency especially common among children and women of childbearing age.

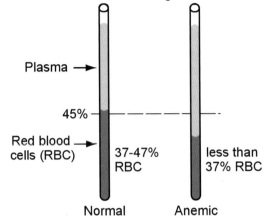

Figure 17-1: Simple lab test for anemia: *Spin blood in specially marked hematocrit tube; red blood cells pack at the bottom; its percentage in blood read on the tube markings.*

Two-thirds of body iron is found in molecules of **hemoglobin**, which are packaged into red blood cells, giving them—and blood—their color. Plentiful hemoglobin adds a pinkish hue to skin. Those who have too little (i.e., are anemic) tend to be pale.

The iron in hemoglobin is essential as a carrier of oxygen. Without hemoglobin, the blood of an average adult (about 5 quarts) would carry only about 1 tablespoon of oxygen. Hemoglobin increases the oxygen-carrying capacity of blood by about 70-fold, to about a quart of oxygen.

Hemoglobin picks up oxygen from the lungs, and carries it throughout the body, supplying it to each cell. When oxygenated, the blood is bright red. When the hemoglobin gives up its oxygen to a cell, it takes on a dark purplish-red color.

Iron-Deficiency Anemia

A person with anemia has fewer red blood cells and/or less hemoglobin in the red blood cells (see Fig. 17-1). This condition can be due to blood loss, impaired production of red blood cells or hemoglobin, or increased destruction of red blood cells. Despite the many possible causes of anemia, the common result is a reduced capacity of the blood to carry oxygen.

Iron deficiency is the most common cause of anemia. Since iron is an essential part of hemoglobin, not enough iron means not enough hemoglobin—and red blood cells that are small and pale (see Fig. 17-2).

Table 17-1: Trace Minerals

Mineral	Function	Source	Deficiency	Possible Toxicity
Chromium	Insulin cofactor	Whole grains, liver, brewer's yeast, nuts, some beers and red wine, mushrooms	Impaired insulin action	None reported, except from occupational inhalation
Copper	Cofactor in making hemo-globin, collagen	Liver, seafood, nuts, seeds, grains, copper plumbing	Rare; anemia, retarded growth, liver damage	Vomiting, diarrhea
Fluoride	Strengthen teeth and bone	Fluoride in drinking water, tea, seafood	Increased tooth decay	Mottling of tooth enamel
Iodine	Part of thyroid hormone	Seafood, iodized salt, dairy products	Simple goiter, cretinism, stillbirths	Goiter, inhibit making of thyroid hormone
Iron	Part of hemo-globin & other key proteins	Liver, red meat, eggs, fortified cereals, legumes, spinach	Anemia, fatigue, infections	Hemochro-matosis, vomiting, diarrhea
Manganese	Cofactor in metabolism	Whole grains, nuts, organ meats	Rare; nausea, vomiting	None reported, ex-cept from occupa-tional inhalation
Molybdenum	Cofactor in metabolism	Beans, grains, nuts	Rare	Gout-like symptoms
Selenium	Antioxidant	Meat, seafood, milk, grains	Heart muscle disorder	Brittleness and loss of hair and nails
Zinc	Cofactor in metabolism	Meat, milk, wheat germ, legumes, shellfish	Retarded growth, reduced sense of smell and taste, fewer white blood cells, skin lesions	Nausea, cramps, diarrhea, fever

An anemic person tires easily and often has such symptoms as weakness, dizziness, head-ache, drowsiness, and irritability. In short, the person has lower physical and mental capacity for work and productivity. Also, anemia can lessen the body's ability to increase heat production in response to cold ("cold intolerance"). Severe ane-mia can cause cessation of menstrual periods, loss of sexual desire, heart failure, and shock.

Iron deficiency can be caused by a greater need for iron (as when growing or pregnant), a dietary deficiency of iron, reduced absorption of iron (e.g., reduced stomach acidity from taking excessive amounts of antacids), or a combination of these factors. As said earlier, iron-deficiency anemia is most common among children and women of child-bearing age.

Children and adolescents need more iron for their increasing blood volume and growing bod-ies. Menstruating women lose iron in menstrual blood. Because women vary in the amount of menstrual blood losses, they vary in the amount of iron that they need for replacement.

It follows that any condition that changes the amount of menstrual blood will also change the iron requirement. Birth-control pills, for example, reduce menstrual blood losses. Menstruation can be scanty or cease entirely with extreme thinness (as sometimes occurs with anorexia nervosa or among ballet dancers) and with extreme exercise (as in competitive runners who train vigorously). Although there are no menstrual blood losses dur-ing pregnancy, more iron is needed for the grow-ing fetus and woman's bigger blood volume.

Iron-deficiency anemia is unusual for men and post-menopausal women, since they have mini-mal iron losses. An exception to this, of course, would be iron losses due to blood donations. Blood banks check for anemia before taking blood, and don't allow donations of more than a pint about

Figure 17-2: Iron deficiency is the most common cause of anemia.

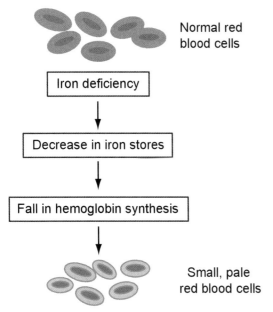

Normal red blood cells

Iron deficiency

↓

Decrease in iron stores

↓

Fall in hemoglobin synthesis

↓

Small, pale red blood cells

every 2 months. When iron-deficiency anemia is seen in men and postmenopausal women who are not blood donors, chronic bleeding—especially in the digestive tract (as in a bleeding ulcer)—is suspected and investigated.

Iron Deficiency and Lead Absorption

Iron deficiency also has a bearing on lead toxicity, particularly among children. During periods of rapid growth, lead is absorbed readily. Infants and young children absorb 5 to 10 times more lead than adults from a given dose. Furthermore, lead absorption and/or toxicity is increased when there is a deficiency of iron (or calcium or zinc).

Unfortunately, iron, calcium, and zinc deficiencies are fairly common among young children and women of child-bearing age. Lead exposure has been falling, but a 2003 Center for Disease Control report suggests that about 2% of children in the U.S. under age 6 still have levels of lead in the blood that indicate substantial exposure to lead's toxic effects.[2]

In slum areas, old peeling lead-based paint has been a major source of lead exposure; young children often ingest the dust or flakes from the paint.

Lead is a potent poison with widespread effects. It can, for example, cause kidney damage (which can result in high blood pressure) and damage to the red blood cells (which can cause anemia). It can also damage the nervous system (which can cause mental retardation or derangement), and the reproductive system (which can cause infertility).

It's been theorized that severe lead poisoning caused infertility and mental illness in the ruling class of ancient Rome, and that this was a factor in the fall of the Roman Empire. Lead plumbing contaminated their drinking water, and lead utensils and vessels (used for cooking, drinking, and storage) contaminated their food and drink.

Iron in Foods

Those with iron-deficiency anemia need to increase their intake of iron and/or increase their ability to absorb the iron in their diet. Compared to other nutrients, iron is poorly absorbed. This is an important natural safeguard, because excessive iron in the body can be toxic.

Aside from blood losses, very little iron is lost from the body once it's absorbed. So the intestine serves as the gatekeeper by adjusting the absorption. Absorption is normally kept low, but increases when the body needs more iron.

Milligram (mg) iron in about 3 oz. lean, cooked portions of animal tissues:

• beef liver 7.5 mg
• hamburger 3.9 mg
• lamb 2.6 mg
• skinless dark chicken meat 1.4 mg
• skinless light chicken meat 1.1 mg
• salmon, swordfish, or trout 1.0 mg

Dietary iron can be categorized into two types. Iron ingested as a part of heme (a complex molecule with an atom of iron in its core) is called *heme iron;* other forms ("inorganic iron") are called *non-heme iron* (see Fig. 17-3).

Heme Iron

Heme iron is found only in animal tissue, mainly in hemoglobin and myoglobin (an oxygen-carrying molecule similar to hemoglobin, but found in muscle). About half the iron in animal tissue is heme iron. The iron in egg yolks, milk, and plant foods is all non-heme iron. Heme iron is generally better absorbed than non-heme iron.

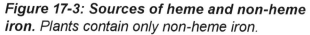

Figure 17-3: Sources of heme and non-heme iron. Plants contain only non-heme iron.

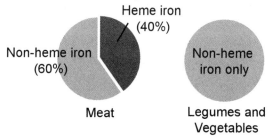

Because of the tell-tale "bloody" color of heme, we can correctly guess that red meat (e.g., beef) has more heme iron than light meat (e.g., chicken, fish), and that the darker meat of a chicken leg has more heme iron than the lighter meat of the chicken breast. Since heme-containing red blood cells are made in the bone marrow and broken down in the liver, bone marrow and liver are rich dietary sources of heme iron. (Bone marrow is eaten more commonly in Europe than in the U.S.).

Non-Heme Iron

We eat a lot of meat, but most of the iron in our diet is non-heme iron (as in fortified breakfast cereals and enriched bread).

Plants contain only non-heme iron, which is generally more poorly absorbed than heme iron. But the absorption of non-heme iron can vary a lot (from about 2% to 45%), depending on whether a person is deficient in iron, the amount of iron in the meal, and the composition of the meal. Thus, compared to heme iron, it's hard to evaluate dietary sources of non-heme iron.

We can't assume that a person will absorb more iron from a half-cup of cooked spinach (2 mg iron) at lunch than from an egg (1 mg iron) at breakfast, because other substances in the meals can affect the amount absorbed. For example, vitamin C-rich food, meat, or fish eaten at the same meal increases the absorption of non-heme iron.

Conversely, substances such as tannins (as in tea), phytic acid (as in wheat bran), and oxalic acid (as in spinach) in the meal can lower the amount absorbed by combining with non-heme iron, preventing its absorption.

We can expect to absorb more iron from the egg if the breakfast also included sausage and a glass of orange juice, and less from a luncheon spinach salad served with a whole wheat roll and tea. The vitamin C in the orange juice and the meat in the sausage increase absorption of the iron in the egg, whereas the oxalic acid in the spinach, the phytic acid in the whole wheat roll, and the tannins in the tea all bind to iron and hamper its absorption.

The spinach salad lunch may not be as good as the egg and sausage breakfast in terms of iron absorption, but it's more in line with dietary advice to eat less saturated fat and cholesterol and more fiber. A breakfast of orange juice and either peanut butter on toast or breakfast cereal would be good, in terms of iron absorption and dietary advice.

Because only a small amount of the iron ingested is actually absorbed, the recommended intake of iron is about ten-fold higher than what our bodies require. Adult men, for example, need about 1 mg/day, so their RDA is 8 mg/day.

Other foods included in the same meal will increase the absorption of non-heme iron: a small amount of meat or fish, and especially foods rich in vitamin C, e.g., oranges, grapefruit, strawberries, melon, broccoli, green peppers.

Foods rich in non-heme iron (have 1 to 2 mg iron):

- ¼ cup peanut butter, raisins, bran breakfast cereal;. or cooked cream of wheat
- ½ cup cooked spinach, chard, lima beans, or peas
- 2 slices enriched or whole wheat bread
- 1 egg yolk
- 3 dried apricot halves
- 5 prunes

Milk and milk products make up a big part of children's diets, and milk contains only a very small amount of iron (about 0.1 mg of non-heme iron per cup). Newborns normally have about a 6-month's supply of iron stored in the liver. This iron "holds them over" until other foods are added to their diet of milk. The iron in breast milk is better absorbed, so it's recommended that infants less than a year old who aren't being breast-fed exclusively, be given iron-fortified infant formula.

Iron Fortification and Supplements: The enrichment of flour with iron, and the fortification of many breakfast cereals with iron has helped reduce the incidence of iron-deficiency anemia in this country. Also, many people take iron supplements.

Iron supplements are generally inexpensive and readily available, but it's still a good idea for those at risk of iron deficiency to work on improving their intake of iron-rich foods. Improving the diet in one nutrient—iron in this case—tends to improve the diet in other nutrients as well. Also, for some people, iron supplements can be constipating.

The form in which the iron is taken affects how well it's absorbed. It's highest for such complexes as ferrous (iron) sulfate, ascorbates, fumarates, and citrates. These latter three forms of iron are sometimes called *chelates,* and there's quite a lot of promotion for unreasonably expensive "chelated iron" supplements. (The same iron complexes are often available at much lower prices in grocery stores, etc.)

There's also a simple way to supplement your diet with iron without pills. That is, by cooking acid-containing foods in old-fashioned utensils— cast iron pots and pans. If the food is somewhat acidic—containing a little vinegar, red wine, citrus juice, tomato juice, or almost anything else that tastes rather sour—small amounts of iron will dissolve out of the pan and into the food. The iron content of tomato-based (acidic) spaghetti sauce, for instance, goes up when simmered in a cast-iron pot.

An old folk remedy for anemia is to put a long iron nail in an apple overnight and then eat the apple—after removing the nail, of course.

One can't say precisely how much iron you'll get from cast iron pots and pans, but some rather casual testing indicates that it's substantial. In fact, people have suffered from iron toxicity when iron vats have been used routinely to store or brew acidic drinks.

Iron Toxicity

Intestinal safeguards normally protect us from an excess of iron, but large amounts can overwhelm the system, and we can absorb too much. There have been many cases of acute and chronic iron toxicity where food or drink was accidentally heavily contaminated with iron.

An accidental overdose of iron supplements is the most common cause of acute iron poisoning in this country. The iron supplements usually belong to the child's mother. Acute iron poisoning requires emergency treatment. Alcoholics and those with certain diseases (e.g., liver disease or thalassemia) are particularly vulnerable to the iron toxicity.

Hemochromatosis

Because iron-deficiency anemia is so common in this country, it's been suggested that more staple foods be fortified with iron. The concern is that this might cause more cases of a disease called *hemochromatosis*. In this disease, excessive amounts of iron are absorbed from normal diets because of a genetic error that impairs the ability of the intestine to adjust iron absorption. The danger is an accumulation of iron to toxic levels in the body.

Sweden fortifies its foods more heavily with iron, resulting in less iron-deficiency anemia, but more hemochromatosis—an example of the challenge presented by a diverse population, and the need to get enough, but not too much.

An estimated 1 of 10 of whites of Northern European descent in the U.S. has inherited the abnormal gene for hemochromatosis from one parent (heterozygotes), and about 1 in 2000 from both parents (homozygotes). It's less common among those of Asian, Hispanic, and Native American descent.[3]

The genetic defect is distributed evenly among the sexes, but hemochromatosis is mainly a man's disease. Men are at substantially greater risk because they can accumulate more iron over the years. Women, in contrast, "get rid of iron" in menstruation and pregnancy.

Treatment for hemochromatosis includes extraction of blood (as in blood donations). As you'd expect, regular blood donors are at lower risk of hemochromatosis.

Hemochromatosis rarely is discovered before middle age, presumably because it's apparent only after many years of accumulating excess iron. Injury from the abnormal deposition of the excess iron occurs in various tissues, e.g., cirrhosis of the liver, arthritis. It can be fatal. Early, mild, and vague symptoms of iron toxicity include joint pain and lack of energy.

Self-prescribed iron supplements taken by men and postmenopausal women are particularly worrisome in this regard. Also worrisome is regularly eating excessive amounts of iron-fortified breakfast cereal (the nothing-else-in-the-cupboard situation faced by many a college-age male). Men and postmenopausal women generally don't need iron supplements except, perhaps, if they're regular blood donors. Even without a genetic defect for increased iron absorption, men and postmenopausal women taking large doses of iron supplements might, over the years, put themselves at risk for iron toxicity. As such, men and postmenopausal women should avoid iron supplements and foods heavily fortified with iron, unless advised otherwise by a physician.

Zinc

In the early 1960s, it was reported that zinc deficiency was the cause of retarded growth and delayed puberty among some 18 to 19-year-old boys in Egypt and Iran. These were the first documented cases of zinc deficiency among humans, establishing zinc as an essential nutrient.[4]

The diets of the zinc-deficient boys consisted mainly of unleavened whole grain bread, which is particularly rich in phytic acid. As we saw earlier for other minerals (e.g., iron and calcium), phytic acid can bind zinc and prevent its absorption. So what little zinc there was in their diet was made less available by the high amounts of phytic acid. Also, other conditions (e.g., parasitic infections) contributed to the deficiency.

Zinc is closely linked to animal protein, and the deficient boys had very little of these "foods of the rich." Rich sources of zinc include shellfish (especially oysters), red meats, and liver. Milk and eggs also provide zinc, but in lesser amounts. For vegans, some fairly rich plant sources of zinc include wheat germ, black-eyed peas, and fermented soybean paste (*miso*).

Zinc is found throughout our bodies—in virtually every cell—and is particularly noted for its role in assisting the activity of numerous proteins,

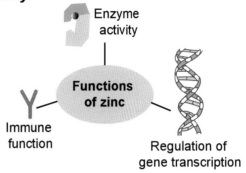

Figure 17-4: Zinc performs critical roles in the body.

Enzyme activity

Functions of zinc

Immune function

Regulation of gene transcription

including many enzymes. Zinc plays a diverse role in a multitude of important bodily functions (e.g., protein synthesis, immune defense), and is needed for the health of all tissues (see Fig. 17-4).

Zinc Deficiency

Since zinc is involved in so many body processes, the list of deficiency symptoms is long. They include impairments of growth, wound healing, immune function, and taste perception. A severe deficiency can also cause acne. But most cases of acne aren't from a zinc deficiency. For acne and other symptoms of zinc deficiency, once again we should remember that if the condition isn't caused by a zinc deficiency, zinc won't help cure it.

Severe zinc deficiency is unusual in this country. But marginal intake may be common among certain segments of the population, particularly people who don't eat much animal protein or whole grains. Unlike iron, zinc isn't commonly added to fortified foods such as breakfast cereals, and isn't a standard component of the enriched flour used to make white bread and other baked goods.

Zinc Toxicity

Excess zinc—typically from zinc supplements—can cause nausea, bloating, cramps, diarrhea, and fever. Zinc taken in amounts not much higher than the recommended amount can cause a copper deficiency by interfering with the absorption and use of that required trace mineral.

Iodine

In anticipation of the fall-out of radioactive iodine from the 1986 Chernobyl nuclear accident, many people in countries downwind from the accident took iodine pills. They did this to protect the thyroid gland.

Thyroid cancer rates rose after the accident among children living in cities near Chernobyl.

The rationale behind their action was that iodine is an essential part of thyroid hormone, the hormone necessary for normal metabolism, and iodine is concentrated in the thyroid gland for the purpose of making this hormone. The iodine pills saturate the thyroid gland with iodine so that very little of the radioactive iodine would be taken up by the gland.

Simple Goiter—The Iodine Deficiency Disease

Iodine is required in the diet for the purpose of making thyroid hormone. Not enough iodine means not enough thyroid hormone, and this results in a condition called *simple goiter*, characterized by an enlargement of the thyroid gland. The thyroid gland enlarges in its attempt to make more hormone. Because the thyroid gland is located in the neck, the enlarged gland protrudes and enlarges the neck.

Until 1924, when iodized salt (iodine added to salt) was introduced, simple goiter—and an enlarged neck—was common in this country. During World War I, the neck sizes of the men drafted from all parts of the U.S. reflected the geographical distribution of goiter.

The effect of simple goiter depends on the extent of the iodine deficiency and also on when the deficiency occurs. A severe iodine deficiency during fetal life can result in physical and mental retardation (cretinism; see Fig. 17-5), whereas a slightly enlarged thyroid gland may be the only

---

Goiter, by definition, is simply an enlargement of the thyroid gland, located in the neck. The enlarged thyroid causes a protrusion in the neck.

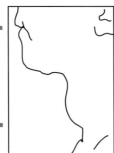

---

noticeable effect of a mild iodine deficiency during adulthood. Intermediate symptoms of inadequate thyroid hormone include sluggish mental activity and weight gain, and "puffiness" due to abnormal retention of water in tissues.

Iodine deficiency is still a worldwide problem, especially in developing countries. Particularly poignant is the story of Jixian village in rural China.[5] In 1978, iodine deficiency was so severe and so prevalent that most of the village suffered from symptoms of severe iodine deficiency, such as mental retardation. Ironically, *Jixian village* means *village of scholars*. An intensive campaign to eradicate iodine deficiency was implemented, and by 1985, there were no longer any cretins below age 7. The physically and mentally normal children helping their impaired parents became a common sight in the village.

Iodine in Food

The most consistent sources of dietary iodine are foods from the sea. As long ago as 3000 B.C., the Chinese used burnt sea sponge to treat simple goiter, even though they didn't know what caused the disease. The treatment was effective because sea sponges contain iodine, and, as a mineral, iodine isn't destroyed when the sponge is burned.

Inland, the iodine in food varies. Plants don't need iodine to grow, so its presence in plants depends on the amount in the soil, water, and environment. Goiter was least common among those who lived next to the sea, not only because seafood is available there, but because the soil next to the sea is rich in iodine.

In the American diet, the main sources of iodine are iodized salt, seafood, and processed foods to which iodine compounds have been added.

Excess Iodine

Moderate excesses of iodine isn't a problem for most people. However, even safe levels for healthy people can be a problem for those with autoimmune thyroid disease (common in older women in the U.S.) and some other conditions.

Ironically, large excesses of iodine can inhibit the production of thyroid hormone and cause goi-

Figure 17-5: Iodine deficiency is the primary cause of preventable brain damage and mental retardation worldwide.

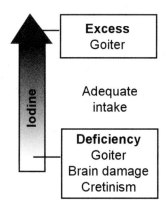

ter (another example of "too much or too little" as a problem). In Japan, for example, some people get goiter from regularly eating large amounts of iodine-rich seaweed. Moderate excesses of iodine are efficiently excreted in the urine.

Selenium

It was selenium's toxic effects that first attracted nutritionists' attention to this trace mineral. When animals grazed on plants high in selenium, they came down with a disease called *blind staggers*; they became stiff and lame, and then became blind and paralyzed before they died.

So it came as a surprise when this "potent poison" was later found to be an essential nutrient. Selenium is part of an enzyme that acts as an antioxidant. (Vitamins C and E also act as antioxidants, as discussed in earlier chapters.) Selenium appears to have other less-defined functions as well.

Selenium is another of the elements in which soil content influences food content. Early reports of both selenium toxicity and deficiency due to soil levels came from rural China. (Even now, rural China is a gold mine for studies of diet and health, because the people there tend to live their entire lives in one area, and eat locally grown foods that can vary substantially from one area to the next.)

In the 1960s there was a major outbreak of selenium toxicity in several rural villages in the Hubei Province of China.[6] It started with a drought that led to a failure of the rice crops. More vegetables

and corn were eaten instead. Although the rice, vegetables, and corn were grown in local soil heavily contaminated with selenium-rich coal, the rice had a lower selenium content. So the switch from less rice to more vegetables and corn meant more selenium in the diet.

The most common symptom was a loss of hair and nails. Other symptoms such as skin lesions, more tooth decay, and abnormalities of the nervous system were also thought to be the direct result of selenium toxicity. (It's hard to pinpoint the symptoms to the selenium toxicity with certainty because the drought brought about other dietary and environmental changes as well.)

In 1979, there was a report of an epidemic in the Keshan province of China of what became known as *Keshan's disease*, a disease of the heart muscle, characterized by an enlarged heart, abnormal heart rhythms, and, sometimes, heart failure and death. The soil there was very low in selenium, resulting in low selenium in the crops. Selenium supplements cleared most of the symptoms. (Deficiencies of other trace minerals and additional sresses may also have contributed to the disease.)

Selenium supplements taken in large doses can cause "garlic breath"—perhaps a safeguard against a temptation to take too much.

Some studies suggest that selenium deficiency increases the risk of cancer, and some people have responded by self-prescribing selenium supplements. Large doses of selenium supplements can be extremely toxic.

Worldwide, the selenium content of plant and animal food largely depends on where the plants are grown and where the animals are raised. Meat has some selenium because it's a required nutrient for animals. Plants, however, don't need selenium, so content reflects the selenium in the soil.

People who don't eat meat because of choice or poverty, and only eat local plant foods grown in low-selenium soil are most at risk for deficiency. In the U.S., animals raised for food have controlled, selenium-containing diets, and we get plant foods from such a variety of locations/soils that selenium deficiency or toxicity is unlikely.

Copper

Copper is needed to make hemoglobin and red blood cells, and is needed for various enzymes, including those involved in the formation of bone and nerve. Deficiencies in this country are seen only in unusual circumstances. For example, copper deficiency can result from a rare genetic disease called *Menkes' steely hair disease* (the hair looks thin and brittle "like steel wool"). Apparent at birth, this genetic disease can be fatal unless promptly treated with high doses of copper. Among adults, anemia from copper deficiency can result from substantial long-term use of zinc supplements. As said earlier, large amounts of zinc can interfere with copper absorption.

Good copper sources include organ meats, shellfish, nuts, and seeds. We usually get plenty of copper. Copper cooking utensils can contribute, as can copper rollers and other vessels and utensils used in the food industry. We can even meet our entire need if our drinking water comes through copper plumbing.

Toxicity symptoms include vomiting and diarrhea. Toxicity rarely occurs from the amounts of copper found in the diet. (An exception is Wilson's disease, a rare disease in which copper accumulates to toxic levels because of an impaired ability to get rid of excesses.)

Manganese

Manganese plays a role in the activity of many enzymes throughout the body. It's also widespread in food, and we need very little. A manganese deficiency isn't anything you need worry about. Its occurrence is so rare that it's hard to confirm symptoms of deficiency.

Manganese in large doses can be toxic to the nervous system, but like deficiencies, manganese toxicity is rare, e.g., toxicity in workers who inhaled manganese dust or fumes. Again, however, people should avoid high-dose supplements.

Fluoride

Fluoride is often thought to be merely an additive which can help prevent tooth decay. It's very

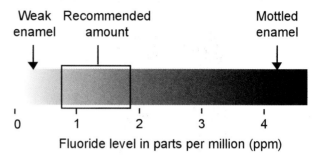

Figure 17-6: Level of fluoride in drinking water affects tooth enamel.

Fluoride level in parts per million (ppm)

effective at doing so, and the cost of adding it to water supplies is much less than the savings in dental care.

Fluoride prevents decay by becoming incorporated into tooth enamel, making it more resistant to the acid produced by mouth bacteria. This process is most effective during the formation of the enamel and the underlying dentin—from birth until the permanent teeth fully erupt at about ages 11-13. (Although some teeth mineralize before birth, there is no proof that maternal fluoride ingestion during pregnancy is protective.)

Fluoride in drinking water, toothpaste, mouth rinse, etc., also helps protect adults' teeth, mainly by promoting the remineralization of enamel (see Chapter 5). Fluoride may also be helpful in strengthening bone.

Fluoride is present in various concentrations in all natural water supplies, and the related variation in levels of tooth decay provided early evidence of fluoride's protective effect. For example, the fluoride content of the water in Quincy, Illinois was no more than 0.2 parts per million (ppm), and they had more than three times as many dental cavities as nearby Galesburg, where the fluoride in the water was 1.9 ppm.

Fluoride at 0.7 to 1.2 ppm in the drinking water is the recommended level. This level provides maximum protection against decay without the mottling (fluorosis) of the enamel of developing teeth that can be caused by excessive fluoride (see Fig. 17-6).

The discovery that mottled teeth in high fluoride areas were highly resistant to tooth decay led to the discovery of fluoride's protective effect. At fluoride levels of 2 ppm or more during tooth development, the enamel can develop small areas that are "extra white." At 4 ppm or more, there may be brown stains.

Other causes of brown stains on the enamel include exposure to the antibiotic tetracycline during tooth development from before birth to about 8 years old.

For water supplies with less than 0.7 ppm fluoride, the addition of fluoride is recommended. Fluoridation substantially reduces the number of decayed teeth. Also, there's substantial evidence that fluoridation of water lowers risk of osteoporosis, by strengthening bone.

For infants who are exclusively breast fed, and for children who don't have access to fluoridated water, daily fluoride drops or tablets are advised, as prescribed by a physician or dentist.

Only about two-thirds of the U.S. population has access to an adequately fluoridated municipal water supply. Unlike most public health measures, fluoridation is voted on by communities. Many people are frightened by being told, for example, that fluoride is a rat poison. In large enough doses, it is, in fact, a rat poison—even a human poison for that matter. The size of the dose determines the hazard. (When water supplies have been naturally excessive in fluoride, and removing fluoride to bring the level down to 1 ppm has been proposed, communities have, on occasion, voted this down, wanting to leave their water "natural.")

The benefits and safety of water fluoridation have been studied for more than 60 years, and has been demonstrated to be safe and effective in about 60 countries.[7]

Chromium

Chromium promotes insulin action and is essential in glucose metabolism. A deficiency can produce diabetes-like symptoms, as seen in some patients who were being fed only by an intravenous solution that lacked chromium. An adequate chromium intake corrects the symptoms if—and only if—they are due to a chromium deficiency.

Brewer's yeast is a particularly rich source of chromium. This yeast comes from brewing beer—making some beers a good source. (Different brands of beer vary a lot in chromium content.)[5]

Other good sources include whole grains, nuts, and some red wines.

Chromium is poorly absorbed from the diet, making toxicity from dietary sources highly unlikely. Toxicity from chromium (of a different form than that normally in the diet) has been caused industrially both through breathing and direct skin contact, resulting in skin ulcers, and liver damage and lung cancer. (This industrial form of chromium is called hexavalent chromium.)

Molybdenum

Molybdenum is a component of several essential enzymes. It's found in a variety of foods, and a deficiency has never been reported for people eating a normal diet. In 1981, the first suspected case of molybdenum deficiency was reported in a surgery patient fed intravenously over a long period with a solution inadvertently deficient in molybdenum.[6] The patient developed a variety of symptoms, including nausea, vomiting, mental disturbances, and coma, and improved when given molybdenum. Molybdenum toxicity is also rare.

Other Trace Minerals

There are other trace minerals that may or may not be required for human health. These include *arsenic, nickel, silicon, vanadium, and boron.* Arsenic, for example, was shown in the mid-1970s to be essential for rats, pigs, and goats. Its need for humans hasn't been firmly established, though it's assumed because it's needed by many animal species.

We needn't worry about a deficiency of these particular trace elements, however. The amounts thought necessary are so small that it's hard not to get enough—thus the scientists' challenge in trying to establish its human need. It's easier to get too much. Toxicities of these minerals (e.g., arsenic as a lethal poison) are much more easily established.

In looking at the realities of food choice, there's little question that certain strategies in planning our meals will deal nicely, not only with the nutrients we know of, but with those we may possibly learn about in the future. Let's now examine how our knowledge of nutrition can shape our strategies for food choice.

Summary

The trace minerals are those that we require in very small amounts, and include iron, zinc, iodine, selenium, copper, manganese, fluoride, chromium, and molybdenum.

Iron deficiency is one of the most common nutritional deficiencies in this country and throughout the world. Iron is critical for carrying oxygen in the hemoglobin of red blood cells, and deficiency leads to anemia. Deficiency can be caused by dietary deficiency, increased need, blood loss, or decreased absorption. Deficiencies are common in children and women of childbearing age. Iron deficiency can also result in increased lead absorption; lead is particularly toxic for children and the developing fetus.

Dietary iron is found in two forms—heme iron (exclusively from animal tissue) and non-heme iron (from animal tissue and exclusively from plants). Heme iron is better absorbed than non-heme iron; other dietary constituents (e.g., vitamin C, oxalic acid) can affect the absorption of non-heme iron.

Iron toxicity can be a problem, particularly in people at risk for the genetic disease hemochromatosis, which results in excess iron being deposited in body tissues. Iron supplements and/or habitually eating foods heavily fortified with iron are ill-advised for these people, as well as for all men and postmenopausal women in general.

Zinc is critical for growth, particularly during pregnancy and childhood. A deficiency can result in birth defects, slow growth, changes in taste, and reduced immune function and wound healing. Toxicity is rare.

Iodine is needed as a part of thyroid hormone, and deficiency causes goiter (an enlargement of the thyroid gland) and cretinism (physical and mental retardation from severe iodine deficiency in the fetus). Other conditions can cause goiter, but goiter caused by iodine deficiency is the most common kind and is called simple goiter.

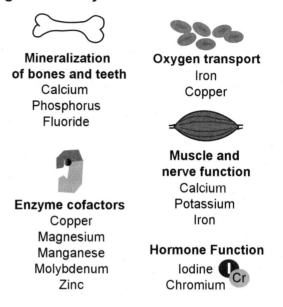

Figure 17-7: Key functions of minerals.

Mineralization of bones and teeth
Calcium
Phosphorus
Fluoride

Oxygen transport
Iron
Copper

Enzyme cofactors
Copper
Magnesium
Manganese
Molybdenum
Zinc

Muscle and nerve function
Calcium
Potassium
Iron

Hormone Function
Iodine
Chromium

Iodine is an essential part of thyroid hormone, and is found in iodized salt, foods from the sea, and in processed foods in which iodine-containing compounds are added.

Selenium is a part of an antioxidant enzyme. Large excesses can be very toxic.

Copper is required for many enzymes and hemoglobin production. Copper deficiency is usually only found in the genetic disease Menkes' steel hair disease, although zinc supplements may also lead to deficiency through competition for absorption.

Manganese is important for many enzymes, and deficiency and toxicity are rare.

Molybdenum is also needed for many enzymes, and it's difficult to become deficient in this trace mineral.

Fluoride increases the hardness of tooth enamel and bone, and is found in adequate amounts in the water supply of about two-thirds of the U.S. population. Fluoridation of water should be considered where it's lower than 0.7 ppm (parts per million). The recommended level is 0.7 to 1.2 ppm.

Chromium promotes insulin action.

There are other minerals which haven't yet been proven to be essential for humans, but it's very unlikely that we'd become deficient in any of these.

Part 7

Balance–Science and the Art of Eating

Chapter 18

Between Food and Health

Dietitians (the group certified as nutrition experts) face a daunting challenge. It's one thing to teach the science, and quite another to provide responsible, realistic guidelines for specific food choices. When you stop to think about it, the challenge is huge.

There's the enormous variety of foods available; there are varying needs of different individuals, to say nothing of their differing likes and dislikes, life styles, and cultural perspectives. And there's the insidious fact that in general we like sweet and fatty foods, the ones we could do with less of.

Too often the nutrition message sounds like a series of "don'ts" and "shoulds," restrictions on the succulent and quotas for the unappetizing.

When the injunction isn't negative, it's still not exciting. Hearing about "balance," "variety," and "moderation" seldom quickens the blood.

For those who take the time to listen and learn a bit, however, there can be an earthly reward of health and good eating. There's room for all the favorite foods, and a balanced diet can be a pleasure.

From the first, nutritionists have had one continuing purpose—to find a balance between the foods we eat and the chemical needs of life.

In the early 1900s, "a balanced diet" seemed simple enough. After all, so far as anyone knew, there were only four nutrients—protein, fat, carbohydrate, and ash (minerals). But when these were fed to growing rats in what was believed the perfect proportion, they stopped growing. It was clear that food contained something more than just these four nutrients. More, indeed.

As we're well aware (having spent four chapters going over the many vitamins and minerals), there are many requirements and a multitude of food choices. The result is often utter confusion.

Imagine walking down the supermarket aisles with a shopping list of required nutrients, trying to choose among the thousands of foods in a way that would provide enough—but not too much— of each nutrient. Think further of having to make these choices in light of what you enjoy—or don't enjoy—eating. Maybe you don't like salads or fish. Maybe you can't pass up the candy counter. Maybe religious or spiritual dictates—from kosher rules to vegetarianism—direct your choices.

Most of us would be overwhelmed. Fortunately, nutrition scientists have provided us with guidelines and shortcuts in diet analysis and planning, and a good diet can encompass a wide variety of preferences.

In this chapter, we first look at the guidelines that deal with getting enough— *Recommended Dietary Allowances* and *A Daily Food Guide*. This will be followed by a look at additional guidelines that are mostly meant to help us avoid dietary excesses. (A balanced diet for a population with a bountiful food supply is one of getting enough, but not too much.) The chapter ends with a discussion of how a good diet can accommodate individual preferences and needs.

Getting Enough

Scientists know about how much of each of the nutrients we need. They also know about how much of these nutrients are in various foods. In rigorously controlled studies, they make precise measurements of the nutrients taken in, and the amounts used, stored, and excreted. They also study how the nutrients interact and function in the body. What they learn leads to the recommendations for the amounts of nutrients we should include in our diet, amounts deemed "safe and adequate"—enough to meet our needs, yet not so much as to risk toxicity (another sort of balance).

Dietary Reference Intakes

Dietary Reference Intakes (DRIs) are a family of four reference values (see Fig. 18-1): Estimated Average Requirement (EAR), Recommended Dietary Allowance (RDA), Adequate Intake (AI), and Tolerable Upper Intake Value (UL). The DRIs are a joint effort with Health Canada, providing a common set of values for both the U.S. and Canada.

We as consumers are most concerned with:

- **Recommended Dietary Allowance (RDA),** the amount recommended in the daily diet to meet the needs of nearly all healthy people. When there isn't enough information to set an RDA for a nutrient, an Adequate Intake (AI)— based mainly on customary intakes of healthy populations—is substituted. For simplicity, RDA is broadened in this book to include AI, since both values are amounts recommended in the diet.

- **Tolerable Upper Intake Value (UL),** the highest daily intake of a nutrient that's unlikely to have adverse effects for nearly all healthy people. (For some nutrients there isn't enough information to set a UL.) The aim is to keep our nutrient intake below this level. In most cases, the UL is exceeded by consuming high doses of dietary supplements (a notable exception is sodium—most of our diets are too salty).

Recommended Dietary Allowance

The first set of Recommended Dietary Allowances (RDAs) was issued in 1941. (Many of the nutrients had just been identified in the previous decade.) The Food and Nutrition Board, assembled as part of the National Academy of

Science's National Research Council, has the responsibility of updating the RDAs. The current set was issued as part of the DRIs in 1997-2005.

The Board's membership, which includes some of our most respected nutrition scientists, changes periodically, both to share the burden of the work, and to infuse a variety of expert opinions. The scientists continually reassess what's known of the nutrients, scouring the newest research reports. They also study the quantities of nutrients in our food supply, their effects on the body, and information about the public's health and eating habits. Their objective is to recommend amounts of nutrients in the diet that will meet the needs of virtually all healthy people in the United States and Canada.

There are different RDAs for males and females, for different ages, and for pregnant women and nursing mothers (see Appendix A).

Are the RDAs Set High Enough for Good Health?

The RDAs are widely misunderstood to be minimums for physical health. They shouldn't be confused with the amounts of nutrients actually required in the body. For one thing, RDAs allow for absorption rates. The RDA for iron, for example, is about ten times higher than the body's requirement, because, on average, we absorb only about 10% of the iron in our diet.

The RDAs aren't daily requirements in the sense that a deficiency will occur if they aren't consumed daily. They include generous safety margins. Also, they're for averages per day, since diets vary day to day. They provide a margin to establish reserves in the body. Practically speaking, it's recommended that nutrient intakes average the RDAs over a 3-day period. Dietary assessments are commonly made on the basis of 3-day diet records.

RDAs, under different names, are also set in other countries and by United Nations agencies, and for some nutrients are lower than our RDAs.

Using vitamin C as an example, we see the extent of the safety margin provided by the adult

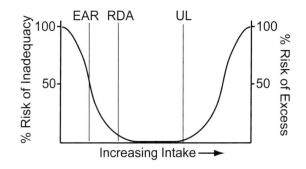

Figure 18-1: Dietary Reference Intakes. *At the RDA, the risk of not getting enough is only 2-3%. At the EAR (Estimated Average Requirement), it's 50%. Above the UL (Tolerable Upper Intake Level), risk of adverse effects goes up.*

RDA: The minimal need for a vitamin is considered to be that level which will prevent physical signs of deficiency. Experimental evidence indicates that 10 mg a day of vitamin C will prevent symptoms of scurvy, the deficiency disease related to this vitamin. The RDA for most adults in the U.S. is 75-90 mg.

The British recommendation of 40 mg a day[1] provides what their scientists consider an ample safety margin for the vitamin. Our RDA of 75-90 mg is thus about twice what the British consider adequate. (On the other hand, some people take thousands of milligrams of vitamin C supplements—2000 mg is the Tolerable Upper Intake Level for adults.)

One can see how misleading it can be to interpret the RDAs too rigidly, treating them as if they were minimums for physical health. Consider a Londoner whose diet averages 40 mg of vitamin C a day. His or her vitamin C intake would fully meet the British standard, but only about half ours.

Aside from what's necessary to meet needs and provide a surplus, is there such a thing as an "optimal intake"? In other words, do amounts higher than the RDAs provide health advantages for the average member of the general population? At the present time, such "optimal intakes," if they actually exist, aren't known. If such evidence were forthcoming, the RDAs would be revised accordingly.

How Useful are the RDAs for Assessing Individual Diets?

The RDAs are now used for such diverse purposes as evaluating diets of various population groups, establishing guidelines for food assistance programs (e.g., school lunch programs) and food-labeling information, and developing nutrition policy and education programs.

For planning and assessing diets, the RDAs are most useful for groups of people, rather than for individuals. A dietitian in charge of the campus cafeteria, for example, would use the RDAs for young adults in planning the menus. On the other hand, since we don't know your exact requirement as an individual, we can only use the RDAs to estimate the likelihood that you're meeting your nutrient needs.

If your diet meets the RDAs, you can be quite certain you are meeting your needs. All that can be said beyond this is that the farther your intake falls below the RDAs, the greater the likelihood that your intake is inadequate.

At any rate, planning a good diet in terms of the RDAs is too tedious a process for most of us—even when run on a computer. We need a shortcut for selecting a good diet. One such shortcut involves grouping foods by their nutrient content, and choosing appropriately from the groups.

Understanding Foods in Groups

In looking at food composition tables, we see a pattern: Animal flesh—whether beef, chicken, or fish—tends to be high in protein. Fruits, vegetables, and whole grains are generally rich in fiber, vitamins, and certain minerals. Milk is a good source of calcium, riboflavin, and protein. By grouping foods according to this pattern, and recommending numbers of servings from each group, scientists have come up with a simple guide for insuring that one gets enough of the essential nutrients.

Such a food-group method of diet planning has been set up by the U.S. Department of Agriculture (USDA). In the 1940s, it was the "Basic Seven" — foods were placed in seven groups, each of which was chosen to furnish certain nutrients.

This system proved too cumbersome. It was hard for school children and adults alike to get a clear view of seven different food groups, together with the recommended number of servings for each. The concept was periodically modified, most recently to *A Daily Food Guide* of five food groups (see Table 18-1).

Originally, the USDA grouped foods to plan crops for the needs of the population.

How can our magnificent array of food and the variety of nutrient needs be reduced so simply to a few food groups? A key assumption in selecting a healthful diet by using the food-group method is that from day to day and season to season, we will select differently from each of these groups, so that over a period of time, the nutritional values of many different foods will be balanced to a desirable average.

For this to happen, **variety is important.** We are assured of some variety by selecting foods from each of the food groups, but it's also important to choose a variety of foods within each food group.

It should be emphasized that each food is unique in its nutritional profile. For example, if one eats a serving of beef instead of pork, one takes in less thiamin, since pork happens to be an especially rich source. Similarly, one sort of apple or orange, nut or bean differs nutritively from others.

Foods are Not Sources of Single Nutrients

Thinking about foods in terms of single nutrients is a popular way of looking at nutrition in our society, and one which has been carefully fostered by commercial interests. They promote foods that are identified with certain glamorized nutrients.

For example, almost everyone knows that citrus is a good source of vitamin C. So a message used in advertising is that an orange-colored powder which contains vitamin C may be mixed with water and substituted for orange juice. The average consumer doesn't realize that other nutrients (e.g., folate) also found in orange juice are absent from this product. In fact, informed consumers know that they don't have to rely on citrus fruits for their vitamin C. They might get the recommended amount from a number of lesser sources during any given day—possibly a banana, some lettuce, a few cherries, some string beans.

A Daily Food Guide

The Daily Food Guide sets out a specified number of portions per day from Grain, Vegetable, Fruit, Milk, and Meat Groups (see Table 18-1). The Guide is part of the 2005 *Food Guide Pyramid* (Fig. 18-2) (www.MyPyramid.gov), which emphasizes the importance of exercise for health and weight control. The previous Food Guide Pyramid published in 1992 (Fig. 18-2) provides a better graphic of the food groups, with the Grain Group at its base, the Vegetable and Fruit Groups on the second tier, the Meat and Milk Groups on the third tier.[2]

We're advised to limit our intake of foods such as fats and sweets. Accordingly, these foods are grouped in a small section at the tip of the pyramid. Although some fats and sweets contribute vitamins and minerals, they mostly contribute calories.

At first glance, the numbers of recommended portions for the Vegetable, Fruit, and Grain Groups may seem high. But it's not unusual to eat 1½ cups of spaghetti (3 Grain portions), drink a 12-oz. cup of orange juice (2 Fruit portions), munch away at a cup's worth of party-platter carrot sticks and other assorted vegetables (2 Vegetable portions), and eat two slices of bread at a time in a sandwich or two halves of a bagel (2 Grain portions).

What Makes the Guide Work —Or Not Work?

Let's examine the Vegetable Group for a moment, as an example of how the food-group concept works. Many Americans don't eat the recommended 3 or more daily servings. (In fact, some people don't regularly eat any vegetables at all.) Instead of a lot of vegetables, we tend to eat a lot of high-fat/low-fiber foods, such as meat, cheese, and pastries. This partly why the American diet tends to be low in fiber and high in fat.

Table 18-1: A Daily Food Guide.

Grain Group: 6 or more portions (including 3 or more **whole grains**) for adolescents and adults; 6 or more smaller portions for children; 7 portions for pregnant or nursing women.

1 portion = 1 small pancake, slice of bread, tortilla; half a hamburger or hot dog bun; half a bagel or English muffin; 5 saltine crackers; 4 graham crackers; 1 oz. dry cereal (= 1 cup* cornflakes, ¼ cup Grape-Nuts); ½ cup cooked rice, pasta, cereal, grits.

Vegetable Group: 3 or more portions for adolescents and adults; 3 or more smaller portions for children; 4 or more portions for pregnant or nursing women. See Fruit Group for portion sizes.

Note: ½ cup* beans or peas can count as 1 full portion of vegetable or as ½ portion in the meat group.

Fruit Group: 2 or more portions for adolescents and adults;* 2 or more smaller portions for children; 3 or more portions for pregnant or nursing women.

1 portion = 1 medium fruit or vegetable (e.g., apple, carrot, banana, potato); 1 cup* raw, leafy green vegetable (e.g., lettuce); ½ cup fruit or vegetable (e.g., broccoli, canned, cooked spinach, chopped fresh fruit or vegetables); ¾ cup (6 fl. oz.) vegetable or fruit juice (for fruit drinks, count only the amount of juice stated on the label, e.g., 1 cup fruit drink of 25% juice = ¼ cup juice).

Note: Include 1 portion of a fruit or vegetable rich in vitamin C (e.g., orange, grapefruit, strawberries, green pepper, broccoli) and 1 portion of a carotene-rich (dark green or orange-colored) fruit or vegetable (e.g., carrot, spinach, pumpkin, broccoli, apricot, cantaloup.

Milk Group: 2 portions for adults age 19-50 and children 1 to 10 years old; 3 portions for ages 11-18, over 50, and for pregnant or nursing women.

1 portion = 1 cup* milk, yogurt, pudding, custard; 1½ cups ice cream, frozen yogurt, 2 cups cottage cheese ¼ cup Parmesan cheese; 1½ oz (1 oz = 1" cube) regular cheese (e.g., cheddar, swiss, monterey jack, mozzarella); 2 oz processed cheese (e.g., Velveeta). Cream cheese doesn't count; it's more like butter.

Meat or Meat-substitute Group: 2 portions for adolescents and adults; 2 smaller portions for children; 3 portions for pregnant or nursing women.

1 portion = 2 to 3 oz.** cooked poultry, fish, meat (including luncheon meats like bologna). (3 oz lean, cooked poultry, fish, meat is about the size of a deck of cards; 1 regular pre-sliced slice of bologna = 0.8 oz.); 2 frankfurters; 2 eggs; 1 cup* cooked peas, beans, lentils or soybean curd (tofu); ½ cup nuts, sunflower seeds; ¼ cup (4 Tablespoons) peanut butter.

*1 cup = 16 Tablespoons = 8 fluid ounces (fl oz).
  a regular can of soda = 1½ cups = 12 fl oz
**3 oz cooked poultry, fish, meat = size of a deck of cards.

Vegetables are generally high in fiber, vitamins, and minerals, and low in fat and calories. Eating the recommended portions of vegetables—and fruits and grains—generally improves our diets. In other words, the food-group method would help nutritionally if it were regularly used.

On the other hand, there are flaws in the system. And these flaws suggest the need for nutrition knowledge and planning beyond this Daily Food Guide. For one, there are now thousands of convenience foods in which "basic foods" are combined. How do you place pizza, or chicken-pot pie, or taco salad, in a food group? In many instances, small amounts from various foods groups may be present, but not enough to constitute a portion of any one group.

Consider a slice of sausage pizza. It has something of the Meat Group, but a high-fat meat in a small quantity. The crust may be suitable as a portion from the Grain Group (though it's unlikely to be made from whole grain), and the cheese may scrape through as a portion from the Milk Group. But what of the tomato sauce? Does it really make a vegetable serving?

Although the Daily Food Guide isn't ideal, it does steer us towards meeting our nutrient needs. It's less helpful in steering us away from excesses that may have a bearing on our risk of chronic disease.

Reducing Risk of Chronic Disease

Although scientists are just beginning to understand the relationships of nutrition to chronic disease, there's already substantial information on how diet affects the risk of such diseases as heart disease, type-2 diabetes, chronic liver disease, and some cancers. We've discussed many of these relationships in earlier chapters.

Unfortunately, we're bombarded with advice from many diverse sources, including advertisements, food labels, diet and health books and websites, and sports and fitness magazines, not all of which is based on scientific evidence. Often, the advice is tied in with products for sale. This—together with a steady stream of news reports of studies that often seem in conflict—can leave us bewildered. What's the consensus of our nutrition experts?

Dietary Guidelines for Americans

The Dietary Guidelines Advisory Committee, established jointly by the U.S. Department of Agriculture and U.S. Department of Health and Human Services, issues a set of *Dietary Guidelines for Americans*. These guidelines are for the general population age 2 and older, and are directed toward reducing the risk of chronic disease.

Originally published in 1980, they are revised every five years to reflect new scientific knowledge. The 2005 guidelines include advice to get adequate nutrients, limit saturated fat and sodium, maintain a healthy body weight, get regular physical activity, drink sensibly and moderately if you drink alcohol, and avoid microbial foodborne illness. For the complete guidelines, go to www.healthierus.gov/dietaryguidelines.

Other Dietary Advice

Many organizations, including the American Heart Association (www.americanheart.org), American Cancer Society (www.cancer.org), American Diabetes Association (www.diabetes.org), and government agencies make dietary recommendations concerning chronic disease. It's reassuring that the experts from these various groups have come up with remarkably similar recommendations (see Table 18-2), most of them covered by the Daily Food Guide and the Dietary Guidelines for Americans.

Practical Applications of Dietary Guides

The dietary guidelines form the basis of a "prudent diet"—There are many reasons to believe that following the advice would be healthful, and there are few, if any, reasons to believe the advice would be harmful. A prudent diet balances benefit against risk.

As said earlier, the Daily Food Guide focuses on providing adequate amounts of essential nutrients. The Dietary Guidelines for Americans and other general recommendations can be used to select foods within the food groups of the Daily Food Guide, For example, if you select low-fat or non-fat milk in the Milk Group, you are following the guideline to choose a diet lower in saturated

Figure 18-2: Two Food Guide Pyramids. The current (2005) one emphasizes the importance of exercise for health and weight control. The previous (1992) one emphasizes a diet rich in plant foods.

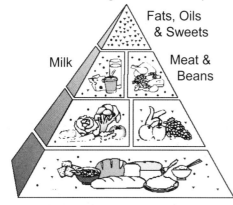

1992 Food Pyramid

- Presents food groups as a hierarhy, with grains as the base of a healthy diet
- Emphasizes limits on fats, oils and sweets, which are shown at the top of the pyramid.

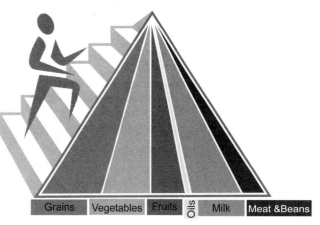

2005 Food Pyramid

- Emphasizes variety by representing food categories as a spectrum
- Introduces the role of exercise in health and weight control

fat, and cholesterol. Also, since non-fat and low-fat milks are lower in calories, this choice helps some people maintain healthy weight, another guideline.

Dietary changes made gradually are more likely to be successful. For example, it's hard to switch abruptly from whole milk to non-fat milk. (Dairy companies have made low-fat and non-fat milks more acceptable by adding either dry or condensed non-fat milk to give the milk more "body" so it has more of the "mouth feel" of whole milk.)

You can make the switch by combining whole milk and low-fat milk, gradually increasing the amount of low-fat milk. Then, you combine low-fat milk and non-fat milk. Once you switch to non-fat milk, even low-fat milk may taste like cream, and you can use it instead of cream in your coffee. Similarly, you can switch from sugared to diet soft drinks by gradually replacing more of the sugared drink in your cup with the calorie-free version.

Toward a More Personal Balance

While food guidelines are useful tools, they can't be depended upon to do the whole job, because really effective nutrition planning should take into consideration more specific characteris-tics of an individual or a group. A fundamental axiom is that food doesn't become nutrition until it passes the lips. Although some cultures view certain worms and termites, for example, as delicious, many of us would say that we wouldn't eat these if our lives depended on them. In fact, some people do refuse unfamiliar foods which could save them from malnutrition.

Many of us routinely refuse to eat familiar foods as well. The first President Bush has said he is familiar with broccoli—and will not eat it.

Dietary guidelines encompass a wide variety of preferences. In selecting from the Meat Group of the Daily Food Guide, for example, one can choose among a variety that includes beef, fish, lentils, eggs, and tofu (soybean curd).

The Calorie Budget

Whatever our food preferences, our choices must be made in light of our energy needs. Our calorie requirement represents a kind of budget, within which we must meet our nutrient needs. Clearly, the smaller our budget, the more careful we must be in how we spend the calories. (Snacks packed in 100-calorie portions make this easier.)

A strenuous athlete, burning perhaps 5,000 calories a day, can live in nutritional luxury. An athlete's need for protein, and most other nutrients,

Table 18-2: Consensus of Diet and Exercise Advice. Dietary Guidelines for Americans (DGA)[2], American Cancer Society (ACS)[3], American Heart Association (AHA).[4]

Aim for a healthy weight (for "healthy weights" see Table 3-1 in Chap. 3):

"Balance calories from food and beverages with calories expended." (DGA)

"Balance caloric intake with physical activity." (ACS)

"Use up at least as many calories as you take in." (AHA)

If you need to lose weight:

"Aim for a slow, steady weight loss by decreasing calorie intake while maintaining an adequate nutrient intake and increasing physical activity." (AGA)

"Achieve and maintain a healthy weight if currently overweight or obese." (ACS)

"Regular physical activity can help you maintain your weight, keep off the weight that you lose, and help you reach physical and cardiovascular fitness." (AHA)

Get regular exercise:

"Engage in at least 30 minutes of moderate-intensity physical activity, above usual activity, at work or home on most days of the week." (DGA)

"Engage in at least 30 minutes of moderate to vigorous physical activity, above usual activities, on 5 or more days of the week." (ACS)

"Aim for at least 30 minutes of moderate physical activity on most days of the week or—best of all—at least 30 minutes every day." (AHA)

Eat a lot of fruits and vegetables:

"Choose a variety of fruits and vegetables each day." (DGA)

"Eat five or more servings of vegetables and fruits each day." (ACS)

"Eating a variety of fruits and vegetables may help you control your weight and your blood pressure." (AHA)

Choose whole grains (e.g., whole wheat, brown rice, oatmeal, barley):

"In general, at least half the grains should come from whole grains." (DGA)

"Choose whole grains in preferences to processed (refined) grains and sugars. Limit consumption of refined carbohydrates, including pastries, sweetened cereals, and other high-sugar foods." (ACS)

"Unrefined whole-grain foods contain fiber that can help lower your blood cholesterol and help you manage your weight." (AHA)

Eat less saturated fat, trans fat, and cholesterol:

"Consume less than 10 percent of calories from saturated fatty acids and less than 300 mg/day of cholesterol, and keep trans fatty acid consumption as low as possible." (DGA)

"Choose fish, poultry, or beans as an alternative to beef, pork, and lamb." (ACS)

"Choose lean meats and poultry without skin and prepare them without added saturated and trans fat. Select fat-free, 1% fat, and low-fat dairy products." (AHA)

If you drink alcohol, do so in moderation (DGA, ACS, AHA define "moderate" the same):

"Those who choose to drink alcoholic beverages should do so sensibly and in moderation—defined as the consumption of up to one drink per day for women and up to two drinks per day for men." (DGA)

"If you drink alcoholic beverages, limit consumption." (ACS)

"If you drink alcohol, drink in moderation." (AHA)

---

isn't much more than that of a non-athlete of the same sex, age, and size. So by eating at least twice as many calories, the athlete can afford some free-spending.

The caloric need of an athlete today is closer to that of the average man living in the early 1900s. In those days, an average man engaged in enough physical labor to burn some 4,000 calories a day. Today, a man of the same size uses only about 2,500 calories because he's far more sedentary.

Some nutrient needs change with the number of calories consumed, but most do not. So most adults today must get much the same quantity of

nutrients from much less food. In terms of a nutrition budget, each calorie we spend must bring a higher nutritive return. Foods which supply many calories, but rather few nutrients, defeat this purpose. In other words, when fat, alcohol, or sugar is a major source of calories, nutritional adequacy can be a problem.

This doesn't mean we can't eat such calorie-dense foods as candy, potato chips, and pastries. It simply means that if we are sedentary, we can't eat as much of them, and must offset their caloric density with nutrient-dense foods. Alternatively, we could be more physically active.

Table 18-3: *Food Guide Comparison*

Food Guide	Description	Purpose
Recommended Dietary Allowances (RDAs)	Recommended daily intake of individual nutrients—amounts deemed safe and adequate for various population groups	Mainly for professional reference in evaluating and planning diets for both individuals and groups
Daily Food Guide/ Food Guide Pyramid	Recommends servings from 5 food groups, based on nutrient content	Simple guide to help consumers choose a diet adequate in nutrients
Dietary Guidelines	General recommendations, focusing mainly on diet and chronic disease relationships	General guideline to help consumers choose a diet thought to reduce risk of obesity, heart disease, cancer, etc.

Eating for Health and Pleasure

Those who grimace at broccoli and salivate at the thought of chocolate should be assured that eating for health can also be eating for pleasure.

Start out by making small and gradual adjustments that make for a better diet. Choose healthier versions of favorite foods: cheese with less fat, canned soups with less sodium, a hamburger instead of a cheeseburger, pepperoni and mushroom pizza rather than a pepperoni and sausage. How about a thick-crust instead of a thin-crust pizza? Add dark-green lettuce and a slice of tomato to your sandwich. Instead of ice cream, choose sherbet, ice milk, or low-fat frozen yogurt. And don't forget the possibility of eating smaller portions of favorite foods.

When nutrition education challenges pleasure, pleasure tends to win. It's perhaps the central thesis of this book that we need not stifle pleasure to survive. We need only be realists when we look at our pleasure and the essentials for good health. For each gustatory joy, there's a balance of good sense.

Chocolate candy and potato chips are not evils; they are foods to be eaten in smaller amounts, or infrequently in larger amounts. Knowledge of nutrition is, in the fullest sense, not an injunction to somber sacrifice. It's a guide to balance, to the use of reason and hard-won knowledge as aids to healthier lives.

Even with good nutrition knowledge, our personal experiences and feelings about food encompass a wide variety. There are those who take no pleasure in eating, and those who take ecstatic, obsessive pleasure in eating. There are those who eat only to satisfy hunger, and those who see food as medicine. And it's hard for one type to undersand the other. The personal stories at the end of this chapter give some insight into such differences.

Summary

A healthy, well-balanced diet provides a variety of foods and the right amount of nutrients—enough but not too much. How do we select such a diet? Expert committees provide us with several guidelines, including the Recommended Dietary Allowances (RDAs), a part of Dietary Reference Intakes (DRIs), A Daily Food Guide, and Dietary Guidelines for Americans (see Table 18-3).

The RDAs are recommended levels of nutrients that are calculated to meet the needs of virtually all healthy people in the U.S. and Canadian population. They have been set for every nutrient for which there is enough information, and they are periodically revised, as new information becomes available. There are many sets of RDAs, to account for such differences as age, gender, pregnancy, and breastfeeding.

The RDAs are not minimum requirements; they are recommended levels of intake. They include safety margins to allow for individual variation, life's normal stresses, and enough to provide for body reserves. All substances will cause harmful effects at some excessive level of intake. As such, ULs (Tolerable Upper Intake Levels) have been set for nutrients for which there is sufficient data to state the highest amount unlikely to have adverse effects for nearly all healthy people.

The U.S. Dept. of Agriculture set up A Daily Food Guide to simplify the process of selecting a diet that includes the recommended amounts of nutrients. The Guide divides food into 5 groups (Grain, Vegetable, Fruit, Milk, and Meat Groups), and recommends eating a certain number of portions from each group. Again, selecting a wide variety of food is recommended, since each food has a unique profile of nutrients.

The Dietary Guidelines for Americans, revised every 5 years, provide help in selecting a diet helpful in reducing the risk of such diseases as heart disease, chronic liver disease, certain cancers, and diseases caused by food-borne microbes.

When making changes toward a more healthy diet, it's better to make gradual changes that will help you make a habit of eating wisely. Adults today generally lead more sedentary lives than our ancestors. Thus, we need to choose foods that are nutrient-dense (more nutrients per calorie), and/or increase our physical activity.

Eating should be enjoyable. We aim for a diet that provides for both pleasure and health.

Personal Story: Nicole & Debra Schlesinger

Anorexia and I

by Nicole Schlesinger

I have lived with this "commander" who tells me what to do, what I can eat, and how much I must exercise, for almost 5 years. In the summer of 1997, when I was formally diagnosed with Anorexia Nervosa, I decided to give this voice a name: I call her, appropriately, Anorexia.

During my first semester at UC Berkeley, in the fall of 1994, Anorexia slowly sucked me into her world. At five feet six inches tall and 139 pounds, I decided to avoid the "freshman 15" by joining Weight Watchers with my mom. It was a mother/daughter "bonding" experience. Instead of following the plan sensibly, I took it to extreme: I counted every calorie, exercised intensely, and wrote everything down in my journal religiously. At this time, I didn't realize that my behaviors were the early signs of the disorder.

After leaving Weight Watchers three months later, weighing only nine pounds lighter, Anorexia became louder; she started to take over my life. I drifted through school between 1995 and 1997, not only convinced that eating an apple and carrots during the day was sufficient, but also that I had to purge those calories through vigorous exercise before I could eat dinner. Although I didn't weigh myself as a measure of my progress (a common practice amongst anorectics), I was losing weight at a rapid pace. When I dropped below 112 lbs, I stopped my period. This is a condition known as amenorrhea and is one of the diagnostic criteria in the DSM IV for Anorexia. I also developed gastrointestinal problems due to the lack of food in my stomach and the build up of acid.

Even though my weight plummeted to 95 lbs, Anorexia blinded me; I literally could not see how thin I was despite the fact that my family and friends expressed great concern about how skinny I looked. In some ways I actually thought I was still too fat. The distorted body image that I had (and still have) is another warning signal of an eating disorder.

The scale says I weigh 89 lbs! I don't believe what the scale says nor do I believe what my clothes show or people say. I know that I am fat and refuse to weigh 115 lbs. I want to be skinny. Skinny. Skinny. I want to lose weight and get to at least 80 lbs, if not lower.

This lifestyle, full of monotony, demands, and rituals, can be so frustrating that sometimes I want to jump out of myself and become someone else. To give you an idea of how bizarre some of these rituals are, I asked a friend how long it takes her to eat an apple. She said it takes her about 15 minutes and that she bites into it (as opposed to slicing it) because it tastes better that way. I, on the other hand, first cut one thin slice, cut that slice in half, and then cut each half into four equal size pieces. Not five, not three, but four. This "process" usually takes about two hours.

In many ways, my life is not really my own. I don't have the freedom to do what many college students do. I don't go out to eat, nor do I socialize with friends at a cafe. However, as strange as this may sound, I often thank Anorexia for her presence. She gives me insight into myself and also into the world of eating disorders.

Eating disorders, in general, are addictions such as smoking or drug dependence. They all serve as coping mechanisisms for the stresses of life. When I escape into Anorexia's world of food, weight, and exercise obsession, I numb out the pain, anger, or sadness that I feel. However, I know that Anorexia's life is a false reality and I am trying to find the key to unlock the handcuffs that tie me to her.

Remembering Nicole

by Debra Hope Schlesinger, Nicole's Mom

Nicole graduated from UC Berkeley in 1999 and that same year, wrote this story. At that time she was only 95 pounds, and yet graduated with a 3.8 with her degree in Molecular Cell Biology. She wanted to be a doctor to help others who are suffering from eating disorders.

She was married in 2000, and then had her baby daughter that following year, a true miracle as the doctors said she would have a very difficult time conceiving, if at all. Nicole was delighted; she wanted to be a mommy, and perhaps her baby would be the key to her recovery. During her pregnancy she ate well so there would be no harm to the baby. It was difficult seeing the pounds pack on, but she did it and was very proud and happy with herself.

Three weeks before Hannah was born, she started to slip, so that is when the doctors decided it was time to have her deliver. Her labor was induced. Hannah was born shortly after and was absolutely perfect!!! However, shortly after her birth and the stress of a newborn, Anorexia stated to take control again. Nicole slowly slipped back into her illness.

Nicole, over the last 8 years of her life, was hospitalized over 10 times. She had the best doctors and psychiatrists, and yet NOTHING nor NO ONE could save my daughter. Our family supported her 100% and did everything humanly possible.

Her illness was out of control and therefore she felt she could no longer fight it. My daughter passed away in her sleep from heart failure due to the Anorexia Nervosa on April 6, 2003. She was my only child/daughter and very best friend. I miss her more than words could ever say.

Anger, rage, depression and sadness is what I feel and that haunts me on a daily basis. Yes, there are some days I can even smile, laugh, or enjoy, BUT inside my heart and spirit are broken. I am so grateful to share this story with others, in memory of my precious daughter, Nicole.

Excerpt from Nicole and Debra's story in The California Woman Magazine, Jan/Feb 2008.

Personal Story: Richard Torregrossa

Respect, Don't Ridicule, Troops in Battle of Bulge

More and more I find myself admiring fat people. In recent days, for instance, on the Iron Mountain hiking trail in Poway—about 25 miles east of San Diego—I passed a large woman who was huffing and puffing on the rocky path that has a peak elevation of about 2,700 feet.

I was on the way down; she was on the way up. Round-trip it's about a 6-mile haul, so she had a long way to go. But although she was huffing and puffing, taking big gulps of hot dry air as the sweat poured down her glistening face, she seemed fiercely determined, and I had to admire that. We nodded hello as we passed, and then I heard her say, "I'm so sick of being fat." The remark was not necessarily directed at me. It was a shout out to the world, a declaration of purpose, a cry of personal motivation.

I silently cheered her on, and suddenly there was an added spring in my step. A fat woman had inspired me.

This had never happened before. Typically, professional athletes such as Michael Jordan, Tiger Woods or Alex Rodriguez serve as the role models for my own fitness routine, not fat women on hiking trails. Or fat women anywhere, for that matter.

In fact, fat people have always irritated me, especially on airplanes when their bulk spills over into my seat, making me feel cramped and uncomfortable. Quietly I would hiss at them, especially on long flights.

But that day I saw how hard at least one woman worked to lose weight, and my perceptions about fat people changed forever.

The "battle of the bulge" really is a battle for people like her, one I've never had to fight. I've always been thin, one of those annoying people who can eat whatever he wants and never gain a pound.

Perhaps even more annoying, I enjoy exercise. It's second nature to me. I've been happily engaged in one form of exercise practically all of my life, starting from the time I was a 12-year-old kid playing Pop Warner football.

Not exercising is more difficult for me than exercising. If I'm sick or injured and unable to work out at the gym or shoot hoops, I become nervous and ill-tempered.

But for many overweight people, exercise is a chore—some might even call it a curse, like my neighbor Jim, or "Jumbo Jim," as he is sometimes called, who suffered a heart attack about eight months ago. He's about 60 pounds overweight, and now exercise for him is an imperative, a matter of life and death, but he hates it. I think he'd rather clean cesspools than do jumping jacks.

Yet he exercises. We often take walks around the neighborhood, looking for steep hills to get his heart rate up, and I see what a struggle it is for him, how much he resists it yet pushes on.

He also has another hurdle that I've never encountered: His love of food is almost religious. I can easily skip a meal, pass up a luscious dessert at a holiday dinner or limit myself to one burger at a backyard barbecue.

He's different. He can launch into lyrical reminiscences about the wonderful meals of yore, when he was a kid growing up in an Italian family and his mother would begin cooking the rich red marinara sauce on Friday for the big meal on Sunday, the smell permeating the entire house for days.

He can recall in Proustian detail the delicious stacks of thinly cut Parma ham, the wonderful wedges of provolone cheese, the heaping mounds of steaming pasta, the long links of grilled sausages and the foot-long loaves of piping hot Italian bread. He can describe a meal he had 20 years ago at a Chinese restaurant he visited on a business trip in some distant city that had the best dumplings he's ever eaten. He visibly salivates when he tells me about a new recipe he's learned. His heroes are chefs—Emeril, Mario Batali and his latest discovery, Sam the Cooking Guy. And he has a huge crush on Giada De Laurentiis, the Food Network hottie.

Since his heart attack, he's dropped about 20 pounds, but he still has a long way to go, at least another 30 pounds. But when I observe how hard he's worked so far, I am filled with admiration.

He's painfully reduced his portions of lasagna, peppers and eggs, and many of the other foods he relishes. Some of his most beloved culinary treats he's eliminated altogether, such as pork fried rice, salami sandwiches and Krispy Kreme doughnuts.

A hike for him used to entail no more than a dash from the sofa to the refrigerator, but now he logs about 3 to 7 miles a week of brisk walking or hiking.

On the face of it, this doesn't seem very impressive to someone like me who is naturally active and athletic and immune to overeating, but when I acknowledge the tremendous willpower and discipline required for someone like Jumbo Jim, his accomplishment is really quite a feat. And once again I find myself inspired by a fat person.

Richard Torregrossa is a journalist and the author of the biography *Cary Grant: A Celebration of Style*. He lectures and writes extensively on style, entertainment, and cultural issues; www.richard torregrossa. com This story is an excerpt from his article in the San Francisco Chronicle (12/16/07).

Chapter 19

Nutrition and the Life Cycle

As we think of the different stages of life from a nutritional perspective, we find that each has its challenges, questions, and sometimes passionate controversies. Does the pregnant woman need supplements, how much weight should she gain, need she totally abstain from alcohol, cigarettes, and caffeine? To breast feed or bottle feed? What to do about the overweight infant or growing youngster? How does one deal with junk food and rampant snacking? And what are the special needs in later life?

In the fast-paced world of working mothers, day care, fast food franchises, and prepackaged microwave meals, there often isn't much time to study up on nutrition needs and resources. And even if there were, the constant siren songs of the pitchmen—on TV and websites, in the overwhelming array of grocery store instant "home cooked" wonder foods—would make objective study a challenge, to say the least.

Fortunately, it need not be as complicated as it often seems to be. Equipped with some basic facts, and the principles of nutrition science already presented, the consumer can make sense out of the over-all confusion, and make choices that are healthy, practical, and satisfying.

We require the same nutrients through-out life, but the amounts vary as we progress from birth to old age. This is reflected in the different sets of the Recommended Dietary Allowances (RDAs), discussed in the last chapter. The broad precepts of good nutrition and well-chosen food apply to all stages of life, but they're applied a bit differently at each stage.

In this chapter, we look at various stages of the life cycle and the special nutrient needs and dietary problems common to each. The emphasis is on the early years—the dietary habits of our childhood are often those we carry with us into adulthood and old age. It's in the later years that we reap the benefits—or pay the penalty—of life-long dietary habits.

The Creation of a New Life

In the nine months of pregnancy, a single cell grows into the multitude that makes up the newborn infant. The unborn child is, of course, completely dependent on a single person—the mother-to-be—not only for the nutrients needed for normal growth and development, but also for a safe haven from toxic substances like alcohol. After birth, the mother who exclusively breast-feeds her child extends her pregnancy role of being wholly responsible for her child's nutrition.

Pregnancy

The Placenta

The woman and her fetus don't share a common blood supply. Instead, substances move between them through the intertwining of maternal and fetal blood vessels in an organ called the placenta (see Fig. 19-1). The placenta develops within the uterus during pregnancy. It connects to the fetus through the umbilical cord, and is discharged shortly after birth (the "afterbirth"). The fetus receives nourishment and discards waste products through the placenta.

For simplicity, "fetus" is used to describe all stages of prenatal development. The technically correct terms are: zygote, for the first 2 weeks; embryo, for weeks 3 to 8; and fetus, from week 8 until birth.

Many medications, including aspirin, can cross the placenta. So can caffeine, alcohol, cocaine, viruses, and substances absorbed into the bloodstream from cigarette smoke. Smoking during pregnancy appears to hinder fetal growth (women who smoke give birth to smaller babies), and may have other adverse effects as well.

The placenta begins to form when the fertilized egg implants itself into the lining of the uterus.

Although the precise effects (if any) of many substances passed to the fetus aren't known, it goes without saying that one should exercise caution. Caffeine, for example, appears to be safe in moderate amounts. To be extra-cautious, however, it's suggested that pregnant women restrict their daily caffeine intake to a small amount (e.g., the amount in one cup of coffee or two 12-oz. cans of caffeine-containing soft drinks).

Fetal Alcohol Effects

Alcohol passes freely through the placenta, so the fetus's blood-alcohol level is the same as the mother's. Exposure to alcohol can affect the fetus's developing brain, and is thought to be a major cause of mental retardation in this country.

Fetal alcohol syndrome is the full-fledged syndrome, characterized by mental retardation, a small head, growth retardation, abnormal facial features (e.g., eye-openings that aren't as wide as normal), and other deformities. Although the full-fledged syndrome occurs in only about 6% of children of alcoholic mothers, milder forms of brain damage occur in many more children.

There's been considerable debate as to whether moderate or low doses of alcohol, especially late in pregnancy, damage the fetus. The controversy exists because of a lack of solid evidence of damage. Unlike deformities of the face or heart, subtle damage to the brain isn't easily measured. Even behavior and learning disabilities are very difficult to assess, since it's nearly impossible to distinguish alcohol effects from those of other environmental or genetic factors.

People sometimes think that if a child doesn't have the characteristically abnormal facial fea-

Figure 19-1: Substances move between mother and fetus through the placenta.

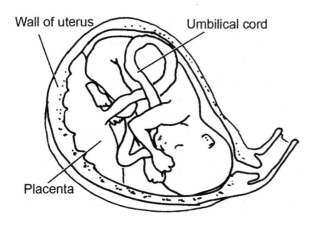

tures of fetal alcohol syndrome, the brain hasn't been affected. But these facial abnormalities are formed only during the first three months of pregnancy, whereas the formation of the brain continues throughout fetal life and into early infancy.

Illogical behavior is common among alcohol-affected children. Those affected literally act as if they aren't properly "connected," perhaps because alcohol interfered with the development of pathways and connections in the brain. Animal studies show that fetal alcohol exposure can cause such effects, but it would be difficult, if not impossible, to pinpoint their causes in human studies.

Given the uncertainties, women who are pregnant or are trying to conceive should **not** drink any alcohol.

Nutrient Needs in Pregnancy

Most women believe that special concern for their diets becomes necessary as soon as they become pregnant. In fact, such concern, and appropriate dietary changes ought to start even earlier. Often, a woman does not realize she is pregnant until she is already a month or two along. Very little growth in size occurs during the first two months, but there are crucial developmental changes. Also, the development of a healthy placenta during the first month of pregnancy is in large part dependent on the nutritional status of the mother when she conceives. A healthy placenta is needed for optimal growth and development of the fetus.

If the mother has eaten a nutritious diet beforehand, she need make little change during her first few months of pregnancy. The obstetrician uses these first few months to correct nutritional problems—such as iron-deficiency anemia—and to see to it that the mother-to-be has adequate stores for the last two-thirds of pregnancy.

A good diet is an important part of prenatal care. Except for iron, the dietary recommendations for pregnancy can easily be met by a sound diet. The RDA for iron during pregnancy is 27 mg—much more than before pregnancy (15-18 mg)—an amount much higher than that found in a regular diet. The reason for such a high iron RDA is that the majority of women come into pregnancy with low iron stores.

Most obstetricians, unsure about the adequacy of their patients' diets, prescribe a prenatal supplement that includes (in addition to iron) vitamins and other minerals.

Folate (folic acid) deficiency in early pregnancy has been associated with neural tube defects. The neural tube (an embryonic structure that develops into the brain and spinal cord) is formed during early pregnancy. Folate deficiency—and neural tube defects—is now less common, because the addition of folate to refined grains (e.g., white flour) has been required since 1998. As an extra precaution, it's recommended that all women capable of becoming pregnant take 400 mcg (100% DV) of folate in a multivitamin pill or in a fortified food product, e.g., a fortified breakfast cereal.

The Need for a More Nutrient-Dense Diet: "Eating for two" does not justify eating with abandon. Although the caloric cost of pregnancy is about 70,000 calories, this is an average of only 260 calories/day over the nine months. The calorie

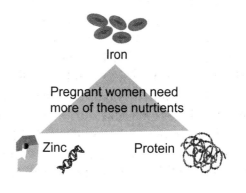

Figure 19-2: Increases in the RDA for certain nutrients during pregnancy.

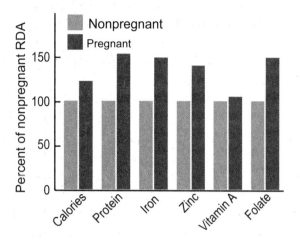

cost isn't distributed evenly over the nine months. The recommended calories doesn't increase in the 1st trimester, is an added 340 calories/day in the 2nd trimester, and an added 452 calories in the 3rd trimester.[1] For a woman who requires 2,000 calories per day when not pregnant, an added 452 calories is only a 23% increase.

The need for many nutrients increases much more. There's a big increase in the folate RDA (from 400 to 600 mcg) and as mentioned earlier, there's a big increase in the iron RDA (from 15-18 to 27 mg). The RDA for other nutrients is increased more moderately (see Fig. 19-2). Because the general increase in RDA for nutrients is more than the increase in calories, a pregnant woman must eat a more nutrient-dense diet. Alternatively, she could be more physically active to further increase her calorie needs.

For women with poor diets, prenatal supplements provide some help. But taking supplements often gives a false sense of security—that the supplement insures adequate nutrition. Supplements don't generally contain protein or fiber or very much calcium, and there may be other missing nutrients. A well-balanced diet, rather than relying on supplements, provides the best safeguard.

Also, excessive amounts of some nutrients can be harmful. Large doses of vitamin A, for example, can cause fetal malformations. One shouldn't be haphazard in taking dietary supplements, especially during pregnancy. For guidance in meeting the nutritional needs of pregnancy, look back at the Daily Food Guide in Chapter 18. The number

of servings recommended from each of the five food groups is higher for pregnancy:

- 7 daily servings in the grain group
- 4 or more in the vegetable group
- 3 or more in the fruit group
- 3 each in the milk and meat groups

Again, because the increase in the recommended number of servings is larger than the increase in calorie need, a pregnant woman should make lower caloric choices (e.g., non-fat milk in the milk group)—or be more physically active.

The Vegan Mother: It's difficult to meet the nutrient needs of pregnancy on a vegan (plant foods only) diet. The most obvious challenge is vitamin B-12, which isn't found in plant foods (see Chap. 14). It must be provided in plant foods fortified with B-12 (e.g., B-12-fortified soy milk) or as a prenatal supplement. B-12 is essential for proper development of the fetal nervous system.

It's also a challenge for pregnant women on a vegan diet to get enough calcium, iron, and zinc. Part of the reason is that minerals from plant foods aren't as well absorbed as they are from animal foods. Extra-special care in planning a vegan diet is important to assure adequate nutrition during pregnancy and lactation. Women who are vegans may want to consult a Registered Dietitian for diet counseling.

Weight Gain During Pregnancy

For a woman of normal weight, a gain of about 25-35 pounds is recommended during pregnancy, with most of the gain taking place during the last 6 months (see Fig. 19-3). Underweight women should gain a bit more, and overweight women a bit less. In no case should a woman—overweight or not—try to lose weight during pregnancy. This can have adverse effects on the fetus. Ideally, underweight and overweight women should attain a normal weight before becoming pregnant.

Birth Weight—A Predictor of Health for the Newborn: A woman's pre-pregnancy weight and her weight gain during pregnancy are often the determining factors in the birth weight of her child. The birth weight, in turn, is a major

Figure 19-3: Components of weight gain during pregnancy.

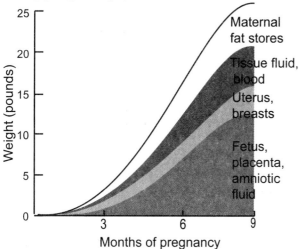

predictor of health and survival of the newborn. Full-term babies weighing 7 to 8 pounds at birth have the greatest chance of infant survival and good health.

A full-term baby weighing $5^{1}/_{2}$ pounds or less at birth is at particularly high risk of developing health problems or not surviving the first year of life. In the U.S., such low-birth-weight babies are more common among blacks and among lower socioeconomic groups.

Although several factors can contribute to low birth weight (e.g., smoking during pregnancy), a mother's health and nutrition during and prior to pregnancy have a major impact. Unmarried young teenagers from lower socioeconomic groups are at greatest risk of delivering low-birth-weight infants. Commonly, these young teens are still growing themselves (increasing their nutrient needs even more), and receive little prenatal care.

The Nursing Mother

For the nursing mother herself, there are physiological advantages of breastfeeding. Among the poor in developing countries, a prominent advantage is that lactation (milk production) reduces a woman's fertility, lessening her chances of becoming pregnant. Where food is scarce, a delay in another pregnancy can make a tremendous difference in her own health, and can be a matter of life or death for her child. The early displacement of an infant at the breast by the birth of a sibling is often a precipitating cause of severe malnutrition and its accompanying ills.

Another advantage in developing countries is that breast feeding is a safe and sanitary method of feeding infants. Bottle feeding may not be, depending on local conditions (e.g., availability of clean water) and the way in which bottles are handled.

In the well-fed U.S. population, a prominent advantage for the mother is that breastfeeding helps her return to her pre-pregnancy weight. She "exports" calories in her breast milk, and also uses energy in producing the milk. The added calorie expenditure of a nursing mother increases in proportion to the amount of milk produced.

The estimated added calorie recommendation is 330 calories/day during the 1st six months. The actual calorie need is about 500 calories per day. The 170-calorie difference (500 minus 330) is expected to come from fat normally stored during pregnancy in anticipation of the added calorie needs of lactation.[1] This extra fat storage amounts to about 8 pounds,[2] enough to provide those 170 calories per day over a 6-month period of lactation.[3] (Conversely, one can see that if a woman doesn't breast-feed, she has to eat less and/or exercise more to lose the added fat stores.)

Kwashiorkor—the severe and often fatal disease of protein-deficiency common in developing countries—is a local term in Gold Coast, Africa for *displaced child*.

An interesting way to look at the added calorie allotments for pregnancy and lactation is this: For the last six months of pregnancy, a woman needs, on average, an extra 400 calories per day, and is expected to gain weight. For the first six months of breastfeeding, a woman needs an extra 500 calories per day, and is expected to lose weight (with 170 of those 500 calories coming from fat she stored during pregnancy). For some women, this is reason enough to breast-feed.

Just as there's a need for a more nutrient-dense diet during pregnancy, so it is during lactation (see Fig. 19-4). Not as much so, however. The extra calorie allotment for lactation is a bit more than for pregnancy, whereas the increases in nutrient requirements are the same or a bit less.

Figure 19-4: Increases in the RDA for certain nutrients during lactation.

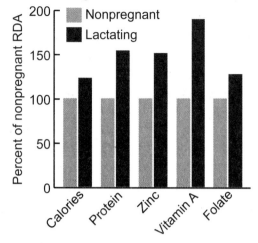

Figure 19-5: Some nutrient needs are much higher for infants, relative to body weight, than for adults.

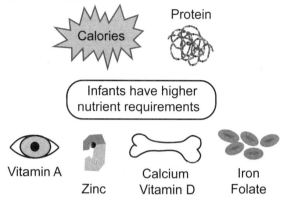

Almost all women are physically able to breast-feed. Breast size isn't a factor. The American Academy of Pediatrics states, "Breastfeeding should be continued for at least the first year of life and beyond for as long as mutually desired by mother and child."[3]

Diet for a Small Life

Babies grow at a tremendous rate. If a 120-pound, 5'4" woman grew as quickly, she'd be about 350 pounds and 8' in a year. Needless to say, newborns need a lot of calories for their body size. An equivalent amount for the baby's father would be about 8,000 calories a day. It's no wonder that newborns spend so much of their waking hours sucking at the breast or bottle. Appropriately, breast milk and infant formula are concentrated sources of calories—about 50% of the calories comes from fat.

Nutrient needs are extraordinary at this stage of life. An infant needs about half the vitamins A and C, and as much vitamin D as the father. The infant-adult comparison of nutrient needs is especially striking when compared per unit of body weight (see Fig. 19-5). Clearly, nutrient deficiencies during this time when infant growth rate is so high can quickly lead to trouble.

The most noticeable result of undernourishment is a stunting of growth. When the undernourishment persists through childhood, the result is a smaller adult. Looking back over the centuries—or even early in this century—we see that

our ancestors were much smaller, a reflection of an inadequate diet and other environmental conditions. We see stunted growth even today in poor children and adults living in developing countries. When people immigrate here from those countries, a marked increase in height in the next generation is common, a reflection of our ample food supply, better sanitation, etc.

Generally speaking, mother's milk is both an adequate and ideal source of all the infant's required nutrients during the first 4 to 6 months of life. This assumes, however, that the infant is born well-nourished, and the mother was well-nourished during pregnancy and continues to be so during lactation.

The well-nourished newborn has stores of such nutrients as iron, copper, and vitamins A and D. Infants meet their nutrient needs from a combination of these body stores and breast milk. For example, infants require a fair amount of iron, and to meet this need they rely both on breast milk and on their liver stores. So if the child is born malnourished, breast milk alone may not provide enough.

Breast or Bottle?

It's hard to find a nutritionist who doesn't emphasize breastfeeding. The psychological and biological advantages of breastfeeding are well documented. For one, breast milk provides immunities against disease, whereas infant formulas do not. Also, breast milk is less likely to cause digestive upsets and allergies. (On the other hand, if a woman can't breastfeed her child,

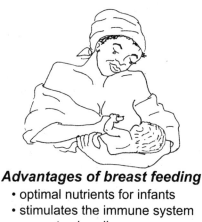

Advantages of breast feeding

• optimal nutrients for infants
• stimulates the immune system
• promotes bonding
• always ready
• at the correct temperature
• sanitary
• inexpensive

be assured that science is now able to provide excellent nutrition for the formula-fed baby.)

In developing countries, infant formula isn't generally a viable option. Breastfeeding is of tremendous importance where malnutrition and poor sanitation are common. Breast milk is often the only regular source of high-quality protein and other essential nutrients.

Aggressive marketing of infant formula in developing countries has often led to misuse, with disastrous results. It's easy to understand why such promotional campaigns have strong appeal. Mothers everywhere want what's most "modern" for their children, and would like them to be as healthy and happy as those pictured in the ads for infant formula.

When free samples of infant formula are given to poor mothers in developing countries, they usually can't afford to buy more. If they stop breastfeeding while using the free samples, they may stop lactating (producing milk). Infants in these countries are often at high risk of developing protein-calorie malnutrition when breastfeeding is cut short because of the short-term use of infant formula.

To make matters worse, the mothers often greatly over-dilute the infant formula (thereby diluting the nutrients) to make it go further. Also, when unsanitary water is added to the formula, it can cause diarrhea (a leading cause of infant mortality in these countries).

Sometimes, when the formula is gone (or there

was none to begin with), liquids of poor nutritional quality with the appearance of milk (e.g., rice water) are used in the baby bottle. World health organizations are doing what they can to encourage breastfeeding in developing countries.

There are circumstances, however, where infant formula is the better choice, e.g., when the mother is infected with HIV, since the virus can be transmitted through breast milk. But where there's no food for the infant, risking HIV infection from breast milk is the only choice.

The advantages of breastfeeding over infant formula aren't so obvious in countries with good sanitation, and where top-quality infant formula is readily available and affordable. There are, of course, instances where breastfeeding is an especially better choice—for an infant who tends to develop allergies, for example.

A mother whose diet is inadequate creates a dilemma in administering food-assistance programs in developing countries: Should the emphasis be on feeding the nursing mother, so she can provide more milk for her child, or should the limited resources be used to feed the infant directly?

Many women have jobs outside the home that make it difficult to breastfeed. A compromise is to breastfeed as long as possible, even if it's only for a few weeks. Thereafter, she can use infant formula exclusively, or combine formula with breastfeeding (directly or by using a breast pump to obtain milk for use when the mother is away.)

The nursing mother must drink plenty of liquids and eat a good diet to adequately nourish her child. Although the mother's diet results in some variation in the composition of the milk, the main variation is in the amount produced. When a mother's diet is inadequate, the main consequence is that she makes less milk.

In addition to eating a good diet, a nursing mother should continue to be cautious about taking in extraneous substances that can pass into her breast milk. For example, small amounts of alcohol can enter the breast milk, and there's some evidence that this small amount can have an effect on the infant's developing nervous system. A nursing mother should also restrict her caffeine intake.

Some flavors in food can pass into the breast milk, perhaps an advance billing for what flavors can be expected when the infant joins in the family meals. On the other hand, some flavors can be a problem if the infant nurses less as a result. If an offending flavor is suspected in breast milk, the mother can try eliminating the food to see if it helps. But she might want to try this more than once to make sure—especially if it means giving up a favorite food.

Balancing Baby Foods and Baby Needs

Infants should be fed breast milk or infant formula through the first year of life. Whole cow's milk shouldn't be introduced until the early part of the second year.

The American Academy of Pediatrics's Committe on Nutrition recommends that solid foods not be introduced until 4 to 6 months of age.[3] Although studies indicate that infants can tolerate cereals, vegetables, etc., at a few weeks of age, there's no need for them so early.

In realistic terms, the amount of solids fed at first is very little; it amounts to little more than training infants to accept and swallow solids. But because this learning takes time, most physicians start babies on such foods as early as four months of age.

The addition of solid food becomes necessary at about six months because nutrient needs are beginning to exceed what milk and body stores alone can provide. The solid foods should be mostly cereals, vegetables, and fruits.

There is no pressing nutritional reason to urge a lot of meat on an often reluctant baby. True, meat is rich in protein. But so is milk (given only as breast milk or infant formula for the first year). Two 8-oz. bottles of whole milk a day furnish the entire protein need for babies up to 20 pounds. Three 8-oz. bottles provides enough protein for a 30-pound baby. True, meat also supplies iron and zinc, but the amount of meat a baby eats is so small that meat is unlikely to be a major contributor.

Cereals, vegetables, and fruits supply a lot of nutrients, especially those in short supply in milk. It would, however, take huge quantities of these foods to meet infant RDAs for iron, so baby cere-als are heavily fortified. The iron deficiency that's common in American children often appears at about the time parents discontinue infant cereals.

Should sugar be eliminated from baby food? As with adults, sugar only really becomes a problem when it becomes too much of a nutritional diluent. Infants are born with an inherent disposition towards sweetness, and a preference for sweets is easy to cultivate—as can be seen by the super-market array of sugary ready-to-eat breakfast cereals made to appeal to young children.

As for sweetening foods or using sweets to entice children to eat, a most important psychological factor enters here. Patterns of coaxing, rewarding, and emotional upset and relief that center on food add life-long emotional connotations to eating, which can cause trouble later on. Parents should keep in mind that infants—and toddlers—have an inherent ability to regulate caloric intake.[4]

From Toddler to Teen

The Slowing of Growth

During the first year of life, the body weight almost triples, and there's about a 9 or 10 inch increase in height. A dramatic slowdown occurs in the second year, and continues (less dramatically) through childhood (see Fig. 19-6). Girls reach a growth peak at about puberty. Boys continue growing for two to six years longer.

The slowdown in that second year of life is dramatic. It's not just growth rate that changes, but the whole pace of metabolism. The newborn's heart beats about 130 times a minute; it slows to 100 at age two. Body temperature increases slightly through the first year, then begins to go down. Breathing goes from 30 breaths a minute in the first year to 25 in the second. These factors all contribute to the baby's very high rate of metabolism, which then drops rapidly as the baby enters the toddler stage.

Toddlers may still eat a considerable amount of food, but less in relation to their size than during that first year of life. This slowdown in eating causes some parents to worry needlessly. But because they're eating less, the nutrient density of their diet is important.

Figure 19-6: Body weight from birth to adulthood.

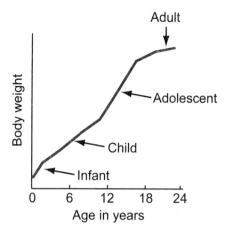

This explains why nutritionists are concerned with the nutritive qualities of children's snacks. Snacks represent such a substantial portion of a typical child's diet that they must be thought of, not as extra treats, but as small auxiliary meals.

Early Childhood— A Time to Start Good Habits

Age two is a milestone of sorts in terms of dietary guidelines. It's at this age, for example, that we're advised to heed the dietary guideline to limit saturated fat (see Chap. 18). But parents shouldn't go overboard. There have been numerous instances where a child's growth has been stunted because of overly strict restriction of fat and calories by well-meaning parents.

Early childhood is a good time to begin instilling the basics of good nutrition—a time to learn about the nutritive value of various foods and the importance of a diet that includes a variety of foods. This is also a good time to start letting children participate in preparing meals, not only to familiarize them with what goes into what they eat, but so that they can develop the skills and enjoyment of cooking.

In the nutrition education of a child, the central aim should be the future well-nourished adult. This is especially important as one begins to deal with the toddler, who is forming and expressing narrow preferences. We shouldn't pass on to our children our culture's esteem for the rich man's diet—centered on meat, and heavy in fat.

Early childhood is when children learn to expect—or not expect—dessert after dinner. To expect—or not expect—a soft drink with the pizza. A bag of chips in the lunch-box. A cookie for being good. Nutrition is a family matter. It's generally found that when a family's food habits are good or poor, so are those of the children.

Variety is important in a balanced diet, and early childhood is a good time to introduce this variety. Although children commonly reject new foods when they are first given a taste, they usually acquire a taste for the foods after repeated tastings.[4] So it is that Mexican children like hot salsa, Japanese children like seaweed, and American children like macaroni and cheese.

Besides establishing eating habits, early childhood is also a time of establishing other health habits, particularly exercise habits. Does the family recreation tend toward watching television together, or does it tend toward early evening walks to the playground?

It's no mystery as to why good eating and exercise habits acquired in early childhood are key to maintaining good health and a healthy body weight throughout one's lifetime.

The Things Kids Eat

It isn't long before we start losing control over what the growing child eats. While we can do our best to see that nutritious snacks and meals are offered at day-care centers and schools, the choices widen for children as they grow older. Nevertheless, a lot of their food is still eaten at home—and they can't eat what's not there.

If a parent's not home when the child comes home from school, there could be a sandwich and cut-up fruit ready for the after-school snack. And for a time, anyway, we have control over how much money they have available to buy food away from home.

We worry about their diet. After all, they tend to make such narrow food choices, with a taste for hot dogs, peanut butter, hamburgers, soft drinks, and whatever is fried, frosted, or suitable for dipping. Yet, with only a few exceptions (e.g., iron intake is commonly low), most of them get enough of the required nutrients.

How can children include so much of what many parents call "junk" in their diet, yet still get enough nutrients to keep healthy and grow? The biggest reason is that the amount of food that children eat *in proportion to their size* is quite different from that of their parents.

For example, let's compare the food intakes of a 10-year-old boy and his 30-year-old mother. He weighs 65 pounds, and she weighs 130—twice as much. Yet, the typical caloric need for each is the same—about 2,100 calories a day.

Next, consider the fact that, although the boy requires more nutrients relative to his body size, most of the boy's RDAs are lower than his mother's. For example, his protein RDA *per pound body weight* is higher than his mom's (0.43 vs. 0.36 gm). But because he weighs so much less, the total amount of protein he needs each day is less: His protein RDA is 28 gm protein (0.43 gm/lb x 65 lb); hers is 47 gm (0.36 gm/lb x 130 lb).

His vitamin C RDA is 45 mg; hers is 75 mg. His iron RDA is 8 mg; hers is 18 mg. And so it goes. Compared to his mother, he needs to use a smaller part of those 2,100 calories to meet his nutrient needs.

He has many more extra calories to "spend" on such foods as candy bars and potato chips. His mother, however, often gets the impression that his diet, replete with "junk food," is really much poorer than it is.

But children this age commonly stretch that extra capacity for luxury foods a bit too far. The delicate job of a parent is to make sure that foods containing the essential nutrients get first priority, and are eaten in adequate amounts. Once this is done, the child should still have plenty of room in the diet for the less nutritious foods.

Even "junk foods" are a source of nutrients. Ice cream has some of the merits of other milk products—and french fries drenched in catsup are derived from the vegetable group. "Junk foods" should not, however, make up a disproportionately large part of the diet, even at this age.

The larger nutritional concerns are those of the "typical American diet"—particularly the problem of excess calories. Alarmingly, obesity (see Chap. 4) and diabetes (see Chap.5) are increasing and occurring at younger ages. One target in

reducing calorie intake is cutting back on the soft drinks ("empty calories") that children drink so much of. Also, drinking one's calories is fast, so even fruit juice should be limited (encourage eating whole fruits). Water and milk should be the beverages of choice.

Children's diets tend to get worse as they enter the adolescent years—all the more reason why it's so important to develop good dietary habits in early childhood. Again, parents still have some control over what their adolescent eats at home.

Convenience is urgently critical to the typical teenager—especially teenage boys who come home from school ravenously hungry. (A published report tells of the teenager who took a jelly donut from freezer to microwave oven, jammed it in his mouth, and suffered a serious burn to the roof of his mouth from the scalding-hot jelly.) Small differences in convenience can change a choice. If the choice is cold water in the refrigerator or unchilled soft drinks in the back cupboard—you guessed it.

Plenty of physical activity can do much to counterbalance the worsening of the diet. Exercise increases the calorie need much more than the nutrient need. The most worrisome combination is a worsening diet and declining physical activity, as one's physical growth comes to an end. This combination is common among adolescent girls as they become more weight conscious, less "tomboyish," and stop growing—all at the same time.

The Adult Years

The general dietary principles that apply during childhood extend into adulthood. But because growth has stopped, it's no longer a factor in determining nutrient need. For men, nutrient needs throughout adulthood vary relatively little—they are based mostly on body size and the amount of physical activity.

In contrast, the nutrient needs of women vary considerably during adulthood, mainly because of childbearing. As discussed earlier, menstruation, pregnancy, and lactation increase nutrient requirements, making women more vulnerable to developing deficiencies.

Women need a more nutrient-dense diet than men. Compared to men, they need fewer calories because they are smaller and are, on average, less physically active. Women also go on low-calorie reducing diets more often. Furthermore, young women are the prime candidates for the eating disorders *anorexia nervosa* and *bulimia* (see Chap. 3), which can cause severe malnutrition.

Women's Special Needs

Nutrients and the Menstrual Cycle

The main nutritional concern with menstruation is the increased need for iron, because iron is lost in menstrual blood losses (see Fig. 19-7). The increased iron requirement of menstruating women and the iron-deficiency anemia that can result were discussed in Chapter 17. The iron RDA of menstruating women is more than twice that of men of comparable ages. At menopause, the iron RDA drops to that of men.

The menstrual cycle also affects caloric needs. A woman's basic caloric requirement starts to rise around the time of ovulation, and peaks just before or at the beginning of menstruation, whereupon it falls and remains at that lower level until mid-cycle when ovulation occurs again.

The fluctuation in the body's base-line energy need is reflected in a fluctuation of body temperature. A woman can find out when she ovulates by taking her temperature upon awakening every morning (before getting out of bed) and looking for the rise in body temperature associated with ovulation.

A woman's appetite often reflects these cyclic changes. Many find that they are hungrier and eat more during the last part of their menstrual cycle, and that their appetite lessens and they eat less when menstruation begins. Body water also fluctuates during the cycle, generally paralleling the fluctuation in basic calorie needs.

Thus, women shouldn't be unduly concerned with increased appetite and weight late in the cycle. The increased hunger is from the body's increased use of calories, and the extra water will be lost early in the following cycle.

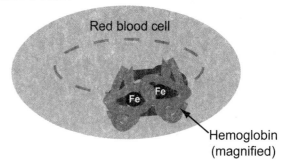

***Figure 19-7: Iron (Fe) is an integral part of hemoglobin**, the oxygen-carrying protein in red blood cells.*

Red blood cell

Hemoglobin (magnified)

Nutrition with Advancing Years

The most basic nutrition problem of many older people is that they eat fewer calories. Part of this decline is appropriately in line with their declining needs. But much too often, caloric intake falls even below need.

With aging, the sense of taste and smell is lost to some extent, and this is thought to be one cause of diminishing appetite. The situation is made worse by false notions that spicy, seasoned foods aren't good for older people. Unless there is some specific digestive disorder, diagnosed by a physician who then prescribes bland foods, there's no reason why an older person can't enjoy seasonings—and spicy foods may perk up the appetite.

The sense of thirst also diminishes for the elderly, and may not be reliable as a guide for water need. So the elderly should make a point of drinking liquids. The precise amount needed varies, of course, depending on such things as climate, physical activity, intake of watery foods (e.g., fruit).

Many elderly eat less because of the social and economic problems which often accompany aging—loss of friends, close family, and income. These can lead to general depression or indifference, and a loss of interest in eating.

Seniors need a nutrient-dense diet. As people age, the decreased need for calories is combined with an undiminished need for nutrients.

One of the most important nutrition problems of our seniors is that promoters commonly single them out to be duped, convincing them that their

Figure 19-8: Age-related changes.

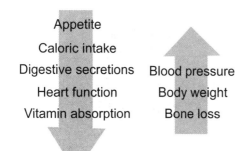

Appetite
Caloric intake
Digestive secretions   Blood pressure
Heart function   Body weight
Vitamin absorption   Bone loss

nutritional needs are unique and can't be met by ordinary foods. There are many pathetic reports of the results. Too commonly, the elderly will spend much of the money they need for ordinary food (not to mention housing, medical care, etc.) on "special foods and supplements" sold to them with special promises.

Because the nutrients must come from less food at this stage of life, there's a greater chance that a false reliance on health foods and special supplements, or experiments with eccentric and unbalanced diets, will be harmful.

Vitamin B-12 in a vitamin pill or a fortified food (e.g., fortified breakfast cereal) is advised for the elderly—not because they need more or eat less, but because their ability to absorb it is often diminished (see Chap. 10).

Improving the Diet

The challenges of aging can be very great indeed, but from strictly a nutritional point of view, the problems aren't really difficult to handle. The usual dietary patterns of the elderly show a disproportionately large intake of breads and cereals, which are cheaper, more easily stored, and more convenient and easier to eat. The intake of meat and milk lessens, and fruits and vegetables are often lacking. Fats, with their concentrated caloric value, tend to hold their place in the diet, as do sweets and desserts.

If one looks at the typical diet of the older person and compares it to the recommended servings in the Daily Food Guide, one quickly sees how the diet can be remedied. Fruits and vegetables add relatively little to the tight caloric budget, but

supply missing vitamins and minerals. A swing away from the over-emphasis on breads and cereals, and toward more animal products also helps. A glass or two of non-fat or low-fat milk a day and a few eggs a week often can improve an older person's diet enormously, at quite small caloric cost. The elderly tend to eat less at meals and to snack, and milk and milk products such as yogurt make very good snacks.

Unless cholesterol is restricted in the diet for medical reasons, eggs have many practical advantages for the elderly. As said in Chapter 9, eggs are inexpensive, keep a long time in the home refrigerator, are tasty, and are easy and quick to cook in a variety of ways. The softness of eggs is desirable for those with missing teeth or ill-fitting dentures. These are significant considerations for the elderly—especially if they are poor as well. Eggs are a major source of cholesterol and can raise blood-cholesterol, but blood-cholesterol levels aren't as predictive of heart disease in the elderly as they are in other adults.

Commonly, however, all that's needed to improve the diet is the company of other people. People young and old tend to prepare more nutritious meals when preparing food for others, and they tend to eat more food in the company of others.

"Move Them Bones"

One of the most important nutritional safeguards of the later years is exercise. Experts on the problems of aging conclude that few of their patients get enough exercise. Yet, as one such doctor puts it, "The longer you keep moving, the longer you'll be able to move."

Aside from the obvious psychological and physical benefits (e.g., osteoporosis, discussed in Chap. 16), exercise gives older people far more room to err in their diet. As with any age group, exercise causes a person to need more and eat more food. An extra couple of hundred calories a day in food can make all the difference in the quality of the older person's diet. The effect is self-perpetuating: The exercise stimulates the appetite, the diet improves, and the resulting sense of well-being encourages one to be more physically active.

Lifelong Habits

We see in the dietary problems of older people the price of poor diet and exercise habits developed in youth and middle age. If people have not become accustomed to fatty, sugary eating, they aren't likely to begin just because they start getting a Social Security check. If they're fond of fruits and vegetables and after-dinner walks in their youth, that fondness tends to stay.

As noted at the start of this chapter, when people favor good health habits in earlier years, they tend to still have them—along with better health—in their later years.

Summary

Each stage in life has special dietary needs and concerns. An unborn child is entirely dependent on the mother for nutrients and for protection against harmful substances. The fetus and its mother do not share a common blood supply. Instead, blood vessels intertwine in the placenta, and nutrients and other substances pass between them.

A good diet should begin before pregnancy to build up reserves and prevent deficiencies. A nutrient-dense diet is required during pregnancy, because nutrient needs increase far more than calorie needs. All women capable of becoming pregnant are advised to take folate/folic acid in a multivitamin pill or fortified food because folate deficiency in early pregnancy (typically before the first doctor's visit) increases the risk of a neural tube defect in the fetus. Pregnant women are typically prescribed prenatal vitamin/mineral tablets, but a good diet is still important.

Alcohol consumed during pregnancy can damage the fetus. Most familiar is fetal alcohol syndrome, which includes mental and growth retardation, and malformations. Alcohol passes freely through the placenta, so women are advised to abstain from alcohol during pregnancy or while trying to conceive.

Women should gain about 25-35 pounds during pregnancy. Weight gain affects birth weight, a good predictor of health in the newborn.

Breastfeeding is the best way to feed a baby. It not only provides the best nutrition, but the moth-

er uses up calories in making the milk. (This can reduce some of the fat stores she has accumulated during pregnancy.) Breast milk also provides protection and immunities against some diseases.

Breast milk (or infant formula) is adequate for the first 4 to 6 months of life, and women should breast feed as long as possible during this time (ideally, at least a year). Alcohol can get into breast milk, and should be avoided.

Solid foods can be started at 4-6 months, and will provide iron and other nutrients that aren't provided in adequate amounts by milk alone beyond 6 months of age. Breast milk and/or infant formula provides the protein that a baby needs, so supplemental foods should be mostly cereals, fruits, and vegetables. After the first year of life, the growth rate slows dramatically, and along with that, calorie needs.

Early childhood is a good time to establish good eating and exercise habits, by providing nutritious foods low in fat and sugar, lots of variety in foods, and by encouraging exercise. Good eating habits should also be encouraged during adolescence, as boys and girls begin making more and more of their own food choices.

When growth stops as adults, calorie needs may be less. Women generally need fewer calories than men, so they need to eat more nutrient-dense foods to get enough nutrients without excess calories. Iron deficiency is particularly common in women of childbearing age because of iron losses in menstruation, and increased needs during pregnancy. Women who may get pregnant are advised to get supplemental folate (folic acid) in a multivitamin tablet or in fortified foods, to prevent a folate deficiency in early pregnancy that increases the risk of a neural tube defect in the fetus.

For the elderly, calorie needs decrease, as does the sense of taste and smell. Combined with the reduced interest in eating that often accompanies reduced social interaction, the risk of nutrient deficiences increase. The elderly need to eat nutrient-dense foods, and are advised to get supplemental vitamin B-12 in a multivitamin tablet or in fortified foods. Exercise can help increase the appetite and the intake of more calories and nutrients.

All through our lives, we tend to follow food habits learned during our early years, so it is important to establish good food habits as early in life as possible.

Guest Lecturer: *Ellyn Satter, MS, RD, LCSW, BCD*

How Much Should My Child Eat?

"How much should my child eat?" is a deceptively simple question. The issue of *how much*, the same as issues related to feeding overall, must be considered in the context of the overall parent-child relationship. Feeding is more than picking out food and getting it into a child. Feeding is about the love and connection between parent and child, about trusting or controlling, providing or neglecting, accepting or rejecting.

Years ago, when I first began consulting in pediatrics, I designed a short guide for introducing solid foods to infants, a guide to be distributed to parents by the nursing staff. The handout made recommendations, by age, for solid-food additions to the baby's diet and told the reasons for the additions. I thought it was a nifty little piece that would answer most of the parents' questions.

However, within a day after the guide was introduced, a pediatric nurse called. "The mothers want to know *how much* they should feed their babies." How much? She had me there. I didn't know *how much*. I had raised three babies and hadn't paid much attention to how much. I just assumed my babies knew how much, and went by what they told me. But the question still intimidated me: How was I to tell those mothers and nurses *how much* when I didn't know it myself? What kind of nutritionist and mother was I?

I thought and thought and read everything I could get my hands on, but I still didn't know. There was nothing consistent on which to base a recommendation. I looked at calorie requirements for infants (which varied), asked for recommendations by pediatricians, nutritionists, and nurses (which varied), and talked with parents about how much their babies ate (which also varied).

About the only thing I came up with that made any sense was a guide to the minimum amounts of solid food that babies need to eat in order to satisfy their nutrient requirements. That wasn't very much—either information or food. Beyond defining the minimums, with respect to saying how much a child should eat, I was stuck. I couldn't possibly answer.

I further realized that for me, or even for the parent, to say *how much* was inappropriate and, in fact, took away a prerogative that belonged to the child. It was not for me to say how much, sitting in my office miles away from where the really important decisions were being made. It was not even for parents to say how much, because they couldn't possibly experience the infant's hunger and desire for food. Parents can only learn to detect and trust the infants' signs of hunger and fullness and use those signs to guide the feeding process. In short, only the child could say *how much*, and that information was not going to fit on my neat little feeding guide.

Dividing Responsibility

Children are extremely tuned in to their internal signals of hunger, appetite and satiety. Provided parents give them appropriate support for their eating, children know how much they need to eat. They pick and choose from what parents have provided. Even though on any one day their food intake appears imbalanced, over time they eat a variety and that variety adds up to a nutritionally adequate diet.

Proper child-feeding depends on a division of responsibility: Parents are responsible for the *what*, *when* and *where* of feeding. Children are responsible for the *how much* and *whether* of eating.

Jobs parents need to do with feeding include:

- Choose and prepare the food
- Provide regular meals and snacks at predictable times
- Make eating times pleasant
- Show children what they have to learn about food and mealtime behavior
- Not let children graze for food or beverages between times
- Let children grow up to get bodies that are right for them

Fundamental to parents' jobs is trusting children to decide how much and whether to eat. If parents do their jobs with feeding, children do their jobs with eating:

- Children will eat
- They will eat the amount they need
- They will eat an increasing variety of food
- They will grow predictably
- They will learn to behave well at the table

Parental Behavior and Children's Eating

Generally, children eat best when their parents are neither over-managing nor over-permissive. In order to eat the amount they need to and to learn to like a variety of food, children need both opportunities to learn and autonomy. They need to have regular mealtimes where they are exposed to a variety of food, and they need to be allowed to determine what and how much to eat at those mealtimes. Studies show that children eat worse when they coerced to eat, whether that coercion is positive as. in cheerleading or rewards, or negative, as in threats and punishment. Appropriate parenting appears to be a factor in obesity as well. Children whose parents give both leadership and autonomy are less likely to be overweight than children of parents who are domineering, permissive or neglectful.

Attempting to manipulate children's food intake simply doesn't work. Children who are forced to eat more or different food that they eat voluntarily become turned off to food and undereat when they get the chance. Children whose food intake is restricted become food-preoccupied and prone to overeat when they get the chance.

Feeding is Parenting

But poor eating habits, undesirable as they are, may not be the worst consequence of interference with food regulation. A child can outgrow a diet that is less than optimally chosen, as long as it is offered supportingly and lovingly. However, outgrowing deeply ingrained attitudes about self and the world is devilishly difficult. If the parent-child relationship around food is distorted, it is likely to distort the whole relationship. Parents' attempts to manipulate or control their child's eating can spoil the parent-child relationship and have a far-reaching impact on a child.

Parents' attitudes about their children are reflected in the way they feed. If parents have an attitude of curiosity, relaxation, and trust, they watch for children's cues and respond to them. They depend on information coming from children to guide feeding and let them develop bodies that are right for them. On the other hand, if parents' attitudes grow out of a sense of responsibility and a need to control, they are likely to closely supervise the child's eating, monitor growth, and attempt to manipulate the child's food intake in order to produce an "acceptable" growth pattern. That pattern is likely to reflect the parents ideas of appropriateness rather than the child's constitutional endowment.

Refusing food to a hungry child or forcing food on a satiated child is miserable for the child and miserable for all but the least tuned-in feeders. But just as bad as the struggles around eating are the lessons children learn from the struggles about themselves and about the world. Children whose size and shape are deemed unacceptable learn that they, themselves, are unacceptable. Children who have to beg and fight in order to get enough to eat learn that the world is untrustworthy. Conversely, if their needs are met in a supportive and consistent fashion, they learn that the world is trustworthy and they can allow themselves to depend on others.

Feeding interactions also teach children whether or not they have the ability to influence others. If they have to fuss and fight and struggle mightily to get their needs met, or if what they get has little or nothing to do with what they want, they are likely to think of themselves as not having much clout in the world. On the other hand, if other people respond to them in a prompt and appropriate fashion, they learn that what they want and need does matter and that other people will respond to them.

Teaching Feeding Teaches Parenting

The way health professionals teach parents to feed children has an impact on parents attitudes about their children. Teaching parents how much to feed children teaches them to be controlling. Being wary about growth and vigilant about preventing fatness teaches parents to be controlling. Worst of all, putting a child on a diet, encourages parents to be controlling in a way that is absolute-ly guaranteed to disrupt the entire family. That is very serious business.

Children have a growth potential that they tend to maintain and defend, and attempting to modify that potential requires the most persistent of efforts. Further, it appears that attempting to modify food intake can backfire and promote the very problems the intervention is intending to avoid, whether it is overgrowth or undergrowth.

Regulation of food intake and appropriate growth depends on a delicately balanced interaction of nutritional, behavioral, physical, and psychological factors. Because the process is so complex, we must be extremely careful about intruding upon it. Changing or overruling the body's ability to regulate food intake and growth potential can only be done against odds, and at a cost that is highly likely to be unacceptable.

Ellyn Satter has Master's degrees in Nutrition and in Clinical Social Work. She heads Ellyn Satter Associates (www.ellynsatter.com), which provides resources for professionals and the public on eating and feeding. She is a therapist, lecturer, and author. Her books include *Your Child's Weight: Helping Without Harming*, and *Secrets of Feeding a Healthy Family*.

Part 8

From Farm to Table

Chapter 20

Agriculture— Realities of Leaf and Soil

The interrelationship of plants and animals (including humans) is fascinating. We often take for granted that plants are just "there," not only filling the yard, shading neighborhood streets, and peeking through cracks in the sidewalk, but providing us with fruit, vegetables, and grain. When we take a closer look, however, we find there is an awesome continuous flow of essential chemical elements between plant and animal worlds, and words like "worldwide ecology" take on a new meaning.

With an increasing respect for our dependence on plant life, it is natural to feel added concern, particularly as science provides us with more and more ways of utilizing biotechnology. There is a perception that we've become too eager to mess with things better left alone in their "natural" state—that economic gain drives the machine in ways that can be shortsighted and ultimately harmful. Thus the understandable attraction of movements supporting "natural" and "organic" methods.

Like so many areas of public concern and advocacy, the facts behind the issues are often poorly understood. A thorough understanding will not of course guarantee universal agreement, but arguments tend to become more specific and logical. Science and technology are not automatically bad guys, and they can be viewed more as potentially useful tools, and less as threats, to health and a bountiful environment.

As consumers have become more interested in nutrition, they have also become more suspicious of the quality of the food supply. They are encouraged in their fears by charges that our crops are grown on depleted soil, making them nutritionally inferior, and that we are being poisoned by pesticides and food additives.

Is our food supply adequate and safe? This is a concern of such importance that government agencies such as the U.S. Dept. of Agriculture (USDA), the Food and Drug Administration (FDA), and the Environmental Protection Agency (EPA) devote considerable amounts of time and money to do the best they can to see that our food supply is, in fact, adequate and safe.

But what our government agencies see as the biggest concerns are quite different from the perceptions of the general public. The public perception is that farm pesticides and food additives top the list of food hazards. In contrast, these experts put these concerns at the bottom, with disease-causing microbes at the top, and environmental contaminants and naturally-occurring food toxicants in between (see Fig. 20-1).

So let's examine the realities of our food supply—from farm to table—beginning with a look at some agricultural concerns: basic plant nutrition; uses of fertilizer, pesticides, and biotechnology; natural toxins in food; and how agriculture today relates to world food production and world health.

The next chapter examines various aspects of food processing, in particular those substances that intentionally or unintentionally get into our food as it's commercially processed, and further processed as we store and prepare the food. These substances include food additives and toxins produced by microorganisms.

The last chapter concerns food labeling, and what the label tells us of the food. We should read these labels in selecting our food. For all our concerns about food adequacy and safety, whether or not our food is healthful depends mostly on what—and how much—we choose to eat.

The Nutrition of Plants

Much of what we've discussed of human nutrition may also be applied to the nutrient needs of plants. Like us, they are organized groups of cells. Like us, their cells must also be supplied with the raw materials of life, and the materials which they require are determined by the DNA in their cells. Their chemical makeup is, like ours, ordained by heredity.

If we think about it for a moment, we realize that the life chemistry of plants must be somewhat similar to our own. For we get our fuel (e.g., fat) and building blocks (e.g., amino acids) from plants, either by consuming them directly, or by eating animals which have fed on them.

Of course, there are also striking differences. One is that plants don't consume other life forms as we do to get their nutrients. Instead, they take in nutrients in very simple form, and use chlorophyll to trap solar energy. Another difference is that, unlike us, plants can't move around to seek food. So they depend on natural phenomena—or on us—to bring them food.

From the beginning of our dependence on agriculture, we've tended to provide plants with a kind of room service. This service was unnecessary while we gathered plants—simply by foraging over the land, seeking out those which were edible. But once we began modern agriculture some 9,000 years ago, by growing plants in batches for a more dependable and convenient food source, "man-made" growing methods became essential to their survival and to ours.

At first glance, it may seem that there's a striking difference between the ways in which we and the plants take in food. But there's a basic similarity. Like us, the plants can absorb and take

Figure 20-1: Microbes are our greatest food hazard.

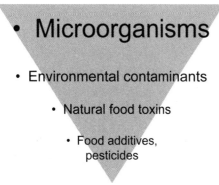

• Microorganisms

• Environmental contaminants

• Natural food toxins

• Food additives, pesticides

into their cells only the simpler structural units of their food.

Of course, our food first has to be processed through our digestive tract, so that our digestive enzymes can break it down into forms that we can absorb and use. But even here, there's some similarity. The roots of a plant may be seen as similar to our intestinal walls. If soil nutrients are in too complex forms, the enzymes of soil bacteria do the work of breaking them apart into forms that plants can absorb and use. This is exactly what happens when we make compost. By mixing complex organic matter (gardening and food scraps, manure, etc.) into the soil, the bacteria can work to "digest" it into plant food.

The Need for Nitrogen

What sort of nutrients must plants take in? Like us, plants mostly need carbon, hydrogen, oxygen, and nitrogen. Plant cells have no problem getting their carbon, hydrogen, and oxygen from water and the carbon dioxide in the air. But they must get their nitrogen from the soil. (We get ours from the protein we eat.)

The plant can't absorb protein or amino acids. It takes up its nitrogen in a simpler form from the soil, combined with oxygen as a nitrate (NO_3). In nature, the nitrogen comes mainly from the protein in decaying plant materials, such as leaves and stems. But it must wait for the soil bacteria to turn the plants' decaying proteins into nitrates, and for rainwater to carry these chemicals to its roots for absorption (see Fig. 20-2). Then, the plant uses the nitrates to make its own amino acids and proteins.

By trial and error, early farmers found that manure and decomposing life materials would keep soils fertile. These materials provide nitrogen. We learned that we must keep the soil supplied with nitrogen, or plants won't grow—without nitrogen they can't form the proteins for new cells. Once we understood this chemistry, we realized that simpler, more concentrated sources of nitrogen supplied these needs faster and more efficiently—resulting in a larger crop in a shorter time.

Our modern "chemical" fertilizers supply nitrates rapidly in a simple, immediately usable (in-organic) form. "Organic" farming, with its compost piles of decaying manure and plants, doesn't directly supply the nitrate. Its nitrogen is tied up in elaborate carbon-skeleton (organic) molecules. The ironic reality of organic farming is that plants can't use nitrogen in organic form.

Industrial production of fertilizer from nitrogen gas uses a lot of energy, whether for the strong electrical currents passed through contained air, or the compression of nitrogen, hydrogen, and oxygen gases at extremely high temperatures. Energy sources for this process (and required technology) are out of reach for many developing countries.

Plants can't use nitrogen in gaseous form either. Ironically, three-fourths of the air we breathe is the nitrogen that both we and plants need so urgently. But in this gaseous state (N_2), it's a chemical loner, reluctant to join with any other element and so is useless to us or plants.

But nitrogen gas can be made ("fixed") into usable form (ammonia, NH_3) by nitrogen-fixing bacteria, which invade the roots of legumes (soybeans, peas, etc.), and provide them with nitrogen usable to make protein. (Recall that legumes are rich plant sources of protein.) The conversion of nitrogen gas to ammonia requires a lot of energy (ATP), which is made by photosynthesis in the legumes. About one-fifth of the ATP made by photosynthesis in the pea plant, for example, is used by the nitrogen-fixing bacteria residing in its roots.

Legumes and the nitrogen-fixing bacteria have a symbiotic relationship: The bacteria provide the legumes with usable nitrogen; the legumes provide the bacteria with the ATP energy to do so.

How did nitrogen get into the soil in usable form before life began on earth? Scientists believe that continual lightning storms struck through the primeval atmosphere. These storms are thought to have supplied the energy for the nitrogen gas to combine with hydrogen gas (forming ammonia, NH_3) and with oxygen gas (forming nitrates, NO_3).

Today, this is the process used by industry to make our fertilizers. In one method, electrical charges are passed through air in closed containers, trapping the nitrogen gas as ammonia and/or

Figure 20-2: Nutritional Sustenance of Plants. Plants take in water and carbon dioxide and, using solar energy, combine the two chemicals into sugar and starch, releasing oxygen. Birds use the sugar and starch for energy by using oxygen to oxidize them. The birds' waste products in this reaction are carbon dioxide and water, which plants use to make sugar and starch, continuing the cycle.

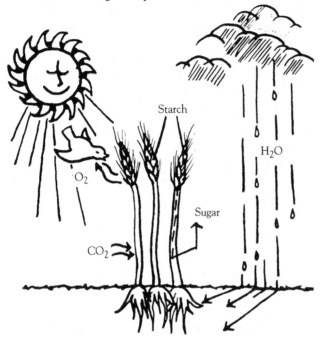

nitrates. These ultimately are added to the soil, often in water, just as primeval rains washed nitrogen compounds out of the atmosphere and into the earth's crust.

The Need for Minerals

Of course, plants need more than nitrogen to grow. They need minerals. These needs are also somewhat parallel to those of humans. The minerals come from the rock and soil of the earth. The plants need as wide a variety as we do—where else would we get ours? Dominant among their needs are phosphorus, potassium, sulfur, and calcium.

Phosphorus is usually incorporated in ammonium phosphates (ammonium, phosphorus, oxygen) or calcium phosphates. Potassium is acquired almost entirely from mined potassium chloride ores. During the last century we began to seek out phosphorus and potassium deposits, grind and modify them into useful form, and return them to our fields to feed the crops.

Calcium sulfate (calcium, sulfur, and oxygen) is another "chemical" fertilizer. And, of course, trace minerals such as iron, which we seek for our own nutrition, are part of the hereditary plant chemistry—how else could we depend on getting iron from eating beans and greens?

Does Agriculture Deplete Soil Minerals?

Certainly. That's why we use fertilizers to supply minerals as well as nitrogen. The plants, responding to their necessities, need minerals just as much as we do. These minerals are called for by the plant's metabolism. If the minerals are missing, the plants can't grow.

What if the minerals aren't entirely missing, but are merely in short supply? Then only as many plants as can be nourished by the available minerals will grow. Or, like undernourished humans, their growth and development will be stunted. As surely as human development is thwarted by inadequate nutrition, so is the development of plants. The farmer who exploits the soil learns the hard way from a crop with very poor yield.

Plants don't need an outside source of vitamins, as we do. Vitamins are used in their metabolism, much as they are used in ours, but plants make their own—and ours too. It's useless to feed plants vitamins.

So plants which exist at all must be complete. They must contain a full complement of substances called for in their genes. Otherwise, they wouldn't exist. All of the elements known to be essential in plant and human nutrition are easily identified in soils by modern analytic methods. Our soils and foods are regularly tested, for good reason.

For one, farmers have an acute economic interest in their soil. It's their most costly and basic asset. A flawed soil, untreated, will produce a poor crop or none at all. The fertilizers which the farmers add are expensive. They can't afford to guess—so they have their soil analyzed.

In addition, the soils are important economic assets to the society, especially in those states which produce most of our food. Governments of agricultural states such as California and Florida have a vested interest in keeping watch over their soils.

No evidence has come to light that our crops are grown on depleted soil, making them nutritionally inferior. Nor has there been any nutritive differences found between plants fertilized "organically" and plants fertilized "chemically."

Are There Unobservable Deficiencies?

A few trace minerals can be low. These are the elements which are essential for animal life, but have little use in plant chemistry. So the plant content of these elements varies, because they are taken up incidentally. These elements are only a few—chiefly iodine, selenium, cobalt, and zinc. Fluoride might be considered another. There are easy safeguards against shortages of iodine and fluoride—iodine through the iodizing of salt, and fluoride through fluoridation of water.

The human needs for some of these trace elements were identified largely through inadequacies in the diets of pasture-raised livestock, mainly sheep and cattle. Nutritionally, our main sources of these elements are animal foods. (Recall, for example, that cobalt is a critical constituent of vitamin B-12, a vitamin not found in plant foods. Since cobalt isn't needed by the plant, it's only there incidentally when it's in the soil.) Where these elements may be lacking in the soil, the deficiency signs are apparent in the animals that graze off the land, and in general they are easily supplemented, by adding them to the soil or to animal feed.

Note that the shortages of such trace minerals aren't due to farming practices, but to regional soil differences. Plants grown in certain areas will, for example, contain little iodine or selenium. If such plants are used for compost, they will obviously not supply any deficiencies of the soil in which they grew.

Unlike us, many of the world's poor only have locally grown produce available. If their soil happens to be low in selenium, the crops grown in them—and the local animals and people eat them exclusively—also will be low in selenium.

Note, also, that plants can incidentally take up undesirable elements as well. Plants grown in lead-contaminated soil, for example, can contain lead, a human toxin. Plants grown in soil contaminated by radioactive fallout (e.g., as from the Chernobyl nuclear accident) can contain radioactive iodine, which can damage the thyroid gland. (Iodine—radioactive or not—concentrates in this gland.) Plants can, in fact, be used in this way for environmental clean up, e.g., to remove toxic metals from polluted ground water.[1]

The Farm in Our Food

One of the more unfortunate terms in the world of food regulation is *filth*. A sure way to arouse reader alarm is with the news that more filth has been found in a food than the law allows. Invariably, some readers write outraged letters questioning why "filth" should be allowed in our food at all.

Filth is really incidental matter which gets into food while it's being grown, harvested, transported, processed, or stored. It's inevitable that there will always be some in the food supply, and it isn't really as awful as it sounds. Consider "insect parts," one kind of filth. Generally these aren't large juicy bug bits, but more often microscopic fractions of tiny aphids, mites, or weevils, members of the insect world which tend to live in and around the soil and food.

Farms are in the country, often near woods and uncultivated lands, and city dwellers sometimes forget that there's an unpaved world of dirt and leaves, and that worms and beetles and bugs make their homes in the soils where our food grows. As neat and clean as farmers may be, some vestige of the country almost invariably remains with the food.

Pesticides—Competing for the Crop

Wherever there's a great deal of food, whether harvested or still growing, there will be a tempting buffet for various creatures. Indeed, our unbalancing of nature—gathering food plants into concentrated growing grounds for convenience and economy—has caused us to turn to pesticides (*pest killers*). We compete with fungi, insects, and such, for the crop. (To them, of course, we are the pests. But a big dose for them is a small dose for us.)

Pesticides are regulated by Federal law. A special Pesticides Amendment to the Food and Drug Act (passed in 1954) sets forth most of our current policies.

We know quite a lot about how to identify pesticides in our food, and quite a lot about how pesticides affect our bodies. So we're able to make some measurements and do a fair job of determining how much we're endangered by them. (Risk assessment will be discussed in the next chapter.)

> Traces of pesticides do appear in our food, but it's not all from the hand of the farmer. Pesticides are used for many purposes, from mosquito abatement to highway weed control, from home gardening to forest conservation.

The Pesticides Amendment requires the Food and Drug Administration (FDA) to monitor pesticides in our food by sampling our market supplies. The criteria for judging safe levels of pesticides in food are determined by our own experts and by expert committees of the United Nations.

It isn't possible to prove a negative (i.e., that there's absolutely no danger), but neither government, nutrition science, nor medicine has seen significant evidence that pesticides in food are causing cancer, birth deformities, or genetic problems. Nor has there been any evidence of illness or death in North America from eating pesticide residues in food. (Accidental overdoses of pesticides inhaled or sprayed onto the skin of farm workers are another matter.)

> Pesticides sometimes can lessen the natural toxins in food. Plants damaged by insects or fungi often make more toxins, e.g., mold damage to some kinds of celery can cause the celery to make 100-times more of a natural toxin—so much, that this "natural celery toxin" can be an occupational hazard for celery pickers and produce checkers.

According to the FDA, the scant amount of pesticide residues in our food supply is safe. In other words, the fear that we have been and are being poisoned by pesticides in our food isn't based on solid evidence. Moreover, no one at FDA has any intention of letting the fear become a reality. Improved controls and greater restrictions come into being with any threat, and scientists continue to look for alternatives to pesticides, and use them when practical.

One such alternative is using the pests' natural predators. But they can take a long time to arrive (just as it took three years for the seagulls to come to Utah to rescue the crops from the plague of locusts in the 1850s), so we usually have to help the situation along. We have, for example, collected parasitic wasps in Iran and brought them to California to successfully combat the olive scale (a pest of olives, plums, apricots, and many other plants) that was damaging many crops.[2]

Another alternative used extensively in the past and present is the use of crossbreeding to obtain plants resistant to particular diseases. More recently, biotechnology has also been used to make the crops more pest-resistant.

Integrated Pest Management

Integrated Pest Management (IPM) takes an ecological and customized approach to pest management. The aim is to minimize pesticide use, and to use that which is needed in the safest and most effective way possible.

> One study (part of a Univ. of Calif. IPM Project) found that releasing certain predator mites on cotton crops in late May and early June was more effective than in late June and early July, and that an efficient and accurate way to release them is to mix them with corn cob grit and use a leaf-blower to dispense the mixture.

IPM integrates various types of controls and strategies, based on the biology of the pests and their predators, the particular crop, local soil and weather conditions, etc. IPM for grapes, for example, might include removal of leaves around developing grape clusters—this has been found to reduce bunch rot and reduce the number of pesticide applications needed to control powdery mildew. IPM for strawberry crops might include:

- Careful monitoring of its pests, for use in deciding if control efforts are needed.
- Using weather information to predict when the pests will be at the most susceptible stage of their life cycle, so that if pesticides are needed, minimal amounts can be used in a timely manner.
- Using weed control to reduce pest reservoirs.

When one considers the variety of crops, pests, predators, and local conditions, it's evident that effective IPM relies on an extensive base of knowledge. Even when one knows, for example, that predator mites can be used to control spider mites in cotton crops, one has to decide when and how to release the predator mites.

Also, when an IPM plan is formulated for a crop, it has to be implemented. Implementation efforts include development of software and databases (e.g., *Database of alternatives to targeted pesticides),* publications (e.g., *IPM for apples and pears),* and hands-on workshops (e.g., how to distinguish between spider mites and predatory mites) for growers and farm workers. IPM research and implementation is supported mainly by state and federal funding.

Biotechnology in Agriculture

Biotechnology is a general term, meaning the use of technology to study or solve problems of living organisms. But the term is commonly used (as it is here) to mean *genetic engineering,* the altering of an organism's genes (its DNA), resulting in a *genetically modified organism* (GMO).

As applied in agriculture, biotechnology is used to create desired genetic characteristics in plants. Ordinarily, this has been (and still is) done by crossbreeding— to get better-tasting vegetables, more drought-resistant plants, watermelon with fewer seeds, roses with fewer thorns, etc.

Genetic engineering or *genetically modified organism* sounds ominous—it sounds like something to automatically be against.

In many cases, biotechnology is simply used as a faster and a more direct and precise method of crossbreeding. (Using crossbreeding, it has sometimes taken decades and over 30,000 painstaking crosses to get a desired genetic change in a plant.) A desirable gene can be selectively transferred into a plant, or an undesirable gene can be inactivated.

Agricultural biotechnology has the potential to make a tremendous impact on the health of many people, especially in countries where food is scarce and the nutritional quality of the staple

diet is inadequate. Often, the scarcity isn't due to inadequate food production, but is the result of losses in the food supply system.

One scientist tried to use crossbreeding to combine the leaf of a cabbage with the root of a radish to get an entirely edible plant. Alas, what resulted was the leaf of the radish with the root of the cabbage.

As examples, there are tremendous losses—particularly in developing countries—because of infestation of crops by pests, loss from harsh weather conditions, and deterioration of the harvest during transport or storage. Biotechnology holds dramatic promise for such problems. By altering the DNA, it's possible to obtain plants that are more nutritious, need less fertilizer, and have increased resistance to viral infection, pests, deterioration, etc. The achievement of a tastier tomato by genetic alteration pales by comparison.

Unseasonably cold weather in California, alone, has caused extensive crop losses due to frost damage, resulting in economic losses to the farmer, the state, and the consumer who pays higher food prices.

The achievement of a tastier tomato provides an example of the use of biotechnology, here to inactivate the gene for a certain tomato enzyme. In 1989, Calgene, Inc. received a patent for a tomato (dubbed Flavr Savr), in which the enzyme that causes it to deteriorate rapidly was "eliminated by genetic engineering" (see Fig. 20-3). Without this enzyme, the tomato lasts longer after picking and thus can be picked when ripe and tasty rather than when green.

Campbell Soup Company helped finance the development of the Flavr Savr tomato. But in response to public fear of scary-sounding *genetically modified food,* they announced that they wouldn't use it in their products.

A tastier vine-ripened tomato isn't necessarily more nutritious than one picked green, but it can make for a more nutritious diet. Presumably, people eat more tomatoes when they are tastier.

A gene can also be transferred from one plant to another, across a wider range of plant species than by crossbreeding. One plant might, for example, make a protein that provides resistance to the formation of damaging internal ice crystals in

Figure 20-3: The decay gene is inactivated in the Flavr Savr tomato.

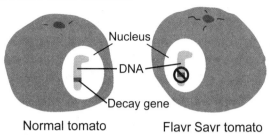

Normal tomato   Flavr Savr tomato

freezing weather. The gene for this protein might then be transferred to other plants, making them resistant to frost damage.

One thing that crossbreeding can't do, but biotechnology can, is transfer non-plant genes into a plant. One can, for example, transfer a gene from a virus into a plant. One such gene is for a protein found in the coat of a virus that infects and damages crops. (In nature, some plant viruses transfer their genes into a plant's DNA as part of their normal disease-causing process.)

Just the protein part of a virus is used in some human vaccines—the protein doesn't cause the disease when injected, nor is it infective. But it causes us to make the antibodies that protect against the virus.

It's been known for some time that crops infected with a mild strain of some viruses aren't susceptible to infection by more damaging strains (similar to the way infection with the cowpox virus protected people against smallpox in the days before vaccines). In investigating this phenomenon, scientists found that one of the virus's proteins, alone, could confer the same protection. Plants, in this way, can be "vaccinated" against a viral infection.

When we eat the "foreign protein," it's digested into its component amino acids. The digestive tract doesn't see it any differently than other proteins in the plant. After all, the plant's native protein is "foreign" to us as well.

Using biotechnology, the gene that provides the directions to make the desired protein can be removed from the virus and inserted into a plant's DNA. This genetically altered plant then makes this "foreign protein" (not the plant's native protein) for its own protection against disease. This method has been used, for example, to create rice varieties that resist infection by a virus that

causes the loss of millions of dollars worth of rice crops each year in China, Japan, Korea, Taiwan, and the former Soviet Union.[3]

Biotechnology might also be used to transplant a set of genes—the genes that provide an organism with the ability to convert nitrogen gas into ammonia, for example. As discussed earlier, the nitrogen-fixing bacteria that reside in the roots of legumes can convert nitrogen gas into ammonia for use by the plant (plants can use ammonia—but not nitrogen gas—to make protein). If these bacterial genes could be transferred into plants that aren't infected by these nitrogen-fixing bacteria, they wouldn't need nitrogen-containing fertilizer —the plants would make their own fertilizer.

Using abundant natural resources—nitrogen from the air and energy from the sun—to make fertilizer "on site" is an attractive alternative to industrial production which, as said earlier, requires energy and technology, limiting its use in developing countries.

The FDA treats bioengineered food as it does any other food. The Flavr Savr tomato, for example, had its "decay gene" inactivated by biotechnology, whereas the DiVine Ripe tomato had its "decay gene" activity bred out. As another example, a plant can be made to produce its own fungicide by the bioengineered introduction of an antifungal gene. Yet, there are many other crop plants that naturally have the genes to produce such agents in even larger amounts (*naturally disease-resistant varieties*).

The Good and Bad of Natural Plant Substances

One can see that it's very hard to separate the "natural" from the "unnatural." It should also be clear by now that, contrary to popular sentiment, "natural" isn't necessarily better than "unnatural."

Plants—like all living organisms—are made up of a huge variety of substances. So many, that it's impossible to test them all. As new varieties of plant life appear, so do new substances. Conversely, as varieties of plant life become extinct, so do some unique substances—including undiscovered medicinal substances.

Plants have long been a source of medicines. Even today, pharmaceutical companies continually search for—and find—novel medications in plants. The bark of the willow tree was known in ancient civilizations as a source of a substance that relieves pain. Based on this substance (salicylic acid), a German chemist synthesized aspirin (acetylsalicylic acid) in 1853. The heart medicine digitalis comes from the leaves of the purple foxglove plant.

Many of our best anticancer drugs also come from plants, such as taxol (for ovarian cancer) from the bark of the Pacific yew tree, and vinblastine (for breast cancer) and vincristine (for leukemia) from the tropical flower rosy periwinkle. As more plants become extinct, particularly those in tropical forests, the worry is that the plants becoming extinct today contain what may have been tomorrow's "miracle drugs."

Many people are severely allergic to peanuts. The peanut proteins responsible for the allergic reaction are being identified, in hope that the genes for these proteins can be eliminated or replaced by genetic modification to create allergen-free peanuts.[4]

Those who like to divide substances into "good" and "bad" would have a very hard time with a plant's constituents. The easiest ones to categorize might be vitamins—but then, again, too much of even these can be toxic. Nutmeg, ginger, cloves, and cinnamon contain a bit of safrole—a carcinogen (cancer-causing substance). Sounds bad. Should we leave out these spices in our recipe for pumpkin pie? What about the caffeine in our coffee? Not so good when it makes the hand of a surgeon tremble during a delicate operation. But good when it keeps a tired surgeon awake on the drive home.

Do we include as plant substances those that form when a plant deteriorates or is cooked? Recall from Chapter 15, that animals that eat spoiled sweet clover can die of hemorrhagic disease, yet the same substance that causes their hemorrhage is used in much smaller doses as human medicine to prevent clots that can lead to a fatal heart attack. Almonds and lima beans are among those foods that produce hydrogen cyanide when cooked or digested—the same poison used in the gas chamber for capital punishment.

But some plant substances are outrightly classified as toxins. Plants contain a variety of these, often in very large amounts. This isn't surprising. To survive, plants must have their own defenses against predators—thorns are the closest they come to having claws to defend themselves, and they can't run from their enemies.

Among these toxins are the naturally-occurring pesticides alluded to earlier. In fact, the amount of synthetic pesticide residues in our food pales in comparison to the amount and variety of naturally-occurring pesticides found in our food.[5,6]

Some of these naturally-occurring pesticides have chemical actions identical to those of the pesticides farmers apply to their crops. For example, some plants contain substances that play havoc with the transmission of nerve impulses. From the plant perspective, this is an ideal toxin— plants don't have nerves, whereas most of their predators do.

Nerve impulse inhibitors are also used in flea collars—a big dose for fleas, a small dose for cats or dogs. During the 1991 Persian Gulf War, we feared that Iraq would use these substances in nerve gases—in large enough doses to kill humans. The substances can stop breathing through a spasm of the respiratory muscles.

Since we have nerves, these substances can be toxic to us as well. But a large dose for an insect is a very small dose for us. Again we're reminded that what's toxic or not is in the size of the dose.

What's Good and What's Bad?

There are valid arguments to be made concerning what and how much of various substances should be allowed in our food. But we confuse rather than enlighten if we focus only on those that we add to food. We do better when we compare these objectively to those that are there "naturally" as part of a native species, or are incorporated by conventional crossbreeding techniques, or are there because of infection by plant microorganisms, the presence of insects, or "natural" deterioration.

Particularly now, when we have more options than in the past, and see agriculture in the context

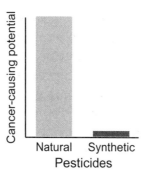

Figure 20-4: Cancer-causing potential of natural vs. residue from synthetic pesticides in our food.[5,6]

of world ecology, there's a much greater need for more objective public dialogue: Is it reasonable to spend more on "organic" produce because of concern about pesticides? What if the particular organic produce happens to "naturally" contain more pesticides than the avoided produce? How much are we as taxpayers willing to support Integrated Pest Management Programs as a way to minimize pesticide use?

There are valid concerns about pesticide sprays. The spray isn't confined to the pests alone and can upset the natural ecology. There's the danger of accidental spills, and worry of the hazards to farm workers. Again there's the potential trade-off with the possible use of biotechnology to make the crop plant more disease resistant so that less or no spraying at all is needed.

In 1970, about 15% of the U.S. corn crop was lost to corn blight. Most of the corn in the U.S. was the same "super variety" of hybrid corn, developed by crossbreeding. The 15% represented over a billion bushels of corn.

Some who argue against genetically modified crops correctly state that the development and widespread use of "super varieties" reduces genetic diversity, making much larger portions of crops vulnerable to a single disease, extreme weather condition, etc. Crops with the same genes have the same genetic susceptibilities.

But we must keep in mind that this isn't a new concern. It has been, and still is a concern in the development of "super varieties" by conventional crossbreeding as well.[7] In large part because of this concern, the National Seed Storage Laboratory in Colorado maintains a stock of wild and "older" varieties of plants.

Non-scientists are understandably uneasy with regard to science and technology. Dramatic changes can seem "unnatural" at first, even those

we later take for granted—the Wright brothers flying through the air, inoculation with a vaccine, the splitting of an atom.

The uneasiness is probably greater today, because of the wide gap between the general public's scientific literacy. and the high level of scientific achievement. When the Wright brothers took off, this gap was narrow, and everyone could make a reasonable assessment of the bright and dark sides of aircraft. Today the situation is far different, particularly in areas like biotechnology—even though we still do share a common goal of doing what's best for our own body, our own community, our own world.

Of Science and Hunger

Eighty percent of the world's population are classified as living in extremely poor societies. Hundreds of millions are malnourished, and tens of millions die each year of malnutrition. An overwhelming number of people are sick and dying for lack of good food.

Although there are gifts of food to the world's hungry, the greater gifts come from the advances in agriculture and food science. Even in our own not-so-distant past, we've come to know the benefits of these advances. There's a sentimental attraction for the days when organic farming on small family farms was the only farming, but the reality is that it was the advent of "chemical" fertilizers, pesticides, and such, that helped make the rapid development of other industries possible.

Increased crop yields became possible with fewer farmers, allowing many to leave the farms for the cities. Even with only a relatively small segment of our population continuing to do our farming, we're able to provide an abundance of food, not only for ourselves, but we have plenty to export as well.

New high-yielding seeds have been developed —seeds which have been said to advance the health of more of the world's people in a shorter time than any other technological advance in history. Plants have been bred which produce less stalk to yield more rice. The development of hybrid corn increased U.S. corn production from 23 bushels per acre in 1936 to 114 bushels in 1982—a 5-fold increase.[8] From all parts of the world came reports of incredible increases in crop yield from the use of such hybrid seeds—and with it the alleviation of much hunger.

In 1964, the opaque-2 gene was discovered, a corn gene that markedly increased the nutrient value of the corn protein. (But the gene was recessive and the crop yield was less, so it was with some difficulty that researchers were finally able, by crossbreeding, to develop it into a commercially useful breed of corn.) This astonishing grain has protein of a quality that approaches that of cow's milk. Even when it's the only protein source in the diet, it meets the hard test of curing kwashiorkor, the tragic protein-deficiency disease which has crippled so many of the world's children.

Many such rabbits have come out of food technology's hat. The new tools of biotechnology have broadly widened the possibilities for agriculture and food technology, promising much faster and more precise contributions. But the goals of agricultural scientists and food technologists remain as before—greater crop yields, the need for less fertilizers and pesticides, more nutritious and tastier plant foods, drought-resistant varieties of staple crops, crops that stay fresh longer from farm to table.

The greatest gains are for the world's hungry. So many can't afford the fertilizers that can result in more food from their plot of land, nor the pesticides that would preserve more of the crop for human consumption. Many live long distances from the farming—with no refrigerated trucks to bring food without spoiling.

A varied diet is a tenet of good nutrition, yet the world's hungry typically have but a few staple plant foods to choose from. For them, new crop varieties can mean the difference between health and disease, between life and death.

But often there's a problem in persuading even the starving and the nutritionally deficient to accept and use what science has to offer them. Often, they can't cross the barriers of old taboos, of unconscious fears and frightening myths, of suspicion of new food forms or tastes. Because they don't understand that science isn't a new magic but merely a way to understand and use the physical realities of nature, they cling to the old folkways, often with closed eyes and ears and minds.

Are we really more advanced? Or are we as often victims of superstition, of an unwillingness to live according to the rational science which may well be the best product of our society and our time?

Let's go on to examine our fears of the food additives that are added in the processing of food.

Summary

Plants require nutrients in simple form. They get their carbon, hydrogen, and oxygen from carbon dioxide and water, their nitrogen from nitrates and ammonia, and their minerals from the soil. Plant growth is limited by the availability of the required nutrients—the quantity of plant produced is affected, not its quality. Fertilizers provide nutrients that increase crop yield.

Some of the minerals we require (e.g., iodine) aren't required by plants. But plants can take these in—and also ones we don't want (e.g., lead)—if they happen to be in the soil. This means the plant content of these minerals vary according to the amount present in the local soil.

Crop yield is also affected by how well we protect our crops from insects and disease. Pesticides are commonly used for this purpose. Alternatively, natural predators of the pests can be used, and plants can be bred to be more pest resistant. Integrated Pest Management customizes pest-control strategies for individual crops and local conditions, using alternatives to pesticides whenever possible—the aim is to minimize the use of pesticides, and to use that which is needed in the safest and most effective way possible.

Plant genes can be altered by biotechnology to create desired characteristics. Biotechnology can be used to transfer desired genes (e.g., ones that provide disease resistance) into a plant or to inactivate undesirable genes (e.g., ones that cause decay).

"Natural" plant substances aren't inherently better or worse than "man-made" ones. Both the natural and the man-made are important to consider in assessing the safety and adequacy of our agricultural products.

Advances in agriculture and food science have had—and are expected to continue to have—the greatest benefit for the world's hungry.

Guest Lecturer*: Peggy G. Lemaux, PhD*

Do We Need Genetically Modified Foods to Feed the World?
A Scientific Perspective

My focus and my area of expertise is that of a practicing scientist—one involved in the genetic engineering of cereal crops and in trying to improve the nutritional quality of sorghum. So my interests in the application of biotechnology are practical—can the technology be used to improve agriculture, and can it improve the lot of the world's poor?

I'm not a governmental official; I'm not an economist; I'm a scientist. What can I do? Of course, the answer as to whether I can make a contribution to agricultural productivity in the developed and developing world depends only in part on the technology. The answer goes far beyond science.

Many forces limit the application of biotechnology in developed countries. We have invented techniques for inserting genes responsible for valuable traits in most crop plants. Major factors affecting the use of genetically engineered crops in developed countries include intellectual property issues, regulatory costs, economic incentives and, in my opinion, the limited ability of the public sector to directly contribute to the development of engineered crops that can be grown in fields by farmers.

The application of biotechnology in developing countries has some of the same limitations, but includes others, such as inadequate infrastructure, unique political and economic hurdles, and societal issues. And, as I can personally attest, lack of funding for scientists and economists to participate effectively. I don't think it is possible to focus on scientific challenges alone without a consideration of the other issues, particularly in developing countries.

In 2001, the United Nations released a report called, Making New Technologies Work for Human Development. The report provided an analysis of the potential of biotech and information and communications technology for developing countries. Summarizing his thoughts on this topic, Peter Rosset of Food First said, "Complex problems of hunger and agricultural development will not be solved by technological silver bullets." I couldn't agree more!

And even if it could be done, biotechnology would not be that bullet. Our world and its increases in population and food shortages are too complex to be addressed adequately with simple solutions—whether they are the application of biotechnology or the use of organic methods to address agricultural problems. The question for me really is, Can biotechnology ease problems of food insufficiency and environmental degradation, due in large part to population expansion?

First, as a practicing scientist in the field of biotechnology and genomics, I remind you that agricultural biotechnology is more than just genetically modified organisms. Based on what we have learned about manipulating plant tissues and DNA, alternative approaches have been developed that don't involve genetic engineering, and some of these are important in developing countries.

A recent example is a new pearl millet hybrid to be released in India that is resistant to downy mildew. In years of severe attack, this organism can cause the loss of up to 30% of the crop.

Another example involves micropropagation methods to rid plants, like banana, potatoes and taro, of viruses and other pests by passing them through tissue culture. This has helped African and Philippino farmers. Although tissue-cultured plants cost more, disease-free plants give higher yields, resulting in more money for farmers.

The last example is Polymerase Chain Reaction (PCR) techniques, which are being used to detect and control pests and viruses in crops like banana and papaya.

But when biotechnology is discussed, most of the focus is on genetic engineering of crop plants

—adding new or modified genes. Here I want to focus on the question of whether this technology holds any hope for developing countries.

I would first like to look at the impact of genetically engineered crops available commercially today. An example is transgenic Bt* plants like corn, potatoes, and cotton. The agricultural economist David Zilberman and his colleagues at UC Berkeley concluded that increases in yields of Bt cotton could be be significant in countries where there are a lot of pests, but minimal pesticide use—like some developing countries. They calculated that, although Bt cotton gains in the U.S. and China would range from 0-15%, gains in South Africa could be 20-40%, and in India 60-80%.

But won't intellectual property issues interfere with deployment of such crops in developing countries, since U.S. companies created them? Zilberman and other agricultural economists claim that, since these crops are generated in developed countries, the companies generally do not patent these inventions in developing countries. They worry most about liability and transaction costs.

Use of genetically engineered crops in Africa, for example, has faced controversy. Some claim that the presently available crops, like Bt corn, do not address small farmers' needs in developing countries and that they will be expensive—only agrochemical companies developing them will benefit. Also, these crops will make farmers dependent on the new varieties, and the biodiversity of the old varieties will be lost. In addition, genetically engineered crops might pose environmental risks by leading to insect resistance, gene flow into wild species, and disruption of non-target organisms.

Most farmers in Kenya use local varieties, and they select varieties based on yield, early maturity and tolerance to drought, field pests and storage pests. One approach is to involve these farmers in testing the new varieties of maize. Working

---

Bacillus thuringiensis, commonly known as Bt, is a bacterium that occurs naturally in soil. Some strains of Bt produce proteins that kill certain insects, but are not harmful to humans, other mammals, birds, or fish. Certain crop plants have been genetically engineered to produce their own Bt.

within the Kenyan regulatory system, existing Bt technology has been found to be effective in the laboratory on leaf samples against all major stem borer species, except one.

The next step is to test the Bt varieties in biosafety greenhouses and in open quarantine facilities. Finally, local farmers will test these crops in the field.

No patents were filed in Kenya restricting the use of Bt genes in maize. Therefore, Bt maize is likely to be commercialized by local Kenyan companies. Since Bt genes are dominant, farmers don't need to become dependent on the seed industry since they can recycle seed. In addition, farmers are free to incorporate the gene into local varieties, if they view it as a valuable trait.

Is this a "magic bullet" solution? No, it is only one approach. Biotechnology must be pursued as part of a portfolio of technologies used to enhance productivity and environmental sustainability of agriculture. Although agricultural technology, like any other technology, will never be "zero risk." If it is carefully considered and introduced, shouldn't farmers and consumers be able to try these products and help develop varieties suited to their local areas?

Is this the only way to address these problems? Certainly not. In many cases the problem is not as simple as pest resistance in maize. Are the food and agricultural problems of poor countries like those of rich countries? No, for the poor in most developing countries, things are different—they live in different ecological zones, face different health conditions, and must overcome agronomic limitations very different from those of developed countries

I believe that science, technology, economics and government policy must all be directed toward solving these problems. Technological gains in developed countries will only be minimally applicable to problems in poorer countries. Technologies directed to poorer countries are not likely to reap economic rewards. Therefore, the private sector is not likely to assume a major responsibility in this area.

This brings me to the last point. What about the role of public sector scientists, both in developed countries and in the developing countries? Finally we come to a topic where I have some personal experience. For years, my laboratory has worked on the genetic engineering of cereal crops. One application focused on reducing wheat allergenicity—a problem of little significance in developing countries. But another application of the same technology appears to improve protein and starch digestibility—a recognized problem with sorghum, a staple in parts of Africa.

For this reason colleague Bob Buchanan and I are attempting to improve the nutritional quality of sorghum. We are focusing on improving its digestibility and its amino acid profile, given that cereals are notoriously deficient in lysine.

We found a U.S. company with a modified barley gene that could improve lysine content, and we approached them for the project. We have worked out the intellectual property issues, and are currently introducing this gene into sorghum. Of course, before this is released to African farmers, liability and environmental and food safety issues have to be addressed, The project is moving forward.

There are potential problems in introducing these crops into developing countries, just as there are dangers in introducing other elements of our agricultural system. Care needs to be taken in releasing genetically engineered varieties in areas where there are wild relatives of the commercially grown crop. But this warning is tempered by the fact that you have to look at the actual genes that will be introduced to see if this might cause problems if they were to escape. In our sorghum project, we are working with a sorghum breeder in the Midwest to assess the possible consequences of the movement of our genes into wild species.

Genes have been flowing back and forth between sorghum and their wild relatives for mil-

lennia. The issue becomes what effect—negative or positive—might the particular genes we are using have? If our approaches are successful and we can address food and environmental safety issues, African breeders will move these genes into local sorghum varieties.

Why did we become involved in this project? For me personally, I believe it is part of my mandate as a public sector scientist to use the skills I have to make a contribution to improve the lot of farmers and consumers in developing countries. Is this the only answer? Is this the best answer? No, it is only part of an answer, but it is something I want to and can do.

It has been said that one-fifth of the world's population is at the bottom of the economic ladder, and over 95% of their food supply is produced locally. Therefore, improving agricultural productivity in developing countries may more directly benefit "consumers," since in many cases they are also "producers." Increasing local food production will also contribute to lower food costs and food security. I hope that I can use my knowledge of science and cooperative extension to make a difference in the developing world.

Dr. Lemaux is Chair, Univ. of Calif. Div. of Agriculture and Natural Resources Biotechnology Workgroup, Cooperative Extension Specialist and faculty member, Dept. of Plant and Microbial Biology at the Univ. of Calif. Berkeley (http://plantbio.berkeley.edu/~lemaux). Her work on sorghum is funded by the Bill & Melinda Gates Foundation. She's also a popular speaker on agriculture and biotechnology. This lecture is an excerpt from the Future of Food Symposium: Value vs. Risk in the Biotechnology Debate at Santa Clara University (4/15/05).

Chapter 21

Food Processing and Food Safety

To some, the terms food processing *and* food safety *may sound like conflicting concepts. There's sometimes the image that processing is something done by commercial interests to make money, and that the best one can hope for is that food will be adulterated as little as possible in the process. Anything that happens between original source and dinner table is going to be for the worse.*

Perhaps the scariest word in the processing vocabulary is additives. *They tend to be "chemicals," and to many people that means they are "unnatural," and generally unwholesome— if not dangerous. We think of the whole process as part of a modern-day trend away from the healthy natural world of yesteryear, toward a world dominated by impersonal technology.*

It's not that simple. Additives aren't a recent invention, and many are in fact applications of substances found in the natural world. Without them, we would have a very different food supply, one that for many would bring a lot less pleasure, as well as some very real health problems.

In this country, most of our food choices are not restricted by season or geography. We grow most of our wheat in the Great Plains, freeze orange juice in Florida, produce fruits and vegetables in California, and import food from all over the world. Consumers across the land take for granted the availability of these foods throughout the year. Most of us don't even think about the origins of a breakfast of California melon, hash browns made from Idaho potatoes, toast made from Kansas wheat, and Brazilian coffee sweetened with Hawaiian sugar.

We can buy foods at virtually any stage of preparation. We can buy raw carrots already washed and ready to eat, or carrots already cooked in a honey glaze, frozen in a pouch, only needing heat to eat. We can buy flour to make our own cookies, or a dry cookie mix, or cookie dough ready to bake, or cookies ready to eat. Overall, food processing provides us with thousands of food choices in our markets, most of which are available continuously through the seasons, at a remarkably constant price.

In this chapter, we start by looking at the objectives and effects of the food processing that makes this possible, and an aspect of most concern to many consumers—food additives and their safety.

When it comes to food safety, microbiological hazards—the subject of the last part of this chapter—are of the greatest concern to our food experts. This aspect of food safety is one that consumers can control quite well, by careful food selection, preparation, and storage.

The Evolution of Food Processing

Imagine what eating must have been like in the days of the caveman. You would feast on meat when an animal hunt was successful. Between times, you'd eat what edible plants could be found. Worrying about your next meal was a constant thing. Too often, it was a cycle of feast and famine. What, you might ask, could you do to save some of the feast to avoid the famine?

We might imagine that the first food preservation discoveries were accidental. Perhaps a scrap of meat or a piece of fruit, leftover from the feasting, may have been overlooked. You find it days later, on a boulder in the sun, all dried out.

Hungry, you tear off a piece with your teeth, and find it quite edible. Ways to preserve food were among our first discoveries.

The Egyptians of the First Dynasty, about 3000 B.C., not only knew much about drying and salting and cooking, but had learned to preserve milk by making cheese. By 2000 B.C. they were baking bread and brewing beer. In the ancient world, alcoholic beverages were as important for food preservation as for revelry. (But keep in mind that beer then was a thick, nutritious brew.) And indeed almost every primitive culture seems to have developed a preservative use for fermentation.

Whole grains of salt were known as "corn" in England, and were used make "corned beef."

The relatively recent American pioneers extended this use for fermentation. In Kentucky and thereabouts, the land along the Ohio River was fine for growing corn. But it grew more than they could use. How could they utilize the left-over corn so it could be transported to a buyer elsewhere? The answer was to make it into corn whisky, which was shipped on rafts down the Ohio and Mississippi Rivers to New Orleans, and thence around the world. Kentucky still produces fine bourbon.

Warfare and empire-building have been important factors in the evolution of food preservation and processing—creating the need to supply armies on the march. Modern food preserving is often said to have begun with Napoleon's forays. In 1810, the French brewer, Nicholas Appert, was awarded a grand prize for developing canning. He had sealed food in jars and then heated them in boiling water, a process which was believed to work because the food was shut away from air. It wasn't until later that science understood that the process actually worked because the heat destroyed microbes present in the food, and the sealing prevented new infections.

During World War II, demand went beyond merely edible food for the troops, to nutritionally adequate food—an impetus for the first set of Recommended Dietary Allowances (RDAs). Then, military demand went beyond nutritionally adequate food, to pleasurable food. In the 1991 Gulf War, the U.S. troops were even provided with chocolate bars specially made for desert eating.

Food processing as we know it today, goes far beyond mere preservation. We have a vast array of such things as *convenience foods* (e.g., frozen dinners), *health foods* (e.g., bran-fortified breakfast cereals), and *fabricated foods* (e.g., meatless "hamburger meat" made from soybeans).

Perhaps the ultimate in fabricated food is the extremely popular diet soft drink. This drink raises the ultimate question asked of some processed foods: Is it *really* food? After all, any nutrient in a diet soft drink is unintentional. We might say that food processing has also given us "fun foods," foods eaten mainly to please our senses.

So we ask a lot of food processing, and sometimes the result is nutrition confusion.

Industry's Desire to Please

Much of our nutrition confusion we blame on the food industry. But industry is in many ways a passive force—amoral but not really immoral, if you will—trying simply to turn out a decent product and make a profit. Basically, industry responds to what we *think* our needs are. It's very expensive to try and create public demands. It's much cheaper simply to find out what people want to buy and give it to them.

For example, the broad food-industry use of added vitamin C is a recognition of the public's distorted idea of the need for this vitamin. *Tang* (an orange-flavored sugar mixture) is sold on the basis that it has "twice as much vitamin C as orange juice." It does so because the public believes that vitamin C is badly needed, and the more the better.

Meanwhile, the Florida citrus industry ballyhoos its oranges as having "natural vitamin C from the Florida sunshine tree." It does this because so many people mistakenly believe that there is a health difference between "natural" and synthetic C.

Taking this consumer confusion a bit further, Sunkist sells tablets of synthetic vitamin C in a colorful box adorned with juicy oranges and emblazoned with *Sunkist Vitamin C*. The implication, of course, is that this synthetic vitamin C is more "natural"—and thus more healthful and desirable—than other synthetic C tablets on the vitamin shelf.

While these sales efforts may not be in the

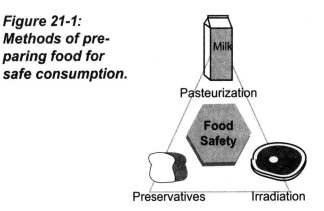

Figure 21-1: Methods of preparing food for safe consumption.

public interest, they are realistic to the extent that they give the public what the public thinks it needs. The industrial reality is that, while production methods are controlled by technologists of great sophistication, the businesses are guided by marketers. Their training is in the economics of producing and selling. Their information about nutrition is minimal. Their primary interest lies in what will sell, and this is determined by what the public wants. Their foremost research effort is to determine public wishes and to meet them.

The industry's promotion people often know even less about nutrition. Their aim is to express as dramatically as possible the idea that the product furnishes what the buyer thinks is important. Essentially their sales message is that "What you want is what we have to sell."

To see how ironically this system works, look at the "natural" cereals. Most are made by the same companies that sell conventional cereals, with the usual additives. But while one part of the company heralds its "natural" cereals by implying that additives and sugar are unhealthful, and "natural" products are somewhat superior, other parts of the company spend millions to convince us that additives and preservatives are valuable and harmless, and that ordinary cereals give us better nutritive content.

In an individual, such behavior might be described as "schizophrenic." In food companies, it's simply a matter of *market identification* and *market penetration*—in two markets.

Objectives of Food Processing
Preparation

One function of processing is the preparation of food for eating. More and more of what used to be done entirely in the home kitchen is now also done by food companies. We can buy entire dinners that only need heating. Much of food processing is really industrialized cookery.

Most of this work centers about two general concepts, just as our home cooking does. First, we select the part of the food we want to eat, and separate it from the part we don't want—as in taking peas from a pod, a banana from its skin, or meat from the bone. And second, we modify the food for a specific eating purpose. Milk may be heated and flavored with chocolate at breakfast, or made into yogurt for lunch, or used to make a pudding for dessert at dinner. Of course, most of this sort of processing has to do with sensory values.

Some processing has to do with consumer demand for "healthier" foods, often at a sacrifice of sensory pleasure. These include low-fat or fat-free modifications (e.g., fat-free salad dressings), low-sodium modifications (e.g., low-sodium cheese), and "fabricated foods" (e.g., margarine).

Preservation

Unlike the home cook who can serve dinner right after making it, the food company must preserve whatever it has prepared, whether a bag of peas out of their pods, a pint of "light" sour cream, or a four-compartment plate of meat, gravy, potatoes, green beans, and apple cobbler.

Preservation has two broad aspects. The first is to combat *deterioration*—changes occurring within the food itself. It may be entirely the result of the food's own chemistry, or it may be caused partly by such outside influences as light, oxygen, heat, and so on. Stale bread and rancid oil are examples of deteriorated food.

To shield foods from light, we use opaque or tinted packaging. (An age-old method is to store foods in the dark—as in the cellar). We do this with the oily potato chips and the mostly-fat bacon, to prevent light-induced rancidity of the fat. We do this with milk, to prevent the destruction of its riboflavin by light. We do this with sacks of potatoes, to lessen light-induced formation of solanine (a nerve toxin found when a green layer forms under potato skin).

To keep oxygen from doing damage, we use vacuum packs and antioxidants. To stop the food's own deterioration-causing enzymes, we blanch (quickly heat) the food. To further slow the food's chemistry, we lower the temperature by refrigeration or freezing.

Sometimes, substances are removed from the food to preserve freshness. Removing the oily wheat germ (the part that goes rancid) to make white flour increases the shelf life of the flour—an especially important factor in the days when flour was stored for a long time, its transport slow, and when bread was our "staff of life." (There was also an esthetic preference for white flour then, as now. White bread is still the generally preferred bread, and cakes and cookies made with whole wheat flour aren't much of a hit.)

The second general aspect of preservation is really a part of our age-old competition with other life forms for food. For just as we must defend our berries from the crows, and our grain from the rats and insects, so must we compete with the microbes which would flourish in our food. *Spoilage* is the term used by food technologists to denote the damage wrought by microbes. Soured milk and moldy bread are examples.

Preventing spoilage (an aspect of microbial chemistry) and preventing deterioration (an aspect of plant chemistry) are similar—life chemistry, whether of food or microbes, is similar. Preservation from spoilage will be discussed further in the section on microbiological food hazards.

Does Processing Affect Nutritive Value?

There's no question that the preparation of food for consumption or storage has some effect on nutritive value. Food begins to change as soon as we take it from the plant. Some vitamin values fall as it goes from farm to store to home. In the cook's domain, cooking time, the amount of water used, and the temperature of the water all affect nutritive value.

In general, the commercial processor has tight controls over all these factors and takes pains to minimize the lag at each step—from the field, to the production line, to the final product available to the consumer. Very few home cooks have direct access to a crop. If they do, they may or may not be so quick or scrupulous with the harvesting, cooking, or preserving.

So the ***nutrient loss*** with home processing is often greater than that of commercial processing. The consumer can minimize nutrient losses at home by storing fresh foods in the cold (to inhibit the chemistry of vitamin deterioration), cooking in minimal amounts of water if the water is to be discarded (to lessen the loss of water-soluble vitamins), and not over-cooking (to lessen the heat-destruction of some vitamins).

Nutrient losses during home storage and preparation mostly involve vitamins. Minerals aren't destroyed by light or heat.

But today's questions of processing and nutritive value are much more than a matter of concern for nutrient losses. With the nutrient ***fortification*** of so many foods (e.g., vitamin D-fortified milk, iodized salt, vitamin and mineral fortified breakfast cereals), modern food processing has, ironically, done more to prevent vitamin and mineral deficiencies than cause them. Some refined foods may even have more vitamins and minerals than the unrefined. Iron and some B-vitamins, for example, are routinely added to white flour in this country, making white flour a richer source of some of these nutrients than whole-wheat flour.

But does this make white flour more nutritious than whole wheat flour? The answer could be yes, because many children and women don't get enough iron, and enriched white flour is a little better source of iron than whole wheat flour. But the answer could also be no, because many people don't get enough fiber in their diet, and whole wheat is a richer source. Also, other nutrients lost in the refining process (e.g., potassium, zinc) are not replaced in enriched white flour. (Nutritionists encourage whole grains in the diet.)

Complicating the processing/nutritive-value evaluation even further, there are food components that have nutritive value, but that consumers want removed by food processing, to make them more "healthful." Just think of the array of "diet foods" available at the supermarket.

Loss of Taste Versus Nutrient Loss

Why do many consumers believe that processed foods are nutritionally lacking? One reason is certainly taste, the idea being that taste and nutrition go hand in hand. The truth is that, although a food gone bad suffers in both nutrient quality and taste, one can't judge nutrition by whether the food is tasteless, moderately tasty, or exquisitely delicious.

Crops are often chosen for their ability to survive processing or for their uniformity of size and color—at a sacrifice of flavor or texture. Also, it's easier to preserve the nutrients than to preserve taste and texture. Frozen berries may seem like a distant relative of the fresh berries you pull off a wild vine along the mountain stream. The frozen berries may leave you wistful, but their nutrients are well-preserved.

A popular comment—made only half in jest—is, "It tastes so good, it surely can't be good for us" or "It tastes so bad, it must be good for us."

Part of the doubt about the nutritiousness of processed food can be blamed on unrealistic advertising. Advertisers often go too far when they try to convince us their cookies, soups, or frozen entrees are "just like mother used to make" (unless, of course, mother was a dreadful cook). When the product fails to live up to the billing, we feel swindled. After all, why should we be expected to accept industry's claims for nutritive concern and care and quality, when its advertising for a dismal, frozen meatball has implied that the poor thing would delight the senses of a Florentine chef?

Processors are constantly striving to improve flavor and texture. The biotech-produced Flavr Savr tomato, mentioned in the last chapter, is but one example. Anyone who thinks that processors don't leap to seize any advantage in flavor or food value grossly underestimates their business sense.

If we want to fix a hot dinner in five minutes, we can have it, and it will be good and safe for survival, but there's often a price in pleasure. The use of convenience foods is a personal choice.

It's perhaps what and how much we choose to eat because of convenience that causes people to associate processed foods with nutritional emptiness. If there's anything "unhealthful" about the advances in food processing, it's that it has brought us an extremely handy variety of food—so attractively packaged, so easily stored, and so convenient to eat, that it is easy to overeat. How often would you eat potato chips if you had to make them yourself from a fresh potato?

What's "Natural" Food?

Consumers often put considerable emphasis on distinctions between "processed" and "natural" foods. The terms are widely used without question. The world "natural" is a powerful stimulus for consumers, who seem to feel that "natural" food is much more healthful, that "processed" means degraded, at least in terms of healthfulness.

Post's *Grape Nuts* are billed as a "Natural Wheat and Barley Cereal." But its long list of ingredients include malted barley (meaning that starch in the barley has been broken down to the sugar maltose) and eight added vitamins.

Kellogg's *All-Bran* is sold as "A Natural Food Fiber Cereal." It's so-called, presumably, because its first listed ingredient is wheat bran. Wheat bran does contain substantial fiber, and it's part of a plant's natural growth. But how natural is it after machines take the bran part of the wheat kernel, mix it into a secret recipe, shape and bake the dough into tiny crunchy cylinders, and package it all into a double wrapper of bag and box? Other "natural" cereals include corn syrup or nonfat dried milk, which certainly don't come directly from cornstalks and cows.

But, clearly, the intent of the consumer is to get food which is as close to its original state as possible. And equally clear is the belief that such food is more healthful. We have seen that this isn't necessarily true in terms of nutrient content, but it's generally true that minimally processed foods tend to be more nutritious. A diet centered around these foods is recommended by nutritionists.

Food Additives—What Did They Put in Our Food?

People correctly associate food processing with food additives. These "chemicals" added to food have been the focus of many scare stories. But even without these stories, there's something a bit discomforting about swallowing down foods that are labeled with long lists of ingredients with forbidding names, vague purposes, and unfamiliar identities.

Whose mouth waters for a diglyceride (an emulsifier)? Who puts butylated hydroxytoluene (an antioxidant) on their grocery list? It's an old

(and accurate) saw that we fear most what we understand least. So let's look a little closer at what additives are.

Suppose we begin by looking at a food's list of ingredients—one that offers us a product containing, "Acetone, methyl acetate, furan, diacetyl, butanol, methylfuran, isoprene, methylbutanol, caffeine, essential oils, methanol, acetaldehyde, methyl formate, ethanol, dimethyl sulfide, and propionaldehyde." The instructions are to soak this stuff in hot water, throw it away, and drink the hot water. Would you do it? Well, would you reconsider if you knew the product was nothing but pure coffee?

All the listed chemicals are merely the natural chemicals found in coffee. Such a list could be made for every food, "natural" or "unnatural," processed or unprocessed.

Coal tar dyes have names like FD&C red no. 40—they're used to color **F**oods, **D**rugs and **C**osmetics.

Many of the substances found naturally in food appear on food labels as additives. For the fact is that many of the feared additives are only food substances taken from other food sources, foods that nature has provided that help preserve, enhance flavor, produce better texture, and so on.

Additives are sometimes fortification and enrichment nutrients of questionable value. Some of these you can recognize and evaluate. For example, you might wonder if the addition of 100% of the Daily Value of so many vitamins and minerals to an energy bar is more for the benefit of sales than the benefit of the consumer.

Hundreds of additives of various kinds are used; some are listed in Table 21-1. Some are such common foods as acetic acid (vinegar). Some are familiar products used to add color, like beta-carotene or chlorophyll. Some are used to change the consistency of the product—pectin from fruit, usually apples, keeps jelly gelatinous. There are stabilizers and thickeners, with the odd names agar, carrageenan, and guar—all are "gums" found naturally in plants.

There are, of course, food additives that aren't found in nature. The most heavily criticized are the ***coal tar dyes*** used to color food. But the approved color additives have survived intensive scrutiny as to their safety. They come under par-

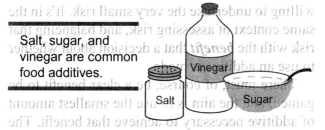

Salt, sugar, and vinegar are common food additives.

ticular attack because their sole purpose is for color—perhaps frivolous, perhaps not.

Ironically, less is known about many of the substances that give plant foods their natural color. Also, color additives didn't come into being with the advent of yellow margarine, orange Kool-Aid, red-striped candy canes, blue Jell-O, and green M&Ms. Even the ancient Egyptians used color additives made from plants—and insects—to color their food.

The public concern with food additives is often based in part on the idea that additives serve only the processors, and that they aren't really needed. But, generally, food additives serve the consumer as much as the manufacturer, in keeping food safe and pleasing.

Preservatives

Although many people recognize flavoring additives on ingredient lists, few recognize the preservatives, and those who do often view them with alarm. What are these chemicals?

Among the most common are calcium and sodium propionate, whose names are often found on labels with the words, "added to retard spoilage." These are intended to keep molds and bacteria from making foods such as bread inedible. They aren't poisons. They are salts of propionic acid, which is produced naturally in Swiss cheese. They are completely metabolized by the body, e.g.; calcium propionate is broken down in the body to calcium, carbon dioxide, and water.

Because of some studies showing that BHA and BHT inhibit cancer in mice and rats, capsules of BHA and BHT ("man-made chemical food additives") are sold as dietary supplements.

Additives used for preserving are often substances present in nature to protect foods. For example, vitamin E occurs naturally with unsaturated oils. It functions in the body as an antioxi-

dant, slowing down the oxidation of the unsaturated fat in our cell membranes. Vitamin E does the same thing on the grocer's shelf; it's added to slow down the oxidation of the oil in foods, and thus helps prevent rancidity. (Even though vitamin E is a natural food constituent, it's still only used sparingly as a food additive.)

Citric acid (found in citrus fruits), and ascorbic acid (vitamin C) are also antioxidants, and both are used to prevent oxidation and discoloration. We use citric acid and vitamin C as antioxidants ourselves, when we combine citrus fruit or its juice with sliced avocados, apples, etc. Sliced oranges in a fruit salad retards the oxidation-caused browning of the sliced apples.

BHA (butylated hydroxyanisole) and BHT (butylated hydroxytoluene) are more commonly added to foods as antioxidants. (BHA and BHT aren't normal food constituents.)

Are Food Additives Safe to Eat?

The public has a single question about these substances: Are they absolutely safe? In realistic scientific terms, the answer to that question can be extremely succinct. No. Then how can we dare to put additives in food? The scientist's answer, and a confusing one for the layman, is, "Because we don't think that they will hurt anyone."

The apparent conflict between these two answers is best understood by looking more closely at the meaning of safety. Webster defines safety as "freedom from danger, injury or damage." In these terms, stop to think of just one thing which you do or eat which is absolutely safe. Remember that, as a measurement, "freedom from" must be considered as zero. Zero what? Zero risk.

Is it safe to cross the street at a quiet intersection with a traffic light and a crossing guard? One can't really say that it is; there's a very low possibility that you'll be hurt, but it's not zero. Is it safe to drink water or eat a banana? In absolute terms, it isn't. Anything we eat or drink can be toxic, if we take enough of it, or take it under certain conditions.

It's hard for many people to understand that the only real measurement of "safety" is *risk*. In crossing the street, we may say that we feel safe, and mean that we think the risk is very low. At

Table 21-1: Some Food Additives

To thicken:	To color:
Agar	Annatto
Calcium alginate	Caramel
Carob bean gum	Carotene
Cellulose	Carrot oil
Gelatin	Citrus red no. 2
Guar gum	Dehydrated beets
Gum ghatti	FD & C blue no. 1
Locust bean gum	FD & C red no. 40
Modified food starch	FD & C yellow no. 5
Pectin	**To prevent oxidation:**
Potassium alginate	Ascorbic acid (vitamin C)
Sodium alginate	BHA (butylated hydroxyanisole)
Tragacanth gum	BHT (butylated hydroxytoluene)
To control acidity:	Citric acid
Acetic acid	EDTA (ethylenediamine
Citric acid	tetraacetic acid)
Lactic acid	Propyl gallate
Sodium acetate	Sulfites
Sodium citrate	Tocopherols (vitamin E)
Tartaric acid	**To enhance flavor:**
To whiten:	Disodium guanylate
Benzoyl peroxide	Hydrolyzed vegetable protein
Calcium bromate	Maltol
Hydrogen peroxide	Monosodium glutamate (MSG)
Potassium bromate	**To make baked goods rise:**
To retain moisture:	Calcium phosphate
Glycerol	Monocalcium phosphate
Propylene glycol	Potassium bitartrate
Sorbitol	("cream of tartar")
To emulsify:	Sodium aluminum phosphate
Carrageenan	Sodium bicarbonate
Diglycerides	("baking soda")
Gum arabic	**To retard microbial growth:**
Lecithin	Benzoic acid
Monoglycerides	Calcium lactate
Polysorbate	Calcium propionate
To prevent caking:	Calcium sorbate
Ammonium citrate	Lactic acid
Calcium silicate	Methylparaben
Magnesium carbonate	Potassium sorbate
Silicon dioxide	Propionic acid
To improve tartness:	Propylparaben
Phosphates	
Phosphoric acid	

rush hour, the risk is somewhat higher, but not really threatening.

And we have something to gain from crossing the street—getting to work, perhaps. So we're willing to undertake the very small risk. It's in the same context of assessing risk, and balancing that risk with the **benefit** that a decision about whether to use an additive is made.

There must, of course, be a clear benefit to be gained, and the aim is to use the smallest amount of additive necessary to achieve that benefit. The hard questions are: What's the hazard (risk), in terms of specific amounts of the additive and the conditions of its use? And what level of risk should we say is acceptable? In crossing our quiet street, one condition we impose is to look both ways for traffic. With this condition we accept the risk without any fear of danger.

Legislating Additive Safety

The safety programs of the FDA began with Dr. Harvey Wiley, a chemist with the USDA from 1883-1930. Dr. Wiley used a volunteer "poison squad" of twelve men, who consumed quantities of food additives to see if they were harmful. Those were the days in which manufacturers could put what they chose in food, and it was up to government agencies to learn if it was harmful, prove that it was, and take action to have the substance removed (this is generally the situation for many dietary supplements today). For the first 52 years of the FDA's existence (from 1906 to 1958), it was the government's duty to prove danger, not the manufacturer's to prove "safety."

In 1958, this process was reversed with the **Food Additives Amendment**. This requires that manufacturers first run extensive tests to prove the safety of an additive, then apply to the FDA for an order permitting use within a specific tolerance of amounts of the substance considered safe.

The amendment outlawed the addition to food of substances of unknown or uncertain toxicity. It established that a newly proposed additive must undergo strict testing designed to establish the safety of the intended use.

This law and its procedures provide protection for the consumer—and a major expense for the manufacturer. Since this amendment, very few additives have been added to the approved list.

Assessing the Risk

A primary step in testing an additive is to determine the **no-effect dose**. Groups of animals are given various doses over their lifetimes. Suppose there's no apparent harmful effect at lifetime doses of up to 100 mg/day, but animals given 1,000 mg/day or more show an impairment of kidney function (doses are commonly tested in 10-fold increments). We've found a "no-effect" dose and an *"effect" dose*. The measurements are important, for usually FDA requires that there be a 100-fold safety factor. In other words, usually the highest expected use of an additive should be no higher than one-hundredth of the no-effect dose.

Vitamin A at RDA levels doesn't cause birth defects. But it can in big doses.

A no-effect lifetime dose of 100 mg/day would mean that the highest expected use should be no higher than 1 mg/day. In many cases, the highest expected use is much lower. If, in this example, the highest expected use was 0.1 mg/day (1/10 of the highest allowed dose), the safety factor would be 1,000-fold.

Some scientists argue that the high doses given to test animals often produce effects unique to the high dosage—effects from the massive amounts exceeding what the body can safely handle.

But to find effects at low doses usually means having to use many more animals over a long time. Using thousands of animals to test each substance over a period of years is extremely expensive and time consuming. So we're left with the alternative of testing substances at high doses on relatively small groups of animals.

Animal tests are extensive. For each proposed additive, studies must be done on both male and female of at least two species of animals, and over at least two generations. Obviously, we aren't biochemically or physiologically identical to the test animals, but the effects on them suggest how we might be affected.

Even with extensive studies, it's clear that estimates of risk have to be made on incomplete knowledge. What's hazardous to an animal may not be hazardous to us; what's safe for an animal may not be safe for us. A substance may be toxic at a given dose for some people and not others; and under some conditions and not others. There may be effects that aren't measurable by current technology.

Because these uncertainties can never be completely addressed, a lot of the assessment of hu-

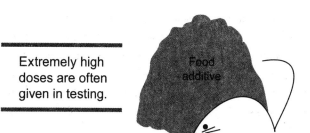

Extremely high doses are often given in testing.

man risk will remain subjective, and there will continue to be arguments about risk assessment among scientists themselves. As a result, industry, consumer and environmental groups, people writing to congress, etc., sometimes have more influence than scientists do in determining whether a particular food additive should be approved or not.

The GRAS List

Most of the additives we use are in a group known as GRAS, or *Generally Recognized as Safe*. The GRAS list came into being with the 1958 Additives Amendment which, as we've seen, emphasizes safety testing for newly proposed additives. The list includes hundreds of substances (including salt, sugar, and some common spices) which had been added to foods for an extended period of time prior to 1958 without apparent harm, on the theory that these substances had been tested by use.

As an extra precaution, these substances were widely accepted as safe by scientists surveyed at that time. And since 1958, the safety of each has been reevaluated. The safety of GRAS additives (and new additives) continues to be reevaluated whenever there's new scientific information—or sometimes when there's a public outcry to do so.

The Delaney Clause

The 1958 Food Additives Amendment also contains what's now popularly referred to as the Delaney Clause, named for Congressman James Delaney of New York. The Clause reads: "No additive shall be deemed to be safe if it's found to induce cancer when ingested by man or animal, or if it's found, after tests which are appropriate for the evaluation of the safety of food additives, to induce cancer in man or animals." In short, it specifies that any substance shown to cause cancer in any amount in any animal can't be allowed as a food additive.

This clause has been the subject of much debate and litigation. The controversy has arisen because no limit or condition was set upon the amounts of a substance or the terms of an experiment which might cause cancer. Several much-publicized bannings of additives have stemmed from this legislation.

In 1969, the artificial sweetener cyclamate was banned because of evidence that it caused bladder cancer in rats. When saccharin also was found to cause bladder cancer in rats, it also was to be banned in 1977. This caused a huge public outcry because, at that time, saccharin was the only artificial sweetener left on the market for use in diet products (e.g., diet soft drinks). (When cyclamate had been banned, we still had saccharin.)

As a result of public pressure, Congress put a moratorium on banning saccharin as a food additive. Thus, saccharin is used as a food additive, whereas cyclamate is banned. It's interesting to note that in Canada, cyclamate is used as a food additive, whereas saccharin is banned. Yet both countries have looked at the same studies in making their decisions.

The Delaney Clause has generated a lot of heated rhetoric. Some argue that the Clause should be modified to allow for an assessment of risk versus benefit, or that an additive shouldn't be banned if its risk of causing cancer is "negligible."

The Delaney Clause stems from a widespread belief that food additives are a major cause of cancer. This belief isn't supported by scientific evidence.

Putting Additives in Perspective

There are reasons to be concerned about additives, but there are also reasons to be unconcerned. As we've seen repeatedly, the same substance can be both "toxic" and "safe," depending on how much is used and how it's used. A very toxic substance given in a small enough dose can be harmless; and a very safe substance given in a large enough dose can be harmful. Because this isn't well-understood by the public, public support for the banning of an additive can often be engendered by merely citing the harm caused by occupational or accidental exposures to large doses of the additive.

We've also seen that there's an overlap between "natural" and "man-made" or "chemical" substances (i.e., a food additive can be exactly the same as that found naturally in food); and that so far as we can determine one isn't inherently better or worse than the other. So it's important to look at food additives in the wider context of all substances found in our food.

There are a large variety and a large amount of natural toxicants in foods. Dr. Bruce Ames, a renowned expert on cancer biochemistry and food toxicants, says that the amounts and effects of food additives and pesticide residues are trivial compared to those of the natural toxicants in our food.[1-3] But this doesn't keep him from eating plant foods—even those he knows to contain large amounts of natural toxins. Dr. Ames emphasizes that plant foods are also an abundant source of substances (e.g., carotenoids, vitamin C) that protect us from toxicants.

Microbiological Hazards in Foods

Each year, millions of Americans are afflicted with food-borne illnesses, most of which are caused by bacteria (see Fig. 21-2). For some people, the result is a day or two of stomach cramps, diarrhea and other familiar intestinal symptoms. For others, particularly infants and the elderly, the result can be deadly.

Most of these cases go unreported. Most people made ill by food think they have "a bug," "a virus," "intestinal flu," or "indigestion." Usually the discomfort goes away and the misery is forgotten; but the more seriously afflicted don't forget so easily. The vast majority of such uncomfortable, wasted days are needless. So let's see what we can do to protect ourselves.

We might begin with one simple but useful fact. By and large, those food-borne infections which can cause us trouble can't be seen, smelled, or tasted in food.

Protecting ourselves requires more intellectual than sensory vigilance, because such infections are carried on foods that our senses tell us are perfectly good. While we can't defend ourselves against all food-borne infections with personal care and hygiene, we can reduce our risk considerably with a little knowledge and effort.

How Food Becomes Infected

Most of us think of microbes in a negative way, and imagine we're getting rid of them with soap and water and smelly solutions. But microbes are more plentiful and pervasive and tougher than most of us suspect. Some exist 18 miles above earth at the edge of space; others are found at the bottom of the sea, in bubbling hot springs, in polar ice or in powerful acids.

We're covered with microbes, inside and out. All of life and food, all of air and soil are replete with them. Despite their tiny size—each is only a single cell—microbes as a group vastly outweigh man. One authority has calculated that the microbes of our planet outweigh all animal life (on land and sea) 25-fold.

So we can forget about trying to get rid of microbes. They are survival experts. Leave one alive and it becomes two, in a matter of minutes to a few hours at most. The consequence of this rapid doubling and redoubling is breathtaking. It's been said that if one cell of *E. coli* had enough food, in three days it could yield a mass of bacteria greater than the earth. And in a matter of minutes, it would double again.

The key phrase here, of course, is "had enough food." What serves as food for microbes is astonishingly varied. Most can live on *our* food; some do so by living in our digestive tract. And some of these give us back such things as vitamins, or join in performing essential functions for us. Microbes are an essential part of life processes on earth.

Our first effort is to keep our food from becoming a growth medium for harmful microbes, and to avoid eating large groups of them—or large amounts of the toxins some produce. The chief ways we can do this are by:

- Not inoculating our food with such microbes
- Rejecting food which has been handled in ways that encourage microbial growth
- Keeping our food in environments which are too hot or cold for microbial growth.

Because microbes are everywhere, they enter food by endless routes. In a few cases we can see them (as in the case of molds), or smell the evidence (as in sour milk). So of course we shouldn't place a new loaf of bread against a moldy one, or allow drops of soured milk to get into fresh milk.

But in most cases, we can't perceive microbes. We must understand where they are likely to be. That is why you shouldn't mix a meat loaf with your hands when you have a cut finger—there may be *staphylococci* in the cut.

Some Kinds of Harmful Microbes

Staphylococci ("staph") are thought to be the most common cause of food poisoning, with millions of cases a year. We don't want them in our food. It isn't so much what the bacteria themselves will do to us. But as they eat and grow, they produce an intestinal toxin. The staph are easily killed by the heat of cooking, but the toxin isn't alive in the first place and is highly heat-resistant. It remains intact and can make us ill.

About half of all humans are thought to carry staph at any given time—on the skin, in nasal passages, and in wounds and skin eruptions. People can transmit the microbe to food by direct handling, or through the air by talking, sneezing, and coughing. Since there's so much staph around, don't leave prepared food at a temperature which isn't hot or cold. Heat or cold slows microbial growth; moderate temperatures encourage it (see Fig. 21-3).

As said earlier, microbes that contaminate food can cause disease themselves or produce harmful toxins. Ingesting *salmonella* bacteria from egg or chicken can result in the digestive upheavals of salmonellosis. On the other hand, *botulinum* organisms aren't the direct cause of the nerve-deadening effects of botulism; what poisons is the toxin they produce.

Again, these organisms are all around us. Bread molds are everywhere. Botulinum is common in soil. So when we undertake the preservation of our food, we must process so as to defend our food and ourselves against a vast microbial world. Some microbes that cause food-borne illnesses are listed in Table 21-2.

Keeping Microbes in Check

Whether or not disease-causing microbes in our food present a hazard is a matter of amount. It's generally only when these microbes are allowed to flourish that there are enough of them or their toxins to make us sick.

Figure 21-2: Causes of Food-Borne Illness.
Bacteria cause more than 90% of food-borne disease.

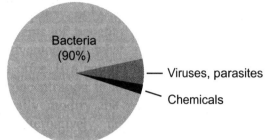

Microbes can be killed outright by **heat or irradiation**, or they can be kept from flourishing by an **inhospitable environment**. Bread can be frozen, apricots dried, beef heavily salted, cucumbers pickled in vinegar, strawberries heavily sugared to make jam. Some methods for keeping microbes in check are:

- Handle foods properly, under sanitary conditions
- Cook foods thoroughly
- Refrigerate foods promptly
- Avoid unpasteurized milk and cheese
- Properly process home-canned foods

The heat doesn't always have to be so high as to kill all the microbes. The heat used to pasteurize milk, for example, kills the disease-causing ones, but isn't high enough to kill the ones that cause spoilage. Much higher heat can be used to kill all the microbes (i.e., sterilize the milk). An "ultra-high" heat treatment is used for "fresh" milk that can be stored for months at room temperature.

A few seconds at very high heat sterilizes the milk without destroying much of the fresh flavor.

Irradiation of food can be used to kill microbes, and also for other purposes. The allowable uses for food irradiation in this country include killing pests in spices and tea, fumigation of certain crops (to replace the post-harvest use of pesticides), killing *Trichinella* worms sometimes found in pork, inhibiting the post-harvest sprouting of potatoes and onions, and delaying ripening or spoiling of some fruits. Irradiating a food does *not* make it radioactive, as some consumers think.

E. coli O157:H7

E. coli (Escherichia coli) is a common microbe normally present in the intestine and feces of all vertebrates, including humans. Most strains are quite harmless; some are even helpful. *E. coli* strain O157:H7 is one of several unusual strains that make a potent toxin that causes serious illness, especially in young children and the elderly.

The first recognized outbreak of *E. coli* O157:H7 was in 1982 when at least 47 people in Oregon and Michigan got sick after eating McDonald's hamburgers. There have been many outbreaks since, including one involving three classes of kindergarten children who drank unpasteurized milk during a trip to a Canadian dairy farm, and another in 1993 traced to fresh apple cider—apples can fall on soil that has animal droppings (feces) or manure fertilizer. The most common route of infection is via fecal contamination, particularly from cows.

A 1993 outbreak in Washington, Idaho, California, and Nevada killed four children and made hundreds of people ill; most cases were traced to Jack-in-the-Box hamburgers. In a 1996 outbreak in Japan, more than 9000 people got sick and at least nine died; most cases were traced to fresh radish sprouts served in school lunches. (When eaten raw, sprouts from contaminated seeds are a problem; seeds won't sprout if heated to kill microbes.) Also in 1996, about 70 people got sick and a 1-year-old girl died from drinking Odwalla juice that contained unpasteurized, contaminated apple juice.

The toxin damages the lining of the colon and its blood vessels, causing severe cramps and bloody diarrhea. In about 5% of the cases, the toxin enters the bloodstream, destroys blood cells, and causes kidney failure. Vaccines and drugs are being developed for humans and livestock.

Hamburger meat is more likely to be contaminated because it's usually made by combining meat from many cattle and from many slaughterhouses to get a homogeneous product with a designated fat content. Suppose 1 of 1000 pieces of beef is contaminated. If all 1000 pieces are ground together, all patties made from that batch will be contaminated. If the pieces aren't combined, as with a steak or roast, the odds of getting the contaminated piece is 1 in 1000.

Symbol for Irradiated Food

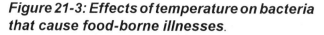

Figure 21-3: Effects of temperature on bacteria that cause food-borne illnesses.

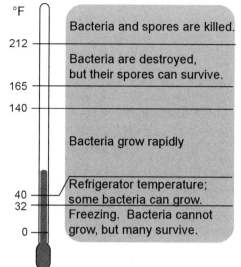

Hamburger chains place huge orders for ground beef (McDonald's buys about half a billion pounds a year). Beef from many sources is combined and the patties shipped to various franchises. If a batch is contaminated, a widespread outbreak can occur (the contaminated Jack-in-the-Box hamburger meat was traced to a single processor).

Contamination won't cause disease if the patties are thoroughly cooked. All parts of the patty must be cooked to 155°F to kill the microbe; 140°F was the standard for Jack-in-the-Box hamburgers. (A contaminated steak would be contaminated only on its surface—only the surface has to be cooked to 155°F.) Consumers should look for hamburger patties that aren't pink inside.

Botulism

Botulism is the food-borne illness caused by the toxin made by *Clostridium botulinum.* Botulism is unusual in this country, but it's worth some discussion because it has some particularly interesting aspects. The toxin is a nerve poison that affects muscle action, and is one of the most potent poisons known. An amount weighing as little as a grain of salt is enough to kill several people within an hour.[10] Botulism poisoning is a medical emergency.

The symptoms usually appear 12 to 36 hours after eating the contaminated food, but the time can vary from 4 hours to 8 days. Neurological symptoms usually start in the head area, and then move downward. Early symptoms include double

vision, dry mouth, drooping eyelids, and speech and swallowing difficulties. The toxin can affect respiration, and cause death by suffocation. Early diagnosis is important. An antitoxin is available, and mechanical ventilation can be used when breathing becomes difficult.

> Local injection of botulism toxin is used medically (to treat facial twitches and excessive underarm sweating) and cosmetically (to deaden facial muscles that cause wrinkles).

In this country, most cases of botulism occur from eating improperly home-canned foods of low acidity (e.g., green beans, corn, spinach). When defective canning methods have failed to kill the botulinum, the conditions are ideal for their growth. They thrive and produce toxin where there's no oxygen (as in the canned food) and where acidity is low (e.g., canned green beans), and they grow best at room temperature (the storage temperature for canned goods).

> Home-canning is actually *home-jarring;* the foods are "canned" in jars.

The presence of the bacteria or the toxin doesn't necessarily make the food look or smell unusual. So if there's even a suspicion of contamination (e.g., haphazard processing, bulging of the canning lid), throw the food out—without tasting. Botulinum toxin (unlike some other toxins) can be destroyed by thorough cooking, but this isn't recommended as a way of ridding the food of the toxin. Throw it out; it's not worth the risk.

Botulism contamination rarely occurs with commercially-prepared foods. Since 1926, there have been only four deaths from commercially canned foods reported in this country. The latest death occurred in 1971 from canned vichysoisse produced by a small company. Vichysoisse is a creamy potato soup (non-acidic), usually served cold. If it had been heated, at least some of the toxin might have been destroyed, and the death might have been avoided.

Nitrite as a Food Additive to Prevent Botulism

In commercially processed food, concern about botulism is mainly confined to frankfurters, sausages, bacon, ham, bologna, etc. Botulinum grows

Table 21-2: Some Microorganisms that Cause Food-Borne Illnesses

Microbe	Symptoms	Onset*	Common Source
Staphylococcus aureus	Vomiting, diarrhea, similar to stomach flu	2-6 hours	Food handler's skin cut or nasal fluid
Salmonella	Nausea, fever, vomiting, diarrhea	5 to 72 hours	Raw poultry and raw eggs
Shigella	Stomach pain/cramps, nausea, vomiting, diarrhea, fever, bloody stool	1 to 7 days	Infected food handler with poor hygiene (fecal contamination)
Clostridium botulinum	Trouble swallowing, double vision, progressing paralysis, medical emergency	12 to 36 hours	Improperly home-canned foods of low acidity
Listeria monocytogenes	Fever, vomiting, headache, can cause miscarriage	4 to 21 days	Soft cheeses, unpasteurized milk
Yersinia enterocolitica	Nausea, diarrhea, fever, flu-like	2 to 3 days	Unpasteurized milk, unchlorinated water
Trichinella spiralis	Fever, weakness, flu-like	Days to months	Inadequately cooked infected pork and wild game
Hepatitis A virus	Flu-like, jaundice, fatigue	2 to 7 weeks	Shellfish from contaminated waters, infected food handler

* Approximate time after eating that symptoms appear.

particularly well in processed meats. (The word *botulism* derives from *botulus,* meaning *sausage* in Latin.) Nitrite added to the processed meats inhibits the production of botulinum toxin, and also gives these meats their distinctive taste and pinkish color.

There has been some concern with this use of nitrite as a food additive. Nitrite can combine with other substances called amines (amines are natural components of food) to form *nitrosamines*, which are very potent *carcinogens* for animals. Nitrosamines in food haven't been proven to cause cancer in humans, but their effect on animals suggests that they might increase the human risk of cancer of the esophagus and stomach. Nitrosamine levels in nitrite-cured meats are low, but these meats are our main dietary source of nitrosamines.

Plant foods contain nitrates and nitrites—recall that these are plant nutrients taken from the soil.

Nitrite as a food additive presents an example of the complexity of risk assessment:

• Nitrite itself hasn't been shown to cause cancer in any animal. (If it had, it would be prohibited as a food additive under the Delaney Clause.)

• The remote risk of cancer from any nitrosamines

formed must be weighed against the immediate risk of botulism, particularly because processed meats often are eaten cold, or may not be thoroughly heated before eating.

• Nitrites and nitrates (which can be converted into nitrites) naturally occur in vegetables and saliva, in larger amounts (but in lower concentrations) than those in processed meat.

• The nitrosamine content of processed meat can be increased by cooking at a high temperature (e.g., frying bacon).

• Nitrosamines can be formed in the stomach from nitrites and amines in food.

Nitrosamines are found in cigarette smoke. Tobacco is a plant (and thus contains nitrates/nitrites). Burning the tobacco provides the high temperature that helps form nitrosamines.

The aim, then, is to minimize the formation of nitrosamines. Vitamin C ("ascorbate") is thus added to nitrite-containing meats, since vitamin C interferes with the chemical reaction that forms nitrosamines. The hazard of nitrite/nitrosamines from processed meats is considered to be very small, but it's prudent to limit the amount we eat —these meats are also high in fat and salt.

Infant Botulism

Infant botulism isn't really considered to be a food-borne illness—it isn't the toxin in food that causes the disease. Rather, the toxin is formed in the infant digestive tract from ingested botulinum. Ingesting the botulinum itself isn't normally harmful, but the infant stomach isn't as acid as the adult's, aiding botulinum growth and toxin production. Also, because the infant is small, a small amount of toxin can be a large dose.

Most cases of infant botulism are in infants 2 to 3 months old. The only food directly implicated has been *honey,* and it's advised that infants less than a year old not be fed honey. (The Center for Disease Control has found botulinum in about 10% of sampled honey.)[4]

Widening the Perspective in Food Safety

In this chapter and the last, a few categories of non-nutritive food substances have been discussed in relation to food safety. It should be clear by now that the categories aren't always clearly defined, and the hazard represented by any one substance can't be assessed in isolation.

The overlap of pesticides, food additives, and natural food substances has been emphasized, as has the importance of dosage. There are many more interactions to consider.

Nutritional status can make a difference in the effects of a toxicant—lead is more readily absorbed by (and thus more toxic for) those who are iron deficient. Also, using several methods of *preservation* allows the use of smaller amounts of preservatives—routine refrigeration of processed meats means less nitrite is needed.

As another example, increasing a plant's drought resistance can help reduce hazards for other foods. The damage to our corn crops wrought by the 1988 drought exposed the corn to greater infection by the molds which make *aflatoxin,* a potent carcinogen. The toxin appeared in milk when cows ate aflatoxin-contaminated corn, and dairies in many states had to dump milk. (Michigan, in 1989 had to dump about 400,000 pounds of milk due to high levels of aflatoxin.)

We apply rigid controls to food additives, sometimes forgetting that the chemical composition of food changes constantly. How else does cheese and fruit ripen and rot? Or beef age? Or cake ingredients combine to make a cake—that later turns stale? How else do we increase the iron content of spaghetti sauce by simmering it in an iron pot? Or form carcinogens by grilling meat? Or release, by cooking, poisonous hydrogen cyanide gas from lima beans? From the moment of food's first creation in plants from carbon dioxide and water to the moment our metabolism returns it to carbon dioxide and water, food's chemical composition is in constant flux.

Our food is rife with natural toxins. Yet these substances are considered safe when consumed in a normal varied diet by healthy people. One reason is that the toxicity of one substance can be offset by another substance in the food. For example, adequate dietary iodine can help prevent the goiter caused by the toxic effect of goitrogens.

Goitrogens, which in large amounts can cause goiter, are a natural component of such foods as cabbage and cassava.

A particularly important factor is that the toxicities of various food *toxicants aren't additive.* Eating small amounts of different toxicants together in the diet is much safer than eating one of them in a larger amount.[5] So the wider the *variety of foods* in our diet, the less the chance that any one chemical will be present at a hazardous level.

Today's varied diet also includes food grown in a variety of geographical locations, as noted at the start of this chapter. It wasn't that long ago that the distribution of goiter reflected the distribution of iodine in the soil, goiter being most common in areas of the U.S. where iodine was lacking. Advances in food processing and preservation removed goiter from our roster of common diseases—by the addition of iodine to salt during processing, and by the preservation that widened the distribution of produce and improved the odds of at least some food rich in iodine arriving at any given kitchen table.

Knowing that there are a lot of natural toxins in food doesn't mean that we should be unconcerned about what's added to food, either intentionally or unintentionally. Rather, we should widen our concern to include the natural toxicants in food and the contributions of the disease-producing microbes that get into our food. (Furthermore, we might weigh food hazards against other health hazards.)

In this way only, can we make reasonable assessments of benefits versus risks, and take best advantage of what advances food science has to offer. If a natural carcinogen is found in high concentration in a plant, we might want to genetically modify the plant's ability to make it—or alternatively, decide against eating the plant altogether. As another example, irradiating produce to kill microbes can lessen the need for post-harvest pesticides. We should balance one "worry" against another.

Worrying about food additives, pesticide residues, and such—whether or not a given worry is justified—is a measure of how fortunate we are in this country. For most of the world's people, the focus is on simply getting enough food to prevent starvation and malnutrition. If all that's available is aflatoxin-contaminated grain, eat it they must.

Summary

Food processing is part of the reason why there's such a large variety of foods to choose from in this country. Many foods are processed in order to make them available year round, to make them safe, and to make them convenient to store, use, and prepare. The food industry is mainly guided by the market, providing consumers with what they want. Many consumers, however, are concerned that processing and the use of additives make foods less healthful.

The loss of nutrients depends in large part on how quickly food moves from the farm to the final product. Commercial processing is often faster than our own procurement and preparation of "fresh" products, resulting in less nutrient loss. Many foods are also commercially fortified, which can provide important nutrients—sometimes just making up for nutrients lost in the processing, sometimes adding more than was there originally.

Processing also affects healthfulness when parts of foods are removed. Removing fat to make low-fat milk is seen as more healthful, and refining whole wheat to make white flour is seen as less healthful. But, generally speaking, foods closest to their original state ("least processed") tend to be the most healthful.

The names of additives are intimidating and seem "unwholesome" and "unnatural," but many of them are substances found naturally in food. They include substances taken from other foods, such as ascorbic acid, or pectins, or gums found in plants. But additives also include chemicals that aren't found naturally in foods, such as certain food colors or some preservatives used to keep microbes under control.

The Delaney Clause prohibits use of any food additive found to cause cancer in any amount in any animal. This Clause has generated a lot of controversy—even among scientists, e.g., arguments as to the validity of animal tests that use extremely large doses of additives, as applied to human usage of much smaller doses. Also, the Delaney Clause doesn't take into account the weighing of benefits against risk, nor does it apply to toxicants found naturally in food.

In reality, nothing is absolutely safe. There are simply degrees of risk, and assessment of that risk is at best a difficult approximation. It's also important to consider such things as, what's the risk relative to other risks, and do benefits outweigh the risk?

The experts put food-borne illnesses at the top of the list of food hazards. Each year, millions of Americans suffer from food-borne illness caused by microbes or their toxins in improperly handled food. Proper food preparation and refrigeration are important in preventing these illnesses. Microbes can be killed by heat or irradiation, and slowed by freezing, salting, pickling, etc.

Nitrite is added to processed meats to inhibit botulinum, but may be a remote cause of cancer, due to formation of nitrosamines in the stomach. This is an example of the need to balance the risk—a possible increase in risk of stomach cancer—against the benefit of preventing botulism.

Eating a variety of foods is a safeguard against ingesting large amounts of any particular toxin, man-made or natural.

Chapter 22

Food Labeling

When it comes to food advertising, many of us can be of two minds: We generally believe that sellers have the right to build up their products. On the other hand, food is important to health, and we don't like to be misled.

Oh, how easily we've been misled. We reached for salad oil labeled "Cholesterol Free!" even though it never contained cholesterol in the first place. And we thought "90% Fat-free!" meant a low-fat product. We've generally come to feel that more regulation has been needed, particularly as our society has come to rely more and more on processed foods.

The basic question of labeling is, what does the food contain? Just the facts, please. But given the facts and even drawing a line on huckstering, there's still the very challenging question of how to meaningfully inform consumers about the many individual nutrients provided by specific products—both those nutrients for which we are at risk for too little and those we are at risk for too much.

The Federal labeling laws have become increasingly complicated and sophisticated, and now require a substantial amount of well-defined information—for those who care enough to do a bit of homework.

Armed with the knowledge that there are nutrient requirements to fill and certain excesses to avoid, choosing healthy foods seems simple enough. But once we get into the grocery store, we're faced with a huge array of choices. The information sources that could help us choose—advertising and label information—can be more confusing than helpful. It isn't so easy to choose.

Labels and advertising purport to tell us whether we want something or not, whether the price is right, and whether or not we will really get what we're led to expect. We know that advertising has only one goal: to sell. We're told we can rely on labels for much of the information we need. But only if we know how to interpret what labels tell us.

Shoppers are forced to rely heavily on labels, if they are to make wise choices. To make intelligent nutrition decisions, we must know how to interpret them correctly—the focus of this chapter.

Supermarket Conflict

In some ways, the food supplier and the nutritionist are at odds. The former is, after all, a business that must make a profit. Nor is the grocer a neutral displayer of foods. Some foods are much more profitable for the grocer than others—generally those which have received the most processing and packaging. Those tend to be displayed in the inner aisles of grocery stores.

In contrast, nutritionists encourage us to do most of our shopping along the far sides and back wall of the grocery store, where fresh produce, bread, dairy, and meat sections are usually located. These sections generally hold the foods which are minimally processed and packaged—foods which tend to have a shorter shelf-life and a smaller profit for the grocer.

Often what beckons most at the supermarket tends to be the least nutritious, and the allocation of prime shelf space may be inversely related to nutritional value. One sees the likes of soft-drink 12-packs, not bags of fresh produce, stacked prominently at the front-of-the-aisle promotion sites.

The Food Label

The food label is the one theoretically objective source of product information in the grocery store. How well it serves this function has been a matter of differing opinion, but the potential is there, particularly as government regulations have required more and more useful information on food labels.

All food labels must identify the product, give the net weight of the food, the name and address of the manufacturer, packer, or distributor, and a listing of ingredients. Not much more than this was required until the 1973 law regarding nutrition information on food labels was implemented.

This law required that nutrition information be given on the label of foods to which nutrients had been added and/or about which nutrition claims were made, either on the label or in advertising. Nutrition information on the label of other foods was optional.

But in the years since 1973, scientific evidence of the relationship between diet and chronic disease has increased dramatically, and there's been increasing consumer interest in nutrition. As consumers have become more concerned about the healthfulness of their diets, food processors have responded by including nutrition labeling on more foods and, at the same time, making more nutrition claims—often misleading ones—on their labels.

As a practical matter, packages with less than 12 square inches for labeling aren't required to carry nutrition information. But the label must give a phone number or address for consumers to get the information.

Advertisers have found that nutrition claims make potent sales pitches. Sales of Kellogg's All-Bran cereal, for example, rose dramatically when the label began suggesting in 1984 that eating this cereal would help prevent colon cancer. Other claims, like "cholesterol-free" and "33% less fat" also proliferated—as did consumer confusion.

How certain is it that fiber protects against colon cancer? Does "cholesterol-free" salad oil mean that cholesterol was removed from this particular brand? Does "33% less fat" really designate a

Figure 22-1: The Food Label

Serving sizes are stated in both household and metric measures.

The general goal is to choose foods that add up to 100% of the DV for total carbohydrate, fiber, vitamins, and minerals, and add up to less than 100% of the DV for fat, saturated fat, cholesterol, and sodium.

Nutrition Facts

Serving Size 1 cup (228g)
Servings Per Container 2

Amount Per Serving	
Calories 250	Calories from Fat 110

	% Daily Value*
Total Fat 12g	18%
Saturated Fat 3g	15%
Trans Fat 1.5g	
Cholesterol 30mg	10%
Sodium 470mg	20%
Total Carbohydrate 31g	10%
Dietary Fiber 0g	0%
Sugars 5g	
Protein 5g	

Vitamin A	4%
Vitamin C	2%
Calcium	20%
Iron	4%

* Percent Daily Values are based on a 2,000 calorie diet. Your Daily Values may be higher or lower depending on your calorie needs:

	Calories:	2,000	2,500
Total Fat	Less than	65g	80g
Sat Fat	Less than	20g	25g
Cholesterol	Less than	300mg	300mg
Sodium	Less than	2,400mg	2,400mg
Total Carbohydrate		300g	375g
Dietary Fiber		25g	30g

% Daily Value (DV) shows how a food fits in your overall diet. Some DVs are upper levels (less than 20 g saturated fat); some are recommended amounts (calcium: 1000 mg).

20% calcium means that 1 serving gives you 20% (200 mg) of what you need to get this reommended amount (1000 mg).

Many women, teenage girls, and less-active men use about 2,000 calories/day.

Many men, teenage boys, and very active women use about 2,500 calories/day.

low-fat product? Many claims did more to mislead than to educate.

Partly for this reason, Congress passed the Nutrition Labeling and Education Act in 1990, mandating that nutrition labels educate about nutrition and health, and that only specified health claims, ones founded on well-established scientific evidence, be allowed.

Nutrition information is now required on most food labels (see Fig. 22-1), except for fresh produce, and fresh and frozen seafood, meat, and poultry. For these exempted foods, nutrition labeling is voluntary.

Some food products, e.g., food produced by small businesses, are exempt from the nutrition labeling requirement.

The regulations came about after much discussion about the best ways to present nutrition information on a label. They aimed to enlarge the amount of required information. But more than this, they also sought to require that this information be presented in a way that showed which

facts were the most important in making healthy choices.

Switching the Emphasis

As we have seen, our nutrition priorities have switched dramatically. It used to be that deficiency diseases were our biggest nutrition problems. And so it was that white flour was enriched, milk vitamin-D-fortified, and table salt iodized. When pellagra, rickets, and goiter were common, enriched flour, vitamin-D-fortified milk, and iodized salt were unquestionably the more healthful choices.

Today, our biggest nutrition problems are related to excess calories, fats, and sodium, and inadequate fiber, as has been discussed in early chapters. So nutrition information on food labels now emphasize these nutrients. The goal is to draw attention to the nutrients of greatest concern for today's consumer—so that a product low in saturated fat, for example, will come to have more "draw" for consumers than one heavily fortified with vitamins and minerals.

Serving Size—A Key to Practical Comparison

The number of servings in a package must be given on the label. Consumers need to know what is in a "typical" serving so they can compare nutrient values between brands. To serve their purpose, it's important that these "typical servings" be well-standardized and reasonable.

Labeling regulations require standard serving sizes for similar foods. For example, one tablespoon must be the serving size for both margarine and butter, so that their nutrition values can be easily compared. But if a package has less than two standard servings or is packaged to be consumed as an individual serving (e.g., snack-sized yogurt and instant ramen, ice cream bars, 12-oz. cans of soft drinks), the entire package must be listed as a serving. (Previously, the label on a 12-oz. can of soft drink or a 8.45-oz. box of juice would list one serving as 6 oz.)

Nutrient Content

Adding nutrition information to food labels would seem to be a simple matter. One had only to analyze the food and then set out the results on the package, in terms of so many grams, milligrams, or micrograms. Then consumers would know what's in the food. Or would they?

For most people, the simple statement that the product has 9 mg of a nutrient is meaningless. Is this a negligible amount or a lot? How were labelers to suggest the importance of a food as a nutrient source? We can't expect the shopper to carry an RDA table and a calculator for every purchase. To be useful, nutrition labeling must convey information simply.

Could the label simply show the nutrient content in terms of percentage of the RDAs? But there are 22 sets of RDAs for the U.S. population (based on age, gender, pregnancy, breastfeeding)—and very little space on the label. Imagine trying to show on a can of soup the percentage of need for more than 20 nutrients for as many population groups.

It was to meet this challenge that the Daily Values (DVs) were created back in 1973 (though they weren't called Daily Values back then). They were based on the 1968 edition of the RDAs, the current one at that time.

The Daily Values were generally established by taking, for each nutrient, the highest RDA for those over age 4 (excluding those for pregnant and nursing women). Thus, some Daily Values can be quite different than the RDAs for your group.

For example, the DV for iron is 18 mg. This is right-on if you're a 19-50 year-old female who isn't pregnant or nursing. But if you're a male over age 18 or a post-menopausal female, your iron RDA is only 8 mg—only 44% of that DV of 18 mg gives you that 8 mg (100% of your RDA).

The nutrient content of a particular food is given as a percentage of the Daily Value for that nutrient. A food that has 9 mg of iron, for example, is listed as having 50% of the Daily Value (i.e., 50% of 18 mg of iron), but if you're a man, this 50% DV is over 100% of your RDA of 8 mg.

The Daily Values were expanded to include reference values for dietary components for which there are no RDAs, e.g., total fat, saturated fat, cholesterol, fiber, and sodium. One intent was to give more emphasis to dietary components known to be related to risk of chronic disease (e.g., the increased risk for susceptible people of high blood pressure from a high-sodium diet). The dietary components for which information is given are listed in Table 22-1.

Again, the simple statement that a product has so many grams or milligrams of fat or sodium is meaningless to most people. So the amounts are also given as percentages of the recommended amount, based on a 2,000-calorie diet.

Women in this country need about 2,000 calories a day; children about 1,800, and men about 2,800.

The food label shown in Figure 22-1, for example, says that the food has 3 grams saturated fat and 15% Daily Value per serving (3 gm fat = 15% of the recommended 20-gram limit for a 2,000 calorie diet).

It's recommended that 10% or less of total calories come from saturated fat: 10% of 2,000 cal = 200 calories, which is equivalent to 22 gm saturated fat (600 cal/9 cal/gm = 22 gm), which has been rounded to 20 gm.

Table 22-1: Dietary Components Listed in the "Nutrition Facts Panel" of Food Labels

Required*	Optional**
Total calories	
Calories from fat	Calories from saturated fat
Total fat	
Saturated fat	Polyunsaturated fat
Trans fat	Monounsaturated fat
Cholesterol	
Sodium	Potassium
Total carbohydrate	
Dietary fiber	Soluble fiber
	Insoluble fiber
Sugars	Sugar alcohol (e.g., sorbitol)
Protein	
Vitamin A	
Vitamin C	
Calcium	
	Other vitamins and
Iron	minerals

* Exceptions allowed in certain circumstances, e.g., soft drink labels don't have to list cholesterol, fiber, etc.

** Exception: required if they've been added, or if label makes claims about them; e.g., zinc's %DV must be given if zinc has been added to the food.

Health Claims

Only certain nutrition-related health claims are allowed on food labels. For example, a claim can be made on a package of frozen vegetables that a diet low in fat and rich in fruits and vegetable may lower the risk of certain cancers. It's scientifically well-established that people who eat a low-fat diet rich in fruits and vegetables have a lower risk of cancer.

A Food and Drug Administration (FDA) website has a continually updated list of *Health Claims that Meet Significant Scientific Agreement* that can be made on labels of food and dietary supplements.[1]

There are strict guidelines for making these health claims. For example, the claim can only use *"may"* or *"might"* in discussing the relationships and must state that other factors play a role, e.g., *"While many factors affect heart disease, diets low in saturated fat and cholesterol may reduce the risk of this disease."*

Also, the health claim can't be made if the food contributes a significant amount of total fat, saturated fat, cholesterol, or sodium. (What constitutes a "significant amount" is clearly defined in the regulations.) For example, the health claim relating calcium to osteoporosis can't be made on an ice cream label. Ice cream is a source of calcium, but it's also high in total fat and saturated fat.

Descriptions like "low-fat" and "sugar-free" have often been used to imply that particular foods are healthier than competing products. So these descriptions have been standardized and given clear definitions (see Table 22-2), and can't be used in a misleading manner. For example, if the box of margarine says "cholesterol-free," it must also say that all margarine is cholesterol-free, e.g., "margarine, a cholesterol-free food."

As another example, a muffin might be high in both fiber and fat. If its label describes the muffin as high in fiber, it must also indicate that it's also high in fat. (It might add "see nutrition information about fat content.")

What Ingredient Lists Can Say About Nutrition

Among the oldest labeling rules are those which require that the ingredients of most foods be listed on the package, in decreasing order of their weight. From this, the consumer can make a number of deductions.

Looking at a package of frozen macaroni and cheese, the ingredients list begins with cooked macaroni, followed by water, followed by cheese. How much cheese can there be? Cheese is the high-priced ingredient in the product—Is the price of the product reasonable?

There are federal regulations about what processed foods can be called. For example, "Chicken and Gravy" must be at least 35% chicken, whereas "Gravy and Chicken" need be only 15% chicken.

In the same freezer case, we see a dish labeled as "gravy and sliced turkey." Water is listed as the first ingredient, turkey as the second. This means that less than half of the dish consists of turkey meat.

A combination of ingredient lists and nutrition labeling can help us to evaluate some other products. Consider fruit "drinks," which may contain as little as 10% fruit juice, but which may boast of high vitamin content. (Juice labels are required to list the percent of juice content). We can see a distorted nutrition profile, often with a lot of one vitamin, such as vitamin C, and little else. Compare these labels with those for real fruit juice, and you can see the difference.

Or take breakfast cereals with high percentages of Daily Values of "essential vitamins and minerals." The list of cereal ingredients, which may read like a pharmaceutical shopping list, can quickly tell us that we're being offered a kind of vitamin pill combined with some grain and sugar.

Foods fortified with 50% or more of the Daily Value for any nutrient must be called a diet supplement, e.g., Total™ breakfast cereal is labeled as a "multivitamin supplement cereal with iron and zinc."

One-hundred percent of some of the day's micronutrients may sound good, but we must remember what it actually is—a serving of "regular cereal" plus a pumped in vitamin pill. If that's what we want, okay—but we should understand that comparison shopping shows that the price of the heavily fortified cereal is more than the combined price of a less expensive cereal and a vitamin pill.

Slipping Sugar Down the List

Prior to the implementation of the 1990 labeling law, what was known as "sugar splitting" became a popular way for manufacturers to avoid the scrutiny of ingredient lists. In selecting cookies, for example, consumers often looked for those with lesser amounts of sugar. Even though the amounts of individual ingredients needn't be given, consumers could see whether sugar or flour was the first ingredient listed, and select the cookies which had flour listed first.

But consumers could still be kept in the dark when the manufacturer used more than one sugar (sugar, honey, corn syrup, etc.) to sweeten

the product. Even when sugar was the principal ingredient, it wouldn't appear first in the ingredient label, so long as no one sugar was the principal ingredient. Flour could be listed first and the sugars listed separately (e.g., sugar, high-fructose corn syrup), further down the list.

Sucrose is listed as sugar in an ingredient list; other sugars (e.g., high-fructose corn syrup, honey) are specified.

To thwart this sleight of hand, the regulations now require that the sugars ("sweeteners") be grouped together.

Enriched Flour

Enriched grain is common on ingredient lists for grain products. It refers specifically to the addition of iron and the B-vitamins thiamin, riboflavin, niacin, and folic acid to refined grains.

Pellagra (the niacin-deficiency disease) was common in the U.S. in 1942. The enrichment program increased niacin intake and lessened pellagra's prevalence and severity. The pellagra death rate was 1 in 100,000 in 1943, and fell to 1 in 500,000 by 1952.

In 1942, enrichment was made mandatory for white flour sold across state lines. At that time, the diets of many Americans were low in thiamin, riboflavin, niacin, and iron, largely because they preferred the refined to the whole grain products that would have provided more of the deficient nutrients.

White rice, corn flour and products made from them might or might not be enriched, depending mainly on state laws. California, for example, doesn't require enrichment of corn tortillas, glucose-coated white rice (the coating makes it look whiter), and oriental-style noodles. To see if a product is enriched, look for the term "enriched" on the label.

In 1998, folic acid was included in the B-vitamins added to refined grains. Folic acid deficiency in pregnant women can lead to birth defects in the spine ("neural tube defects"), and these defects have indeed fallen since 1998.[2] Canada has also had a fall in these birth defects since folic acid fortification.[3] Virtually all of the white flour found in our grocery stores is enriched, as is food made from enriched flour (e.g., bread, pastas, cereals).

What Do the Grades Given to Foods Mean?

Many people believe that grades like *Grade A* or *Choice* on a food label have nutritive significance. In general, this isn't true. Mainly, such ratings show esthetic (e.g., appearance, texture), not nutritive values. As such, the government gradings (given by government graders) are optional and paid for by the processor or packer. (In contrast, food inspection for safety and healthfulness is required, and paid for by the government.)

Sometimes packers and stores use labels with terms like *Super* or *Excellent*. Don't confuse these "grades" with official government grades.

Many of these grades are given under U.S. Dept. of Agriculture (USDA) standards, recognizable by the appearance of the grade designation in the shield of the USDA (see Fig. 22-2).

A USDA poultry "wing tag" shows three marks at once. First, it shows the age of the bird (a frying chicken is younger than a stewing chicken). Second (lower left), it shows the inspection mark for all poultry, fresh, frozen, canned or dried, indicating cleanliness and safety. Third (lower right), it shows the mark for quality, showing meatiness, for example.

The high-fat content of "Prime" beef, for example, is in large part responsible for its increased tenderness, juiciness, and flavorfulness, giving it its "Prime" grade. Each succeeding lower grade is generally lower in fat and price. People who need to restrict fat intake do well to buy the cheaper grades of beef.

The lower grades of beef are generally lower in fat, so it could be said that in this case, the grades have nutritional significance. But this isn't the intent. If it were, the lower fat meats would be given the higher grades, since these would be the healthier choice.

Practically speaking, we don't have much choice among grades of meat, so it's not some-

Figure 22-2: Government Grade Marks.

a) Fresh fruits/vegetables; packed under supervision of U.S. government grader; shows quality, but not nutritional, differences. (b) Fresh and cured meat; health inspection of food and packing plant. (c) Butter, cheddar cheese grading mark, (d) Meat quality stamps. (e) Food can't meet its standard; reason why; still good nutrition. (f) USDA grade for canned, frozen, dried fruits and vegetables; also for jam, jelly, honey, similar items. (g) Egg grading mark. (h) Canned, frozen, dried or packaged meat products passed sanitation inspection. (j) USDA poultry "wing tag" (see text).

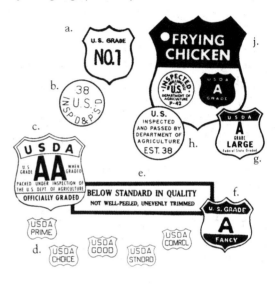

thing we really need to consider in our shopping. The top grade of meat is mostly sold to fancy restaurants; the next two grades are what we're most commonly offered at the meat counter. The lowest grades are commonly sold to food processors.

The grade mark appears in a purple USDA shield, stamped on the cut (usually a side) of meat delivered to the butcher. But we seldom see even a glimpse of the stamp, since most of the meat we buy has been subdivided by the butcher into steaks, chops, etc., and the edges trimmed of some of the fat.

Choosing Eggs By Size and Grade

The USDA sets three grades for eggs AA, A, and B. AA eggs look prettier. If you break one into a hot skillet, it will stay in a smaller space, instead of spreading out. Eggs graded A cover a moderate area when broken, and are fine for all purposes. B eggs aren't as attractive, spreading thinly over the pan, and so are commonly used when they're

Table 22-2: Some Labeling Terms, Definitions

Free (e.g., sugar-free, cholesterol-free): The amount of the substance in a serving is nutritionally and physiologically trivial. If *free* is used to describe a food normally free of the substance, the label must state this (e.g., "vegetable oil, a cholesterol-free food").

Fresh (e.g., fresh orange juice): Unprocessed, uncooked foods. (Approved treatments for fresh fruits and vegetables, such as washing or coating, are allowed.) Food can't have been previously frozen. But recently harvested foods that are quickly frozen can be described as fresh frozen or frozen fresh (e.g., fresh-frozen fish).

Freshly (e.g., freshly squeezed orange juice, freshly roasted peanuts): Recently prepared from fresh (i.e., can't have been previously frozen, or processed).

Good Source (e.g., good source of vitamin E): A serving has 10 to 19% of the Daily Value of a beneficial nutrient.

High (e.g., high-calcium): A serving has 20% or more of the Daily Value of a beneficial nutrient.

Less (e.g., less fat, less sodium): Has at least one-fourth less of this nutrient than the stated food to which it's compared (e.g., has less sodium than regular cheddar cheese).

Low (e.g., low-fat, low-sodium): Eating the food frequently won't increase the amount of this substance to more than the Daily Values specify. If *low* is used to describe a food normally low in the substance, the label must state this (e.g., milk, a low-sodium food). Maximum amounts per serving are specified (e.g., low-fat means 3 gm fat or less, low-sodium means less than 140 mg, low-calorie means 40 calories or less, etc.)

More (e.g., more vitamin C): A serving has at least 10% more of the Daily Value of a beneficial nutrient than the stated food to which it's compared (e.g., more vitamin C than orange juice).

to be beaten or mixed into a recipe. The nutritive values for all three grades of eggs are the same. (The nutritive value of brown-shelled eggs and white-shelled eggs are also the same.)

When egg prices are between one and two dollars per dozen, a general rule of thumb is: If the price difference is less than 20¢ per dozen between neighboring sizes in the same grade, you get more for your money by buying the bigger ones.

Egg sizes are based on minimum weight, and vary by a quarter-ounce per egg as follows: Jumbo (2.5 oz); Extra-large (2.25 oz); Large (2 oz); Medium (1.75 oz); and Small (1.5 oz).

Fruits and Vegetables

There are standards of quality for canned and frozen fruits and vegetables: *Grade A* or *Fancy, Grade B* or *Extra Standard,* and *Grade C* or *Standard.* But nutritive quality is again not the issue; the grading is for *esthetic quality.* Knowing this, there isn't much point in paying for perfect shape and appearance if you're going to puree the fruit or vegetable.

When grades appear on labels, many consumers are suspicious of anything that doesn't sound absolutely tops in quality, but such suspicion can cheat you of good buys in canned and frozen produce.

Fresh fruits and vegetables are easier for most people to judge, so there isn't as much grading. When government grades are given, they're put on the crates, so we don't usually see them (the top grades are *U.S. Fancy* or *U.S. No. 1*). But this doesn't matter much. We select fresh produce by price, sight, feel, and smell, and when the produce deteriorates, the store throws it out.

Changing Labels for Changing Times

What's in a Name?

There was once a time when unscrupulous food companies would add water to cheeses. Or they'd mix a bit of fruit with a lot of water and pectin and artificial color and flavor—and a bit of grass seed—and call it jam. So in the late 1930s, certain foods (e.g., ice cream, mayonnaise, jelly) were given *standards of identity,* which specified amounts of mandatory ingredients. Cheddar cheese, for example, could have no less than a certain amount of milk fat and no more than a certain moisture content. Add water beyond this limit, and you could no longer label it cheddar cheese.

In those days, a lot of people still made many of these foods at home. They were familiar with their recipes, and when they bought any of these foods ready made, they expected them to contain the ingredients they had used.

Beat up a bit of egg and vinegar with a lot of oil, and you have mayonnaise. Buy it in a store, and that's what you expected it to be. The content of these foods was so commonly agreed upon that their labels required an ingredient list only if optional ingredients were added.

Today, there aren't many people who make their own mayonnaise, ice cream, cheese, and such. In fact, many are quite surprised to learn that mayonnaise is mostly salad oil, and that cheese is so high in fat. Today's typical consumer needs an ingredient list on the labels of these "standard foods," and unlike before, the law requires it.

Recent times have also brought a consumer awareness that many of us are eating more fat and calories than is good for us. So food makers responded by giving us lower-fat and lower-calorie versions of ice cream, cheddar cheese, and the like. They provided healthier food options, but created marketing problems for themselves.

A low-fat cheddar cheese could no longer be labeled cheddar cheese, since it didn't conform to its standard of identity. It could be called "cheese food," "cheese substitute," "imitation cheddar cheese," etc., but it couldn't be called cheddar cheese. And these new descriptions weren't attractive to consumers.

Consumers were torn, particularly because so many have become enthusiastic about anything "natural," and repelled by "unnatural." What could sound more "unnatural" or "chemical" than an "imitation"? The consumer was lured by the lower-fat concept, yet repelled by the idea that these must not be "real foods."

Lower fat versions of familiar foods are the more healthful choices for most of us. In fact, now we want water added to cheeses, to replace some of the fat! Thus the regulations designed to prevent consumer deception in the 1940s became a problem of consumer perception in the 1980s.

As a result, the 1990 law did away with standards of identity, allowing low-fat versions of cheese, mayonnaise, ice cream, sour cream, and such, to be called "low-fat sour cream," "cholesterol-free mayonnaise," etc.

What About the Unprocessed Foods?

The irony of the major revamping of food-labeling regulations is that nutrition information isn't required on fresh vegetables and fruits—foods that are generally low in fat, saturated fat, and sodium, high in fiber, and devoid of cholesterol—the very foods that nutritionists encourage us to eat. And wasn't getting us to make more healthful choices an aim of the 1990 law?

Of course, it isn't that fresh fruits, vegetables, meat, poultry, and fish (and alcoholic beverages) were purposely overlooked in the labeling reform. Guidelines are given for voluntary labeling of these foods, and labeling may become mandatory. Mandatory or not, there are unique challenges.

For one, the labeling of most of these foods aren't under the jurisdiction of the Food and Drug Administration (as most other foods are). Fresh fruits and vegetables and fresh and frozen meat and poultry are regulated by the Dept. of Agriculture, fresh and frozen fish by the Dept. of the Interior, and alcoholic beverages (except for wine beverages with less than 7% alcohol) by the Bureau of Alcohol, Tobacco, and Firearms. This is but a minor hurdle. There have already been some coordinating efforts by these organizations to establish a system for consistent labeling.

The biggest hurdle is the most obvious one. How do you label a bunch of grapes? Do you change the label of a banana as the sugar content increases as it ripens? Is the 5-oz. steak one serving, and the 7-oz. steak in the package underneath also one serving (each is, after all, packaged as an individual serving)? If so, which do you use to compare the nutrient content of a serving of steak to a 6-oz. chicken leg? Should they be compared cooked or uncooked? If cooked, how cooked? Trimmed of fat or not?

Clearly, the likes of Oreo cookies are much easier to label—they're consistent in size, weight, and composition, and stay the same for a long time. The same is true of the many drinks that are essentially water, to which precise amounts of sugar, vitamins, flavor, and color have been added before bottling.

What about comparative shopping? We already know "you can't compare apples and oranges." But we can't conveniently compare fresh apples with canned apples either. In comparing sour creams, the various brands of regular sour cream are there next to the low-fat and fat-free versions.

We can compare prices and nutrient content, and even factor in our taste or distaste for various versions. In comparing peaches, those canned in syrup are shelved next to those canned in juice—but a long way from the fresh peaches. Some stores do provide nutrition information for these foods on leaflets and the like—portable information that facilitates comparative shopping.

Organic Foods

Labeling a food as *Organic* has marketing value, and so it was that many foods were labeled *Organic* without a uniform definition of what that meant. This led to a push for national standards, enacted in 2002 as the National Organic Program of the U.S. Dept. of Agriculture (USDA).

Certain claims (or similar ones) can now be used on packaged products and are precisely defined:[4]

100% Organic: contains only organically produced ingredients, not counting added water and salt.

Organic: contains at least 95% organically produced ingredients by weight, not counting added water and salt; remaining ingredients are ones not commercially available as organic and/or other allowed substances. Cannot contain sulfites.

Made with organic ingredients: contains at least 70% organic ingredients, not counting added water or salt; remaining ingredients are ones not commercially available as organic and/or other allowed substances. Cannot contain sulfites, except sulfur dioxide in wine, as specified.

Has some organic ingredients: contains less than 70% organic ingredients, not counting added water or salt; remaining ingredients are ones not commercially available as organic and/or other allowed substances.

Products that are 95-100% organic can display the *USDA Organic* seal. Organic farms must comply with USDA standards, as must organic meat, poultry, eggs, and dairy products.

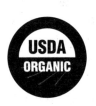

Eating Out

The labeling regulations don't apply to restaurant food, but there's more nutrition information here, too. As part of the trend towards less cooking "from scratch," we not only buy more processed foods, but also eat out more often.

Many fast-food chains offer nutrition information on their products on-site and/or on their websites, and an increasing number of restaurants provide some general nutritional guidelines, such as putting a heart symbol ("heart healthy") next to low-fat, low-salt items on their menus. (But there aren't yet standard definitions for these symbols and terms.)

Realities of Nutrition Labeling

When labeling was voluntary for a food product, nutrition information wasn't expected, unless it helped sell the product. Thus voluntary labeling appeared most often on such "nutritious" foods as bread and canned fruits and vegetables.

But there were some surprises—surprises to nutritionists, anyway. Nutrition labeling started appearing voluntarily on such foods as potato chips and cookies. Fig Newtons, one can understand, but Oreos?

The food makers realized that nutrition labeling might not affect the popularity of Oreos. One's mind is usually made up before the package is taken from the market shelf. Oreo buyers probably don't read labels carefully. Even if they ordinarily do and are generally concerned about nutrition, one expects that if they want their Oreo fix, they wouldn't look in this instance. The nutrition information might spoil their pleasure.

Ultimately, Wise Food Selection Is a Personal Matter

Ah, pleasure! Let's not forget that a healthful diet doesn't mean giving up favorite, not-so-nutritious foods. Individual foods aren't good or bad. As with individual nutrients, it's the amount that matters most.

Nutrient labeling of foods focuses on the nutritional merits and demerits of individual foods. So it's perhaps ironic that we should circle around to say that individual foods aren't necessarily good or bad. It's one's overall diet that counts.

For all that's been said about nutrition labeling, and all the healthier choices nutritionists hope consumers will make because of them, we know all too well that consumers first need to be motivated to make the changes.

What good is nutrition information on a label if it isn't read? Moreover, the information is only useful in the hands of a nutritionally literate consumer. Only if there's some real understanding of the roles of the various nutrients will nutrient content be meaningful.

As consumers become more knowledgeable about food and nutrition, there's less of a need to read labels. One develops a comfortable familiarity with foods, and is able to choose wisely without having to rely much on labels. Also, the most nutrition-conscious are those who tend to eat fewer processed foods and more fresh foods—foods without much labeling.

The hope is that those who have read this book are now more knowledgeable about food and nutrition, and will increasingly find pleasure in diets they know to be healthy. As we're freed from the spell of food rumor and fantasy, we can confidently choose from the wonderful variety of foods—fresh and processed—available in the marketplace.

Summary

Food labels can help informed consumers make wise nutrition choices. Until 1973, little more than the product name, weight, manufacturer, and list of ingredients were required on the labels. A 1973 law required nutrition information if nutrients had been added or where claims had been made about the food's nutritive value. But the nutrition information and claims were often confusing and misleading, and many foods didn't carry any nutrition information at all.

The 1990 Nutrition Labeling and Education Act was enacted to require nutrition information on almost all food labels, and to make the information more consistent and relevant to current nutritional concerns. For example, calorie and fat content heads the list of Nutrition Facts on the label. Whereas nutritional deficiencies used to be our biggest dietary problem, our main concern now is with excesses (e.g., excess calories, fat, sodium) and too little fiber.

The nutrients are expressed on the label as *% Daily Value*, and reference values for total fat, saturated fat, cholesterol, fiber, and sodium are included. The Daily Values for vitamins and minerals are based on the 1968 edition of the RDAs, set at the highest recommended amount for those over age 4 and not pregnant or nursing, For dietary components like saturated fat (*get less than 10% of calories from saturated fat*), the Daily Values are based on a 2,000 calorie diet.

Among the other food-label changes, standard serving sizes have been established (nutrition information is given per serving), terms such as *low-fat* are precisely defined, and only certain health claims are permitted. As before, ingredients must be listed in decreasing order of weight.

Nutrition labeling is voluntary for many raw foods, such as fresh fruits, vegetables, meat, poultry, and fish. Labeling may soon be required on these foods as well.

"Enriched" refers to the addition of iron and the B-vitamins thiamin, riboflavin, niacin, and folic acid to refined grain. Virtually all of our white flour is enriched, as would be the pasta, cereal, etc., made from enriched flour. Enrichment is indicated in the ingredient list (e.g., *enriched flour*).

Grading of food by the U.S. Dept. of Agriculture refers to the esthetic appearance and texture of food, not the nutritive value. A lower grade of meat, for example, may not be as tender but may be "healthier," because of a lower fat content.

Similarly, canned peaches that are less firm and are unevenly cut can be just as nutritious as those of a higher grade.

Consumers knowledgeable in nutrition can use the nutrition information on food labels to choose a healthful diet. As informed consumers, we know that we don't have to exclude foods high in fat, salt, sugar, etc. Rather, we know that food labels help us identify these foods more easily, so that we can eat them in smaller amounts or not as often. The food labels help us select a diet that's both healthy and pleasurable.

Guest Lecturer: *Judy Fitzgibbons, MS, RD, LD*

Nutrition Label Zone: Thinking Required

Nutrition labels give us the facts about the foods, but we still must make the buy or not-buy decision, based on the information provided and our knowledge of our nutritional needs and goals. Here are three ways you can use your nutrition knowledge to be a wise consumer:

1. Develop your sense of the nutritional value of basic, minimally processed foods
2. Beware of decision-making based on single nutrients
3. Control the "problem potential" of "fun foods"

Learning About the Nutrients in Foods

Knowing the nutrients we should expect in foods guides us over the first decision hurdle of whether a food will help meet our basic nutrient needs or whether to relegate it to the "fun food" category that adds mostly calories.

For example, snack crackers are basically flour and shortening or oil. "Multi-grain" or "wheat" crackers in yellow or brown packaging give the impression they're made from whole grain flour and so should be a good snack choice. By checking the ingredient list and reading the nutrient content on the label, we can tell whether or not they are the nutritious snack we expect.

A slice of whole wheat bread, containing a little more than 2 grams of fiber, as well as B-vitamins and iron, gives us a reference point. We should expect about the same from an ounce or so of whole grain crackers. If the ingredient label shows that whole wheat (or other whole grain flour) is in the top two ingredients and the nutrition facts label shows the nutrients we expect, the crackers offer a healthy choice. On the other hand, if the fiber content looks acceptable, but there is no whole grain flour listed (or it falls low on the list), we will probably find a refined fiber, such as oat fiber, listed. This increases the fiber content, but doesn't bring along with it the other nutrients we expect from whole grains. High fiber in foods does not guarantee whole grain.

Learning what to expect from basic foods improves our ability to make smart food choices.

Beware of Single-Nutrient Decision-Making

Table A shows the top 10 pieces of information consumers said they look for on nutrition facts labels, according to a 2007 survey conducted by the Food Marketing Institute. Fat, cholesterol, sugar, and sodium have been in the top ten for the past 20 years, and the percentage of consumers indicating their concern for them continues to grow. More recently, whole grains and trans fat became top-of-mind for consumers.

Various foods and nutrients go in and out of favor, running the gamut from "miracle cures" to "evil curses." In the late 1980's, oat bran was the miracle cure, and fat became the evil curse. In the mid-2000's, the antioxidant-rich value of blueberries and pomegranates (along with major marketing efforts) catapulted these fruits and their products into shoppers' carts for their purported potential to prevent heart disease, cancer and diabetes. Trans fat, the by-product of the hydrogenation of vegetable oils, became the "evil curse".

Table A. Top 10 Items Food Shoppers Check on Nutrition Facts Labels

Food Label Item	% of Food Shoppers
Total Fat	57
Saturated Fat	57
Trans Fat	55
Whole Grain	47
Cholesterol	45
Salt/Sodium	45
Calories	45
Chemical Additives	43
Sugar	42
Fiber	40

—from Food Marketing Institute, U.S. Grocery Shopper Trends, 2007

Table B. Estimating Fat and Sugar Budgets

To calculate the maximum fat and sugar recommendations in grams, first decide what would be a "healthy" weight for you. To estimate your grams of sugar limit, divide your weight by 3. To estimate your grams of fat limit, divide your healthy weight by 2. If you lead a sedentary life, subtract 10 grams from the fat total.

For example:

$\frac{150 \text{ lbs}}{3}$ = 50 grams of sugar per day (approximately 10% of calories)

$\frac{150 \text{ lbs}}{2}$ = 75 grams of fat per day (approximately 30% of calories)

If sedentary, 75 grams - 10 = 65 grams fat per day

(Although the underlying facts are valid,) the problem with the cure-or-curse mind-set is that we can become so focused on obtaining or avoiding a certain nutrient that we lose perspective.

For example, you can now find hundreds of foods made with pomegranate and blueberry. Juices containing them line the grocery shelves. Yogurts are flavored with pomegranate juice and cereals contain dried blueberries. If you decide to substitute pomegranate juice for a daily serving of orange juice, you've just dropped an important source of vitamin C and folic acid from your diet. Pomegranate juice contains neither in significant amounts.

How about avoiding trans fat, a new trend? There are plenty of margarines, cookies and crackers with "trans-fat-free" labels. However, in order to maintain expected texture and shelf life, some manufacturers have gone back to using palm oil, increasing the saturated fat value of the food. (Palm oil had its turn as an "evil curse" at one time.) Paying attention to BOTH trans fat and saturated fat needs to guide choices for people concerned about heart disease.

Balancing our choices over several meals, even over several days, protects us from the single-nutrient focus. Blueberries are a great fruit, but so are oranges, kiwi fruit, and bananas. Trans fat is a problem, but we can handle a little of it in a commercial oatmeal cookie when we choose to use an olive oil-based dressing on a salad.

Dealing with "Fun Foods"

The preparation and eating of a good diet can and ought to be fun and pleasurable. The trick is to control what I like to call the "problem potential" of foods such as candy, pastries, soft drinks—"fun foods."

Fat and sugar are the chief contributors to the "problem potential." Both can either add excessive calories or fill us up so we don't feel like eating foods that make important nutrient contributions. And, of course, there are the concerns about excess fat contributing to the development of obesity, cardiovascular disease, and cancer.

Current recommendations call for fat to contribute no more than 30% of our total calories and for using sugar only in moderation. Many dietitians recommend that added sugar contribute no more than 10% of total calories. For the typical adult, this translates to 50 to 70 grams of fat per day and 40 to 60 grams of added sugar (see Table B for how to estimate your personal fat/sugar limits).

Once you have a perspective on your fat and sugar "budgets," you're equipped for comparison-shopping. Knowing these numbers allows you to decide whether the Hershey's Milk Chocolate bar staring you down in the grocery checkout line is really "worth" the 13 grams of fat and 22 grams of sugar it will take out of your fat and sugar budgets.

Another factor in controlling the "problem potential" is to consider how much of a food you will eat over a period of time. The special sale on the 13-ounce bag of Doritos from the end-of-aisle display brings 104 grams of fat into your household (grams of fat or sugar/serving x servings per container). If your daily fat budget is 60 for the day and you single-handedly eat the whole bag in a couple of days, its "problem potential" is high. If, on the other hand, you stretch the chips out over several days or share them with others, their "problem potential" is greatly reduced.

There are many issues relating to nutrition labeling. But the concepts of evaluating nutrient value, avoiding single nutrient decision-making, and assessing "problem potential" will provide good starting places for nutritionally sound shopping.

Judy Fitzgibbons is a Registered Dietitian who has worked in the field of nutrition for 30 years, 10 of them writing the syndicated column *On the Label*. She is now an in-store dietitian for Hy-Vee, Inc., an Iowa-based regional supermarket chain, helping customers find foods that fit their individual nutrition concerns through supermarket tours, nutrition workshops, and personal nutrition coaching.

Appendix A: Adult Recommended Intakes, Daily Values, Upper Levels
Recommended Intake/day

	Women (age) 19-50	Women (age) 51+	Men (age) 19-50	Men (age) 51+	Daily Value	Upper Level[a]
Biotin (mcg)	30	30	30	30	300	b
Choline (mg)	425	425	550	550	-	3500
Folate (mcg)	400h	400	400	400	400	1000
Niacin (mg)	14	14	16	16	20	35
Pantothenic acid (mg)	5	5	5	5	10	b
Riboflavin (mg)	1.1	1.1	1.3	1.3	1.7	b
Thiamin (mg)	1.1	1.1	1.2	1.2	1.5	b
Vitamin A (mcg)[c]	700	700	900	900	1000	3000
Vitamin B-6 (mg)	1.3	1.5	1.3	1.7	2	100
Vitamin B-12 (mg)	2.4	2.4[n]	2.4	2.4[n]	6	b
Vitamin C (mg)	75[f]	75[f]	75[f]	90[f]	60	2000
Vitamin D (mcg)[d]	5	10/15[e]	5	10/15[e]	10	50
Vitamin E (mg)[g]	15	15	15	15	22	1000
Vitamin K (mcg)	90	90	120	120	-	b
Calcium (mg)	1000	1200	1000	1200	1000	2500
Fluoride (mg)	3	3	4	4	-	10
Iodine (mcg)	150	150	150	150	150	1100
Iron (mg)	18	8	8	8	18	45
Magnesium (mg)	310/320[k]	320	400/420[k]	420	400	350[m]
Phosphorus (mg)	700	700	700	700	1000	4000/3000[e]
Selenium (mcg)	55	55	55	55	-	400
Zinc (mg)	8	8	11	11	15	40

a Tolerable Upper Intake Level: the maximum intake at which an adverse effect is unlikely

b Not determinable due to lack of data; caution advised as to excessive intake

c 1 mcg vitamin A (retinol) = 1 Retinol Equivalents (RE) = 5 International Units (IU)

d 1 mcg vitamin D (cholecalciferol) = 40 International units (IU). Can get vitamin D via sun exposure

e 2nd value is for ages 71+

f Recommended amount for smokers is 35 mg more vitamin C

g 22 mg vitamin E = 30 International Units (IU)

h Women capable of pregnancy advised to get 400 mcg from supplements or fortified food

k 2nd value is for ages 31-50

m Applies to magnesium from pharmaceutical agents only

n 10-30% of elderly may malabsorb B-12; age 51+ advised to get B-12 from fortified food or supplements

Appendix A: Recommended Intake/day

Age	Infants (months)		Children (years)			Male	Female	Pregnant	Nursing
	0-6	7-12	1-3	4-8	9-13	14-18	14-18	19-30*	19-30*
Biotin (mcg)	5	6	8	12	20	25	25	30	35
Choline (mg)	125	150	200	250	375	550	400	450	550
Folate (mcg)	65	80	150	200	300	400	400	600	500
Niacin (mg)	2	4	6	8	12	16	14	18	17
Pantothenic acid (mg)	1.7	1.8	2	3	4	5	5	6	7
Riboflavin (mg)	0.3	0.4	0.5	0.6	0.9	1.3	1.0	1.4	1.6
Thiamin (mg)	0.2	0.3	0.5	0.6	0.9	1.2	1.0	1.4	1.4
Vitamin A (mcg)	400	500	300	400	600	900	700	770*	1300*
Vitamin B-6 (mg)	0.1	0.3	0.5	0.6	1.0	1.3	1.2	1.9	2.0
Vitamin B-12 (mg)	0.4	0.5	0.9	1.2	1.8	2.4	2.4	2.6	2.8
Vitamin C (mg)	40	50	15	25	45	75	65	85*	120*
Vitamin D (mcg)	5	5	5	5	5	5	5	5	5
Vitamin E (mg)	4	5	6	7	11	15	15	15	19
Vitamin K (mcg)	2.0	2.5	30	55	60	75	75	90*	90*
Calcium (mg)	210	270	500	800	1300	1300	1300	1000*	1000*
Fluoride (mg)	0.01	0.5	0.7	1	2	3	3	3	3
Iodine (mcg)	110	130	90	90	120	150	150	220	290
Iron (mg)	0.27	11	7	10	8	11	15	27	9
Magnesium (mg)	30	75	80	130	240	410	360	350*	310*
Phosphorus (mg)	100	275	460	500	1250	1250	1250	700*	700*
Selenium (mcg)	15	20	20	30	40	55	55	60	70
Zinc (mg)	2	3	3	5	8	11	9	11*	12*

*Recommendations vary for some nutrients for younger (<19 years) or older (>30 years) pregnant or nursing women: Pregnant age <19: vit A 750, vit C 80, vit K 75, calcium 1300, magnesium 400, phosphorus 1250, zinc 12. Pregnant age >30: magnesium 360. Nursing age <19: vit A 1200, vit C 115, vit K 75, calcium 1300, iron 10, magnesium 360, phosphorus 1250, zinc 13. Nursing age >30: magnesium 320.

Appendix B: Study Questions

Chap. 1. Nutrition Myths and Tests of Reality

1. Why was the 18th century revelation that "life is a chemical function," such a milestone in nutrition science?

2. John tells Laurie that without a vitamin pill with his breakfast coffee, he lacks energy the whole day. Laurie looks doubtful. What might she be doubtful about, and how could she go about testing whether the vitamin pill has the effect John says it has?

3. What are some reasons for the persistence of some myths about diet and health?

Part 1: Energy and the Human Machine

Chap. 2. Food Power—Use and Storage

1. Thinness is a part of our cultural concept of womanly beauty. Yet, in many cultures throughout history and in some cultures today, obese women are the beautiful ones. What are some explanations?

2. Where in our bodies do we store most of our fat? Besides fuel storage, what other purposes are served by these fat deposits?

3. When a slice of bread is said to contain 70 calories, what does this mean, and how is calorie content measured?

4. Vince would like to know exactly how many calories he uses when working out for a half hour. A scientist will use one of two methods to make this measurement. Describe the two methods.

5. Jay and Juan are the same in age and weight. Yet, Jay has a higher basal (minimum) energy requirement. What are some likely explanations?

Chap. 3. Putting the Laws of Energy to Work

1. What are some ways of measuring body fatness? Discuss the accuracy of these methods.

2. We eat for many reasons besides satisfying physical hunger. Discuss some of these.

3. Explain why so many weight-loss diets are successful only in the short term. What are the components of a sensible diet program for long-term weight control?

4. Marie has been off and on "'crash" diets since she was 20 years old. She would usually go off these diets by bingeing. She now finds, 25 years later, that she is having a harder and harder time losing weight. Explain the probable reasons for this.

5. Many of us are having trouble keeping off the extra pounds and would like to increase our basal metabolism so that we could eat more without having to exercise more. What are some ways in which we could increase our basal metabolism?

Part 2: Carbohydrates and the Foundations of Food

Chap. 4. The Trapping of the Sun

1. What is the connection between photosynthesis and metabolism? How does this explain the statement that the energy our body uses comes ultimately from the sun?

2. Which single sugars make up the common double sugars sucrose, lactose, and maltose? Which double sugar is common table sugar?

3. In what form do we store carbohydrate in our liver and muscles? What aspect of its structure is very important to its function as a storage form of carbohydrate?

4. Why does a banana get sweeter as it ripens?

5. Food companies use a lot of high-fructose corn syrup in food products. Why might they prefer to use this rather than regular table sugar? How is high-fructose corn syrup made?

6. NutraSweet is not a sugar (it is made of two amino acids linked together). Why is it sweet?

Chap. 5. Of Carbohydrates and Health

1. How might fiber help prevent diverticulosis, constipation, colon cancer?

2. What is the role of sugar in tooth decay?

3. What are the two types of diabetes? Which is related to obesity?

4. It is popularly believed that sugar causes hyperactivity. Carefully controlled studies, however, suggest that sugar has a calming effect. Explain this effect in terms of the amino acid tryptophan and the neurotransmitter serotonin.

Part 3: Proteins—The Masters of Life

Chap. 6. The Protein Confusion

1. What is meant by "essential" and "non-essential" amino acids?

2. Only 20 different amino acids are used to make a seemingly endless variety of proteins. How can this be?

3. What does it mean to denature a protein? Does this change its nutritional value?

4. Maria takes an amino acid supplement that contains 22 amino acids. Kay boasts that her supplement is superior because it contains 25. Maria asks you if Kay is right. What would you say?

5. Explain why eating two sources of plant proteins together can improve the quality of protein.

6. In developing countries, protein deficiency is more common in young children than in adults, even when both eat the same diet. Why is this?

Chap. 7. *Putting Amino Acids to Work*

1. List the steps of protein synthesis, beginning with DNA.

2. Sue eats a "typical American diet," and is thinking of switching to a strictly vegetarian diet. What are the nutritional advantages and disadvantages of this switch?

3. Joe's diet contains about four times the amount of protein he needs. In addition, he takes amino acid supplements. He complains of excessive urination and thirst. What is a possible explanation?

4. Why is the promotion of breast-feeding particularly important in developing countries?

5. If the typical American diet (diet A) could be "mixed with" a diet typical of a developing country (diet B) to form a composite diet (diet C), diet C would be a healthier diet for both countries. Do you agree with this statement? Why or why not?

Part 4: Fats—The Mysteries and Simplicities

Chap. 8. *Fats Seen and Unseen*

1. Explain why an ounce of salad oil has almost 10 times more calories than an ounce of cooked brown rice.

2. How is margarine made?

3. Tom learned that cholesterol is necessary to make some hormones and cell membranes. As a strict vegetarian, he is concerned that he is not getting enough cholesterol in his diet. Does his diet provide much cholesterol? Should he be concerned?

4. Marie thinks that fat is really bad, and has decided to cut fat out of her diet. Explain how this might be good and/or bad for her.

5. What is a partially hydrogenated oil? Why do packaged cookies, for example, commonly contain such an oil?

6. What is meant by the statement that lecithin is essential in the body but not in the diet?

7. An advertisement heralds corn oil as "Cholesterol-free!" Why is this misleading?

8. How do saturated fatty acids differ chemically from unsaturated fatty acids? Which kind is found mostly in animal fats? In plant oils? 'What are some exceptions?

Chap. 9. *Fat and the Doctor's Dilemma*

1. What is atherosclerosis; why can it cause more than one disease?

2. What changes in our diet and lifestyle can we make to lower our risk of atherosclerosis? Explain how these changes lower risk.

3. What's the difference between LDL-cholesterol and HDL-cholesterol?

4. Although extraordinarily high amounts of nicotinic acid (a B-vitamin) can lower LDL-cholesterol, why is it unwise to take such high doses on one's own?

5. Al had a heart attack at age 55 even though he ate a low-fat diet his entire life. List possible risk factors that could have contributed to his heart attack.

6. The rate of cancer is increasing in the United States. It is popularly believed that this is due to more cancer-causing substances in our food and environment. What are other reasonable explanations for this increase in cancer?

7. Explain why lowering the amount of fat in the diet may lower risk of both heart disease and cancer.

8. The label states that 1 serving of mixed nuts (1 oz.) has 180 calories and 16 gm fat. What % of the calories come from fat?

Part 5: Fueling the Body

Chap. 10. *The Digestive System*

1. Why is the top part of the small intestine (the duodenum) a susceptible site for developing an ulcer?

2. What is the cause of lactose intolerance and its symptoms? In which ethnic groups is this condition more common?

3. In what form are carbohydrates, protein, and fat absorbed from the digestive tract?

4. What is the function of bile in digestion? Where is it made, and where is it stored?

5. What is "heartburn"? How might it be prevented?

Chap. 11. *Metabolism and the Vitamin Key*

1. Why are low-carbohydrate diets popular?

2. What is the difference between aerobic and anaerobic metabolism? Which is used predominantly in which type of exercise? Explain why.

3. What role do B-vitamins have in metabolism?
4. Why is it that glucose can be made into fat, but fat cannot be made into glucose?
5. A crocodile spends most of its time being very still. Small animals (and children) become meals when they come to the water edge and don't see the hungry crocodile with its eyes barely above the water line. When the crocodile makes its move, it moves extremely fast. It can't run fast for long, but can probably outrun you for the first 20 yards. Ordering a crocodile burger in Australia, would you expect the meat to be dark meat or white meat?

Chap. 12. Water—The Body's Inner Sea

1. On a summer day, why do we feel hotter when the air is more humid?
2. How does body water content change with age?
3. A weight loss of 5 pounds during an endurance event represents about how many pints of water loss?
4. Discuss several major functions of body water.

Part 6: Micronutrients

Chap. 13. Some Practical Realities of Vitamins

1. What is meant by the statement that vitamins in massive doses function as drugs rather than vitamins?
2. Although Bill eats a good diet and is generally in very good health, he takes large doses of vitamin C because his gums have a tendency to bleed. Why is it doubtful that his gums bleed because of a vitamin C deficiency?
3. Why is it preferable to get vitamins from food, rather than dietary supplements?
4. Do you think dietary supplements should continue to be classified as "food," or should they be classified as drugs?

Chap. 14. Water-Soluble Vitamins

1. What are some general characteristics of water-soluble vitamins?
2. Why would including citrus fruits in a meal increase iron absorption?
3. Why do deficiencies of several of the B-vitamins cause similar symptoms?
4. A deficiency of either of two B-vitamins can cause anemia. What are these two B-vitamins? Describe the most common circumstances in which each deficiency occurs.

5. Why is it that a diet low in niacin and rich in animal protein does not cause a niacin deficiency?

Chap. 15. Fat-Soluble Vitamins

1. What are some general characteristics of fat-soluble vitamins?
2. Food composition tables show carrots to contain large amounts of vitamin A. Why, then, don't we get vitamin A toxicity from eating a lot of carrots?
3. Why are vitamin D and calcium deficiencies intertwined?
4. Why is vitamin K deficiency uncommon, even among those who have low levels of vitamin K in their diet?
5. Why are drugs that interfere with vitamin K activity used to treat someone with a previous heart attack?

Chap. 16. The Major Minerals

1. Sara is 13 years old and has a grandmother with osteoporosis. Sara wants to know if there is anything she can do now to lower her own risk of osteoporosis. What recommendations might you give her? Explain.
2. Why can't we assess a dietary deficiency of calcium by measuring the amount of calcium in the blood?
3. Milk is the main source of calcium in the typical American diet. What are some other good sources of calcium?
4. Our typical diet is quite salty. Why is this a health concern?
5. Which foods are rich in potassium?

Chap. 17. The Trace Minerals

1. How do heme iron and non-heme iron differ in terms of their distribution in foods and their absorption from the digestive tract?
2. Why is it that iron deficiency is uncommon among adult men?
3. Why does iron deficiency cause anemia?
4. Why is it that iron deficiency and lead toxicity often go hand in hand, particularly among U.S. children living in poverty?
5. Why is iron overload more common among men than women?
6. Why does an iodine deficiency cause an enlarged thyroid gland?
7. Milk is not naturally rich in iodine, yet milk as purchased in the grocery store can be. Why is this?
8. How does fluoride help prevent tooth decay?

Part 7: Balance—Science and the Art of Eating

Chap. 18. Between Food and Health

1. What are the RDAs? What was their original purpose, and how are they used today?
2. What are the food groups of the Food Guide Pyramid? How many daily servings from each group are recommended for you?
3. What are dietary guidelines relating to chronic diseases? For each, which disease(s) might be affected, and how might following the guideline help in prevention?
4. One dietary guideline is: If you drink alcoholic beverages, do so in moderation. What is a moderate amount?
5. What are some changes you can make to improve your own diet, considering your own likes and dislikes, lifestyle, etc.?

Chap. 19. Nutrition arid the Life Cycle

1. What effects can alcohol have on the developing fetus?
2. What are some advantages of breast-feeding, as compared to infant formula?
3. Explain why encouraging the use of infant formulas in developing countries can seriously downgrade infant health.
4. Why is it that a low-fat, low-cholesterol, high-fiber diet is not recommended for children under age 2?
5. Why is it that children can generally get away with eating more "junk food" than their mothers?
6. What general changes in nutrient requirements occur from birth to old age?
7. Continual dieting and obsession with thinness are most common in young, upper middle class white women. In raising a daughter, what might you do to avoid this? Anorexia nervosa and bulimia are also common among these women. Describe these disorders.

Part 8: From Farm to Table

Chap. 20. Agriculture—Realities of Leaf and Soil

1. Are crops grown on "depleted soil" nutritionally inferior? Why or why not?
2. Why is it that for some minerals, plant content varies according to local soil content?
3. What are some alternatives to pesticide use in controlling crop pests and disease?
4. How is biotechnology used in agriculture, and what is its advantage over traditional plant crossbreeding?

Chap. 21. Food Processing and Food Safety

1. What is meant by: "The dose determines the poison"?
2. What are some functions of food additives?
3. What are some general rules for preventing or avoiding microbial hazards in foods?
4. Why is nitrite added to foods such as frankfurters, bacon, and ham? What are nitrosamines, and why are they of concern? How can we lessen the formation of nitrite into nitrosamines?
5. A basic tenet of good nutrition is to eat a varied diet. Why does a varied diet also tend to be a less hazardous diet?
6. How does the public perception of food hazards differ from that of the experts?

Chap. 22. Food Labeling

1. What are Daily Values? Why is fiber, for example, given as a % of Daily Value, instead of only in gram amounts?
2. What nutrients have been added to enriched flour?
3. Prior to the implementation of the 1990 food-labeling regulations, what were some of the ways in which food labels misled consumers?
4. What are your own suggestions for improving the presentation of nutrition information on food labels?

Appendix C: **Glossary**

A

Absorption: The taking in of substances, as when nutrients are taken from the digestive tract into the bloodstream.

Aerobic metabolism: The oxygen-requiring reactions occurring in mitochondria which produce energy from the breakdown of acetyl CoA into carbon dioxide and water.

Aflatoxin: Toxin(s) formed by the growth of a fungus (especially Aspergillus flavus). The fungus can contaminate certain crops (e.g., peanuts, corn) and flourish under hospitable conditions. Aflatoxin is thought to be a cause of liver cancer.

Albumin: A protein found in the plasma portion of blood which helps transport substances, regulates acidity of blood, and regulates the amount of fluid held in blood. A deficiency of albumin can lead to edema.

Alcohol: A fermentation product of carbohydrate that has a high caloric content (7 calories per gram), is essentially devoid of nutrients, and acts as a drug.

Amino acid: The structural unit ("building block") of protein; contains an amino group and an acid group.

Anemia: A lower-than-normal amount of red blood cells or hemoglobin. Dietary deficiencies of iron and folate, and lack of intrinsic factor (for vitamin B-12 absorption) are common causes.

Anaerobic: Able to function in the absence of oxygen.

Anaerobic metabolism: Energy-producing reactions which break glucose into pyruvate without the need for oxygen. Also known as glycolysis.

Aneurysm: An outpouching of a weakened portion of the arterial wall. Usually caused by a defect in the affected artery and/or high blood pressure. Rupture of an aneurysm in an artery in the brain causes a hemorrhagic stroke.

Angina [pectoris]: Chest pain caused by inadequate oxygen delivery by coronary arteries to the heart muscle.

Anorexia: A loss of appetite.

Anorexia nervosa: A psychological eating disorder characterized by a dramatic reduction of food intake for fear of becoming fat, resulting in extreme weight loss and sometimes death.

Antibody: A blood protein made in response to a foreign substance (e.g., measles virus), creating a defense and immunity against it.

Antioxidant: A substance that prevents or retards oxidation. BHA (butylated hydroxyanisole) and BHT (butylated hydroxytoluene) are common antioxidants used in foods. Vitamins C and E can also function as antioxidants in food and in the body.

Appetite: A learned response which causes the desire for food.

Artery: A thick, muscular blood vessel that carries blood away from the heart. Blood carried in arteries is oxygenated (except for the pulmonary artery, which carries blood from the heart to the lungs to be oxygenated).

-ase: A suffix used in forming the name of an enzyme, such as lipase, sucrase, and lactase.

Atherosclerosis: An accumulation of fatty material in the lining of the arterial wall, resulting in the thickening, hardening, and loss of elasticity of the arteries.

Atom: The smallest particle that can no longer be subdivided without losing its characteristic properties. Atoms contain protons, neutrons, and electrons.

ATP (adenosine triphosphate): The high-energy molecule a cell makes by breaking down the energy-providing nutrients.

Autoimmune disease: A disease that occurs when a part of the body is mistakenly seen as foreign and is destroyed by the immune system, e.g., insulin-producing pancreatic cells destroyed by the immune system resulting in childhood-onset diabetes.

Axon: An extension of a nerve cell that conducts a nerve impulse away from the body of a nerve cell.

B

Basal metabolic rate (BMR): The rate at which energy (calories) is used for a person's involuntary functions. It is measured under standard conditions, directly by the heat expended, or indirectly by the amount of oxygen consumed.

Bile: A fluid made by the liver and stored and concentrated in the gallbladder. It is released into the upper part of the small intestine (the duodenum) and serves to emulsify fats, aiding fat digestion.

Bile acids: A component of bile made in the liver from cholesterol.

Biotechnology: The use of technology to study or solve problems of living organisms, e.g., the production of human proteins by bacteria that have had the human gene for that protein inserted into their DNA ("recombinant DNA"). The term biotechnology is often used interchangeably with genetic engineering and recombinant *DNA*.

BMR: See Basal metabolic rate.

Bomb calorimeter: An apparatus used to determine the energy value of food by measuring the amount of heat produced by complete oxidation ("burning") of a food sample.

Bulimia: A psychological eating disorder characterized by a compulsion to eat large quantities of food in a short period of time and then "purging," usually by inducing vomiting or taking large amounts of laxatives.

C

Caffeine: A stimulant found in coffee, which makes the nervous system more excitable. Also refers to related substances found in tea and chocolate which act as stimulants.

Calorie: The amount of heat needed to raise the temperature of one liter of water one degree Celsius. A calorie as used in nutrition is actually a kilocalorie—1,000 times the calorie of physics/chemistry.

Cancer: The uncontrolled overgrowth of cells which can lead to death.

Capillary: A small, thin-walled blood vessel. Reaching every living cell in the body, capillaries provide the means for exchange of substances between the blood and each cell.

Carbohydrate: One of the three classes of nutrients in food that provide energy to the body. Carbohydrates (e.g., sugar, starch) have an energy value of 4 calories per gram.

Carbohydrate loading: A regimen used by endurance athletes to temporarily increase muscle glycogen to higher-than-normal levels by emptying the muscle of glycogen by exercise, and then, in the days immediately prior to competition, resting and replenishing muscle glycogen by eating a high-carbohydrate diet.

Carcinogen: A substance that causes cancer.

Catalyst: A substance that increases the rate of a chemical reaction. (Enzymes are biological catalysts.)

Cell: The basic structural unit of an organism.

Cell membrane: The outside layer of a cell.

Cholesterol: A fat found in all cell membranes, where it helps regulate membrane fluidity. It is found in animal fat and animal tissue, but not in plants. Excessive amounts in the blood can lead to atherosclerosis.

Chromosome: Structures in the cell nucleus that are made of protein and DNA (the cell's genetic information).

Citric acid cycle: A series of chemical reactions occurring in the mitochondria in which molecules are oxidized to produce ATP (energy). Also known as the Krebs cycle or the TCA (tricarboxylic acid) cycle.

Coenzyme: A non-protein substance which works with enzymes in chemical reactions. Coenzymes often contain B-vitamins as part of their structures.

Cofactor: A non-protein substance, often a mineral, that can be required for enzyme action.

Collagen: A protein found in bone, cartilage, and connective tissue.

Constipation: Difficult or infrequent passage of stool. Insoluble dietary fiber helps prevent constipation by absorbing water, making the stool bulkier and softer.

Covalent bond: The connection of two atoms that occurs because they share one or more electrons.

Cytoplasm: The fluid in a cell.

D

Delaney clause: Adopted in 1958, it prohibits the Food and Drug Administration (FDA) from approving food additives that have been shown, in any dose, to cause cancer in any animal.

Denaturation: A change in the 3-dimensional shape of a protein molecule.

Dental plaque: Soft patches, containing bacteria and debris, that cling to teeth. Involved in tooth decay and gum disease.

Deoxyribonucleic acid: *See* DNA.

Dextrose: *See* glucose.

Diarrhea: Rapid movement of fecal matter through the colon, producing watery stool.

Diabetes: A disease characterized by high blood sugar, resulting from a deficiency or ineffectiveness of insulin.

Dietary fiber: *See* fiber.

Digestion: The breakdown of foods by digestive enzymes into smaller units that can be absorbed by the body.

Digestive tract: The series of organs (including the mouth, esophagus, stomach, small intestine, and colon) responsible for the digestion and absorption of nutrients. Also called the gastrointestinal (GI) tract.

Direct calorimetry: A method for determining the amount of calories expended by an organism by measuring the amount of heat produced.

Disaccharide: A carbohydrate consisting of two monosaccharides linked together. Disaccharides and monosaccharides are also called double sugars and single sugars, respectively.

Diverticulosis: An outpouching of the colon wall. Dietary fiber is believed to reduce the risk by providing bulk to contents of the colon.

DNA (deoxyribonucleic acid): The double-stranded molecule, located in the cell nucleus, that encodes an organism's genetic information.

Double-blind study: A study in which neither the subjects nor the investigators actively involved know whether a particular subject is in the experimental group or the control group used for comparison.

Duodenum: Uppermost region (about the first 12 inches) of the small intestine. Site where pancreatic and liver secretions enter the small intestine through the bile duct.

E

Edema: Swelling in the body caused by excess fluids in body tissues. Seen in severe protein deficiency and some other medical conditions.

Emulsifier: A substance which finely divides and suspends fat in a water-based solution.

Enrichment: The addition of specific nutrients (thiamin, riboflavin, niacin, and iron) to refined grains such as white rice and white flour.

Enzyme: A biological catalyst, usually a protein, that speeds biochemical reactions.

Epidemiology: The study of the factors associated with diseases in populations, e.g., comparing populations world-wide, low-fiber diets are associated with higher rates of colon cancer.

Estrogen: The main female sex hormone.

Esophagus: The muscular tube, serving as a passageway for food, that extends from the throat to the stomach.

F

Fat: One of the three classes of nutrients in food that provide energy (9 calories per gram) to the body. Fats dissolve in organic solvents but not in water.

Fat-soluble vitamins: The vitamins (A,D,E,K) that dissolve in fat.

Fatty acid: A chain of carbon (and hydrogen) atoms with an acid group (—COOH) on one end; the main component of triglycerides.

Fiber: Indigestible material found in plants. Insoluble fibers (those that don't dissolve in water) help prevent diverticulosis, constipation, and possibly colon cancer. Soluble fibers may help lower blood-cholesterol levels.

Fructose: A single sugar (monosaccharide) found in such foods as honey and fruit and a part of the double sugar sucrose.

G

Galactose: A single sugar (monosaccharide) that is a part of the double sugar lactose.

Gastric juice: An acidic secretion from the stomach lining that kills bacteria ingested along with food, denatures proteins, dissolves minerals (enabling their absorption), etc.

Glucose: The most common single sugar (monosaccharide), also known as dextrose. It is found in various foods, is the sugar found in blood, and is a part of the double sugars sucrose, maltose, and lactose.

Glycogen: A starch-like carbohydrate (a polysaccharide made of glucose) found in animal tissue (muscle and liver). Provides for the storage of glucose in the body.

Glycolysis: The production of ATP energy from the anaerobic breakdown of glucose in the cell cytoplasm.

Goiter: Enlarged thyroid gland caused by any of several factors. When caused by a deficiency of dietary iodine, it is called simple goiter.

Goitrogens: Substances found in foods and some drugs which, when ingested in large amounts of over a long time, can cause goiter.

Ghrelin: A hormone produced by the cells lining the stomach that stimulates appetite.

H

HDL (high-density lipoprotein) -cholesterol: The blood cholesterol carried in the protein-rich lipoprotein that is associated with a lower risk of cardiovascular disease. It is dubbed "good cholesterol" for this reason.

Heme iron: Iron that is part of the iron-containing molecule called heme. Heme is found in the oxygen-carrying molecules hemoglobin and myoglobin; found only in animal tissue.

Hemoglobin: The iron-containing protein found in red blood cells; carries oxygen and carbon dioxide.

Hormone: A chemical messenger, typically secreted in one location, carried in the bloodstream, and having specific effects elsewhere, e.g., the hormone glucagon is secreted by the pancreas and causes the liver to release glucose.

Hydrogenation: The addition of hydrogen to unsaturated fat. This changes the double bonds in fatty acids to single bonds, resulting in a more solid (i.e., more saturated) fat.

Hypoglycemia: An abnormally low blood-glucose level. An excess of insulin is the usual cause.

I

Indirect calorimetry: Measurement of oxygen consumption to determine the calories expended by the organism.

Insulin: A hormone made in the pancreas that allows glucose to enter cells.

Intrinsic factor: A protein secreted by the stomach that is essential for the absorption of vitamin B-12. An insufficient secretion of intrinsic factor leads to a B-12 deficiency and pernicious anemia.

Ion: A positively or negatively charged atom or molecule.

K

Ketone: A chemical formed from acetyl CoA when there is an accumulation of acetyl CoA (from the breakdown of fatty acids) in metabolism.

Ketosis: An abnormal condition in which ketones are produced in large amounts because of a lack of carbohydrates for fuel. This can happen in starvation, untreated diabetes, and low-carbohydrate diets.

L

Lactase: The digestive enzyme that breaks the double sugar lactose into galactose and glucose.

Lactic acid: An acid formed by glycolysis when oxygen is limited (e.g., in sustained, strenuous physical activity).

Lactose: A double sugar (disaccharide) found in milk; made of galactose and glucose.

Lactose intolerance: The reduced ability to digest lactose (because of insufficient lactase enzyme in the small intestine), resulting in symptoms such as diarrhea and gas.

LDL (low-density lipoprotein)-cholesterol: The blood cholesterol carried in the fat-rich lipoprotein that is associated with an increased risk of cardiovascular disease. It is dubbed "bad cholesterol" for this reason.

Lecithin: A phospholipid (a type of fat) found in food and body tissues. In food products, it is commonly used as an emulsifier. In the body, it forms the basic structure of cell membranes.

Leptin: A hormone produced by fatty tissue that plays a key role in regulating energy intake and energy expenditure, including the regulation (decrease) of appetite and (increase) of metabolism.

Lipoprotein: A fat and protein combination used to carry fat in the plasma portion of blood.

M

Malnutrition: A condition of too much or too little of a nutrient, resulting in poor health.

Maltose: A double sugar (disaccharide) made of two glucose molecules linked together.

Menopause: The permanent cessation of menstruation that occurs normally between about age 40 and 50.

Messenger RNA (mRNA): A copy of the genetic information needed to make a particular protein.

Metabolism: The sum total of the chemical changes or reactions occurring in the body. Energy metabolism is the process by which cells release energy from food.

Microvilli: The ruffled portion of the membrane of the cells lining the small intestine.

Mitochondria: Cell components in which all oxygen-requiring reactions occur.

Monounsaturated fatty acid: A fatty acid with one double bond in its carbon chain. Olive oil is a rich source.

Mutation: A change in the sequence of bases in DNA.

N

Non-heme iron: Iron that is not part of the molecule called heme (an oxygen-carrying molecule found in blood and muscle). All plant iron is non-heme iron.

Nucleus, cell: The cell component that holds genetic information.

O

Obesity: Excess accumulation of body fat. Generally defined as exceeding ideal body weight by 20% or more.

Obestatin: A hormone produced by the cells lining the stomach; it drastically reduces appetite.

Organism: Any living plant or animal.

-ose: A suffix used in naming of carbohydrates such as glucose, maltose, and lactose.

Osteomalacia: Vitamin D deficiency in adults, resulting in bone demineralization and easily fractured bones.

Osteoporosis: A loss of bone calcium such that the bone is easily fractured. Occurs most commonly in postmenopausal women.

Oxidation: The addition of oxygen atoms to (or the removal of hydrogen atoms from) a substance.

P

Pectin: A dietary fiber which can help lower blood-cholesterol levels. It is also used to "gel" jams and jellies.

Peptide: Two or more amino acids joined together. The bond that joins them together is called a peptide bond.

Periodontal tissue: The gums, periodontal ligament, and other tissue surrounding the teeth.

Peristalsis: The wave-like contractions of the digestive tract muscles that move the digestive material downward.

Phenylalanine: One of the 9 amino acids required in the diet. The inherited inability to break down phenylalanine is the cause of the disease phenylketonuria (PKU**).**

Phospholipid: A phosphorus-containing fat (lipid) made of glycerol, two fatty acids, and one phosphorus-containing substance. Phospholipids are the basic unit in cell membranes and are used as emulsifiers in foods. Lecithin is a common phospholipid.

Photosynthesis: The process whereby plants use the energy in sunlight to make carbohydrates and oxygen from carbon dioxide and water.

Placebo: An inert substance which seems identical to the real substance to be tested in an experiment; used to control for nonspecific effects.

Placebo effect: An effect that results from, but is not caused by, the test substance or procedure (e.g., feeling better simply because you expect to).

Plasma: The fluid portion of blood in which blood cells are suspended.

Platelets: Small blood cells which cluster at the site of injury to a blood vessel, acting immediately to stop the bleeding until a clot forms.

Polysaccharide: A carbohydrate of 3 or more monosaccharides (single sugars) linked together. Digestible polysaccharides are commonly called complex carbohydrates.

Polyunsaturated fatty acid: A fatty acid with two or more double bonds in its carbon chain. When these fatty acids predominate in a fat, the fat is liquid at room temperature.

Protein: An energy-providing nutrient (4 calories per gram) made of a chain of amino acids.

Protein complementation: Combining plant proteins to increase the quality of protein in the diet. A protein low in one essential amino acids is complemented by another protein that is low in another amino acid.

Protein-energy malnutrition: A severe deficiency of both protein and calories. Young children are particularly vulnerable because of their heightened need for calories and high-quality protein.

Pyruvate: The end-product of anaerobic metabolism (glycolysis) that can be made into acetyl CoA, to proceed onto aerobic metabolism. When oxygen is limited, pyruvate is made into lactic acid instead.

R

Rancid: Having the disagreeable taste and/or smell of decomposed fat, caused by oxidation of double bonds in unsaturated fat.

Rhodopsin: The vitamin-A containing molecule that plays a crucial role in vision.

Ribosome: A cell component that is the site of protein synthesis.

Rickets: Bone deformities caused by vitamin D or calcium deficiency in children.

Risk factor: A condition or circumstance thought to increase the chance of developing a disease or injury, e.g., smoking is a risk factor for lung cancer; high LDL-cholesterol is a risk factor for cardiovascular disease.

RNA (ribonucleic acid): *See* messenger RNA and transfer RNA.

S

Satiety: Feeling of fullness or of being satisfied. Fat provides a longer satiety than carbohydrate or protein.

Saturated fatty acid: A fatty acid that does not contain any double bonds in its carbon chain because it is saturated with hydrogen atoms.

Scientific method: The standard procedure used to acquire scientific knowledge, involving a hypothesis, experimentation, evaluation, discussion of results and conclusions, all subject to peer review.

Serotonin: The brain chemical (neurotransmitter) made from the amino acid tryptophan; has a calming effect.

Sickle cell anemia: A severe and painful inherited anemia caused by defective hemoglobin in red blood cells.

Stroke: Brain damage stemming from an interruption of oxygen delivery to the brain, because of a blockage or bleeding (hemorrhage) in an artery that supplies the brain.

Sucrase: The digestive enzyme that breaks sucrose into fructose and glucose.

Sucrose: A double sugar (disaccharide) made of fructose and glucose. Commonly known as "table sugar."

Sugar: The general name that includes single sugars (e.g., glucose, fructose, and galactose) and double sugars (e.g., sucrose, lactose, maltose), "Table sugar" is sucrose.

Skinfold thickness: A measure of fatness, based on the fact that body fat is mostly stored under the skin and adheres to the skin when the skin is pinched (skinfold).

T

Thyroxine: An iodine-containing hormone made by the thyroid gland that is important in maintaining normal rates of metabolism.

Transfer RNA (tRNA): Carries the amino acids used to make protein in the cell.

Triglyceride: A fat made of three fatty acids attached to glycerol; makes up most of the fat in food and in our body.

Tryptophan: One of the nine diet-essential amino acids; can be made into the B-vitamin niacin and the neurotransmitter serotonin.

U

Umami: One of the five basic tastes sensed by the tongue. It describes the flavor common to savory foods such as meats and cheeses.

Unsaturated fatty acid: A fatty acid which contains one or more double bonds in its carbon chain.

Urea: The waste product made up of discarded amino groups from amino acids (as when amino acids are used for energy or made into body fat). Urea is excreted in the urine.

V

Vegan: A person who eats only plant foods.

Vegetarianism: Consuming a diet of only plant foods and plant products. Some vegetarians, however, eat some animal foods, e.g., a lacto-ovo-vegetarian diet includes milk (lacto-) and eggs (ovo-).

Villus: Finger-like projection in the inner lining of the small intestine that is covered with a single layer of intestinal cells. The projections (villi) markedly increase the surface area of the small intestine.

Vitamin: An essential molecule required in the diet. Of the 13 vitamins required for human health, 9 are water-soluble, and 4 are fat-soluble.

W

Warfarin: An anticoagulant that works by interfering with vitamin K's role in the formation of blood clots.

Water-soluble vitamins: Vitamins that dissolve in water; vitamin C and the 8 B-vitamins.

X

Xerophthalmia: A dryness of the eyeball caused by vitamin A deficiency, which can progress to blindness.

Appendix D: References

Chap. 1: *Nutrition Myths and Tests of Reality*
Cited Sources
1. Calverton, VF. ed. 1931. *The Making of Man,* Modern Library, New York.
2. Childe, C. 1946. *What Happened in History?* Pelican, New York.
3. Lowenberg, M, et al. 1974. *Food and Man.* Wiley, New York.
4. Weyer, E. 1961. *Primitive Peoples Today.* Dolphin, New York.
5. Frazer, JG. 1971. *The Golden Bough,* Macmillan, New York.
6. Temkin, O. 1960. *Nutrition from Classical Antiquity to the Baroque,* in *Human Nutrition, Historic and Scientific,* N.Y. Academy of Medicine, New York, pp. 78-97.
7. National Center for Health Statistics, Centers for Disease Control, U.S. Dept. of Health and Human Services (DHHS). 2006. *Health, United States, 2006.* DHHS Publication #2006-1232.
8. Bieler, HG. 1973. *Food is Your Best Medicine,* Vintage Books (Random House), New York.
9. Morrill, J, et al. 2003. *Are You Eating Right? Compare your diet to the official recommendations using the nutrient content of 5000+ foods.* Orange Grove Publishing, Menlo Park, CA www.orangegrovepub.com
10. Deutsch, RM. 1977. *The New Nuts Among the Berries,* Bull Publishing, Boulder, CO, p. 282. www.bullpub.com
11. Dosti, R. 3/20/86, *Book May Remain No. 1 Among Readers, But Nutritionists Don't Agree,* Los Angeles Times.
12. Diamond, H, Diamond, M. 1985. *Fit for Life.* Warner Books, Inc., New York.
13. Center for Disease Control and Prevention. 2007. *Crude and Age-adjusted prevalence of diagnosed diabetes per 100 population, United States, 1980-2005.* www.cdc.gov/diabetes/statistics, 3/26/2007 update, accessed 10/28/07.

Other Sources
Herbert, V. 1990. *Separating Food Facts and Myths,* in The *Mount Sinai School of Medicine Complete Book of Nutrition.* Herbert, V, ed. St. Martin Press, New York.
McCollum, EV. 1957. *A History of Nutrition—the Sequence of Ideas in Nutrition Investigations,* Houghton Muffin Co., Boston.
Todhunter, EN. 1984. *Historical Landmarks in Nutrition,* in *Present Knowledge in Nutrition,* 5/e, The Nutrition Foundation, Inc., Wash. DC.

Chap. 2: *Food Power—Use and Storage*
Cited Sources
1. Diamond, H, Diamond, M. 1985. *Fit for Life.* Warner Books, Inc., New York, p. 7.
2. Kreider, RB et al. 1998. *Effects of creatine supplementation on body composition, strength, and sprint performance.* Med. Sci. Sports Exercise 30: 73-82.
3. Mead, M. January 1971. *Why Do We Overeat?* Redbook, p.28.

4. Mayer, J. 1965. *Genetic Factors in Human Obesity.* Ann. N.Y. Acad. Sci. 131: 412.
5. Stunkard, AJ, et al. 1990. *Body-Mass Index of Twins Who Have Been Reared Apart.* New Eng. J. Med. 322:1483.
6. Bouchard, CA, et al. 1990. *The Response to Long-term Overfeeding in Identical Twins.* New Eng. J. Med. 322: 1477-1482.
7. Stunkard, AJ. 1988. *The Salmon Lecture. Some Perspectives on Human Obesity: Its Causes.* Bull. N.Y. Acad. Med 64: 902-923.
8. Stunkard AJ, et al. 2006. *A paradigm for facilitating pharmacotherapy at a distance: sertraline treatment of the night eating syndrome.* J Clin Psychiatry. 67(10):1568-72.

Other Sources
Flier, JS, Maratos-Flier, E. 2007. *What fuels fat.* Scientific American 297(3): 72-81.
Food and Nutrition Board, Institute of Medicine. 2005. *Dietary Reference Intakes for Energy, Carbohydrates, Fiber, Fat, Fatty Acids, Cholesterol, Protein, and Amino Acids (Macronutrients).* National Academies Press, Wash. DC. www.nap.edu
Food and Nutrition Board, Institute of Medicine. 2006. *Dietary Reference Intakes: The Essential Guide to Nutrient Requirements.* Editors: Otten, JJ, et al. National Academies Press, Wash. DC.

Chap. 3: *Putting the Laws of Energy to Work*
Cited Sources
1. NIH (National Institutes of Health) Publication #00-4084. October 2000. *The Practical Guide: Identification, evaluation, and treatment of overweight and obesity in adults.* www.nhlbi.nih.gov/guidelines/obesity/prctgd_c.pdf
2. Stubbs, RJ et al. 2004. *A decrease in physical activity affects appetite, energy, and nutrient balance in lean men feeding ad libitum.* Am. J. Clin. Nutr. 79:62-69.
3. Pomerleau, M et al. 2004. *Effects of exercise intensity on food intake and appetite in women.* Am J. Clin. Nutr. 80: 1230-1236.
4. Ledikwe, Rolls, BJ et al. 2007. *Reductions in dietary energy density are associated with weight loss in overweight and obese participants in the PREMIER trial.* Am J Clin Nutr 85:1212-121.
5. Ledikwe, J.H. et al. 2006. *Dietary energy density is associated with energy intake and weight status in US adults.* Am J Clin Nutr 83:1362-1368.
6. Rolls, BJ et al. *Reductions in portion size and energy density of foods are additive and lead to sustained decreases in energy intake.* Am J Clin Nutr 83:11-7.

Other Sources
Bulik, CM, et al. 2007. *The Genetics of Anorexia Nervosa.* Ann. Rev. Nutr. 27:263-275.
Food and Nutrition Board, Institute of Medicine. 2005. *Dietary Reference Intakes for Energy, Carbohydrates, Fiber, Fat, Fatty Acids, Cholesterol, Protein, and Amino*

Acids (Macronutrients). National Academies Press, Wash, DC. www.nap.edu

Food and Nutrition Board, Institute of Medicine. 2006. *Dietary Reference Intakes: The Essential Guide to Nutrient Requirements.* Editors: Otten, JJ, et al. National Academies Press, Wash. DC www.nap.edu

Ode, JJ, et al. 2007. *Body Mass Index as a Predictor of Percent Fat in College Athletes and Nonathletes.* Med Sci Sports Exerc. 39:403-409.

Wenten, M., et al. 2002. *Associations of Weight, Weight Change, and Body Mass with Breast Cancer Risk in Hispanic and Non-Hispanic White Women.* Ann Epidemiol. 12:435-444.

Chap. 4: The Trapping of the Sun
Cited Sources

1. Chang, T-T. 2002. *Rice.* In: *The Cambridge World History of Food.* Kiple, KF, Orelas, KC, editors. Cambridge University Press.

2. Benzoni, G. 1656. *History of the New World.* Translation by W.H. Smyth. Hakluyt Society, London, 1857.

3. Goldemberg, J. 2007. *Perspective: Ethanol for a Sustainable Energy Future.* Science 315: 808-810.

4. Service, RF. 2007. *Cellulosic Ethanol: Biofuel Researchers Prepare to Reap a New Harvest.* Science 315:1488-1491.

Other Sources

FDA Consumer Magazine. July-Aug 2006. *Artificial Sweeteners: No Calories...Sweet!* www.fda.gov/fdac/features/2006/406_sweeteners.html

Food and Nutrition Board, Institute of Medicine. 2005. *Dietary Reference Intakes for Energy, Carbohydrates, Fiber, Fat, Fatty Acids, Cholesterol, Protein, and Amino Acids (Macronutrients).* National Academies Press, Wash. DC. www.nap.edu

Food and Nutrition Board, Institute of Medicine. 2006. *Dietary Reference Intakes: The Essential Guide to Nutrient Requirements.* Editors: Otten, JJ, et al. National Academies Press, Wash., DC. www.nap.edu

Chap. 5: Of Carbohydrates and Health
Cited Sources

1. National Institute of Diabetes and Digestive and Kidney Diseases. 2005. National Diabetes *Statistics fact sheet: general information and national estimates on diabetes in the United States, 2005.* Bethesda, MD: U.S. Department of Health and Human Services, National Institute of Health. http://diabetes.niddk.nih.gov/dm/pubs/statistics/index.htm

2. Center for Disease Control. 2005. *National Diabetes Fact Sheet, United States, 2005.* www.cdc.gov/diabetes/pubs/pdf/ndfs_2005.pdf

3. National Institute of Diabetes and Digestive and Kidney Diseases. 2006. *Diverticulosis and Diverticulitis.* Bethesda, MD: U.S. Department of Health and Human Services, National Institute of Health. http://digestive.niddk.nih.gov/ddiseases/pubs/diverticulosis/index.htm

4. Willett, W, et al., 1990. *Relation of Meat, Fat, and Fiber Intake to the Risk of Colon Cancer in a Prospective Study Among Women.* New Engl J Med. 323:1664.

Other Sources

Coleman, E. 2003. *Eating for Endurance,* 4/e, Bull Publishing, Boulder, CO. BullPub.com

Coleman, E, Steen, SN. 2000. *Ultimate Sports Nutrition,* 2/e. Bull Publishing, Boulder, CO.

Food and Nutrition Board, Institute of Medicine. 2005. *Dietary Reference Intakes for Energy, Carbohydrates, Fiber, Fat, Fatty Acids, Cholesterol, Protein, and Amino Acids (Macronutrients).* National Academies Press, Wash. DC. www.nap.edu

Food and Nutrition Board, Institute of Medicine. 2006. *Dietary Reference Intakes: The Essential Guide to Nutrient Requirements.* Editors: Otten, JJ, et al. National Academies Press. Wash., DC.

Chap. 6: The Protein Confusion
Cited Sources

1. Tannahill, R. 1973. *Food in History.* Stein and Day, New York, p. 300.

2. News and Comment. 1991. *Gene Mapping Japan's Number One Crop.* Science 252:1611.

3. National Research Council, National Academy of Sciences. 1989. *Recommended Dietary Allowances,* 10/e. National Academies Press, Wash., DC, p. 70.

Other Sources

Clark, J, Goldblith, S. January 1976. *Processing of Foods in Ancient Rome.* Food Tech., p. 30.

Food and Nutrition Board, Institute of Medicine. 2002. *Dietary Reference Intakes for Energy, Carbohydrates, Fiber, Fat, Fatty Acids, Cholesterol, Protein, and Amino Acids (Macronutrients).* National Academies Press, Wash. DC. www.nap.edu

Food and Nutrition Board, Institute of Medicine. 2006. *Dietary Reference Intakes: The Essential Guide to Nutrient Requirements.* Editors: Otten, JJ, et al. National Academies Press, Wash. DC.

Hale, W. et al. 1968. Illustrated *History of Eating and Drinking Through the Ages.* Vol. 1, Horizon Cookbook, American Heritage, New York.

Jacob, H. 1944. Six *Thousand Years of Bread,* Doubleday, New York.

Jones, W. 1946. *Philosophy and Medicine in Ancient Greece,* Johns Hopkins Press, Baltimore, MD..

Lewis, H. 1952. *Fifty Years of Study of the Role of Protein in Nutrition.* J. Amer. Diet. Assoc., 28: 701.

Lowenberg, M. et al. 1974, *Early Times through Roman Times and Medieval Times through the 19th Century,* in *Food and Man,* Wiley, New York, pp. 1-27.

McHenry, E. 1960. *From Lavoisier to Beaumont and Hopkins,* in *Human Nutrition Historic and Scientific,* NY Acad Med.

Pariser, E. 1976. *Foods in Ancient Egypt and Classical Greece.* Food Tech., Jan. 1976, p. 23.

Petronius, A. 1913. *The Satyricon.* Modern Library, New York.

Pyke, M. 1958. *Food and Society,* Murray, London.

Simon, A. 1949. *Food,* Burke, London.

U.S. Dept. of Commerce. 1960. *Historical Statistics of the U.S.: Colonial Times to 1957.* Wash DC.

Chap. 7: Putting Amino Acids to Work
Cited Sources

1. Food and Nutrition Board, Institute of Medicine. 2006. *Dietary Reference Intakes: The Essential Guide to Nutrient Requirement.* (pp.144-150). Editors: Otten, JJ, et al. National Academies Press, Wash DC.

2. Hadas, M., *Imperial Rome,* Time, Inc., New York, 1965.

Other Sources

Apolzan, JW, et al. 2007. *Inadequate Dietary Protein Increases Hunger and Desire to Eat in Younger and Older Men.* J Nutr. 137:1478-1482.

Food and Nutrition Board, Institute of Medicine. 2005. *Dietary Reference Intakes for Energy, Carbohydrates, Fiber, Fat, Fatty Acids, Cholesterol, Protein, and Amino Acids (Macronutrients).* National Academies Press, Wash DC. www.nap.edu

Layman, DK, et al. 2005. *Dietary Protein and Exercise Have Additive Effects on Body Composition during Weight Loss in Adult Women.* J Nutr. 135:1903-1910.

Smith, NJ, Worthington-Roberts, B. 1989. *Food For Sport,* Bull Publishing, Boulder, CO.

Watson, J. 1968. *The Double Helix,* Atheneum Publ., New York.

Chap. 8: Fats Seen and Unseen
Cited Sources

1. Stefansson, V. 1960. *Food and Food Habits in Alaska and Northern Canada, in Human Nutrition, Historic and Scientific.* N.Y. Acad. of Med., International Universities Press, New York.

2. Food and Nutrition Board, Institute of Medicine. 2006. *Dietary Reference Intakes: The Essential Guide to Nutrient Requirement.* (p.150). Editors: Otten, JJ, et al. National Academies Press, Wash DC.

3. Cheskin, LJ et al. 1998. *Gastrointestinal Symptoms Following Consumption of Olestra or Regular Triglyceride Potato Chips.* JAMA 279: 150-153.

Other Sources

Fillmore, R. Spring 2007. *Shining Some Light on the Sunflower.* Univ. of Calif. Research Magazine. www.researchmagazine.uga.edu/spring2007/shiningsome5.htm

Food and Nutrition Board, Institute of Medicine. 2005. *Dietary Reference Intakes for Energy, Carbohydrates, Fiber, Fat, Fatty Acids, Cholesterol, Protein, and Amino Acids (Macronutrients).* National Academies Press, Wash DC. www.nap.edu

Food and Nutrition Board, Institute of Medicine. 2006. *Dietary Reference Intakes: The Essential Guide to Nutrient Requirements.* Editors: Otten, JJ et al. National Academies Press, Wash DC.

Chap. 9: Fat and the Doctor's Dilemma
Cited Sources

1. National Center for Health Statistics. 2007. Health, United States, 2007.

2. National Heart, Lung, Blood Institute, National Institutes of Health. *National Cholesterol Education Program:* www.nhlbi.nih.gov/about/ncep/index.htm, www.nhlbi.nih.gov/health/public/heart/chol/wyntk.pdf (accessed 12/6/07).

3. Grundy, SM et al. 2005. *Diagnosis and Management of the Metabolic Syndrome. An American Heart Association/National Heart, Lung, Blood Institute Scientific Statement.* Circulation 112: 2735-2752.

4. Grundy, SM et al. 2004. *Implications of Recent Clinical Trials for the National Cholesterol Education Program Adult Treatment Panel III Guidelines.* Circulation 110:227-239. (Also: J. Am Coll. Cardiol. 44:720-732.)

5. Food and Nutrition Board, Institute of Medicine. 2006. *Dietary Reference Intakes: The Essential Guide to Nutrient Requirements.* Editors: Otten, JJ et al. National Academies Press, Wash DC. p. 139.

6. Rosenberg, I. 2002. *Fish—Food to Calm the Heart.* New Engl J Med. 346:1102-1103.

7. Valenzuela, TD. 2000. *Outcomes of Rapid Defibrillation by Security Officers after Cardiac Arrest in Casinos.* New Engl J Med. 343: 1206-1209.

8. Jemal, A et al. 2007. *Cancer Statistics, 2007.* CA Cancer J. Clin. 57:43-66.

9. American Cancer Society. 2007. *Cancer Facts and Figures—2007.*

10. Parkin, DM et al. 2005. *Global Cancer Statistics, 2002.* CA Cancer J. Clin. 55:74-108.

11. Kushi, LH et al. 2006. *American Cancer Society Guidelines on Nutrition and Physical Activity: Reducing the Risk of Cancer with Healthy Food Choices and Physical Activity.* CA Cancer J. Clin. 56: 254-281.

12. Hamajima, N et al. 2002. *Alcohol, tobacco and breast cancer—collaborative reanalysis of individual data from 53 epidemiological studies, including 58,515 women with breast cancer and 95,067 women without the disease.* Br. J. Cancer 87:1234-1245.

Other Sources

Food and Nutrition Board, Institute of Medicine. 2005. *Dietary Reference Intakes for Energy, Carbohydrates, Fiber, Fat, Fatty Acids, Cholesterol, Protein, and Amino Acids (Macronutrients).* National Academies Press, Wash DC (www.nap.edu).

Food and Nutrition Board, Institute of Medicine. 2006. *Dietary Reference Intakes: The Essential Guide to Nutrient Requirements.* Editors: Otten, JJet al. National Academies Press, Wash DC (www.nap.edu).

Manson, J et al. 1992. *The Primary Prevention of Myocardial Infarction.* New Eng. J. Med. 236: 1406.

Mosca, L, et al. 2007. *Evidence-Based Guidelines for Cardiovascular Disease Prevention in Women: 2007 Update.* Circulation 115:1481-1501.

National Heart, Lung, Blood Institute, National Institutes of Health. 2006. *Your Guide to Lowering your Blood Pressure with DASH.* NIH Publication 06-4082. http://www.nhlbi.nih.gov/health/public/heart/hbp/dash/new_dash.pdf

Chap. 10: The Digestive System
Cited Sources

1. Grundy, D, Schemann, M. 2006. *Enteric Nervous System.* Curr. Opin. Gastroenterol. 22:102-110.

2. Chandrasekharan, B, Srinivasan, S. 2007. *Diabetes and the Enteric Nervous System.* Neurogastroenterology & Motility (OnlineEarly Articles). doi:10.1111/j.1365-2982.2007.01023.x

3. Frezza, M et al. 1990. *High blood alcohol levels in women. The role of decreased gastric alcohol dehydrogenase activity and first-pass metabolism.* New Eng. J. Med. 322: 95-99.

4. Wall, TL et al. 2000. *Hangover symptoms in Asian Americans with variations in the aldehyde dehydrogenase (ALDH2) gene.* J. Stud. Alcohol 61:13-17.

5. Yokoyama, M et al. 2005. *Hangover susceptibility in relation to aldehyde dehydrogenase-2 genotype, alcohol flushing, and mean corpuscular volume in Japanese workers.* Alcohol Clin. Exp. Res. 29:1165-1171.

6. Almy, TP et al. 1949. *Alterations in colonic function in man under stress. II. Experimental production of sigmoid spasm in healthy persons.* Gastroenterol. 12:425-436.

7. Suarez, FL et al. 1995. *A Comparison of Symptoms After the Consumption of Milk or Lactose-Hydrolyzed Milk by People with Self-Reported Severe Lactose Intolerance.* New Engl J Med 333:1-4.

Other Sources

Allen, OE. 1982. *Secrets of a Good Digestion.* Library of Health, Time-Life Books, Alexandria, VA.

National Digestive Diseases Information Clearinghouse website, a service of the National Institute of Diabetes, Digestive, and Kidney Diseases (NIDDK), National Institutes of Health (NIH). http://digestive.niddk.nih.gov

Chap. 11: Metabolism and the Vitamin Key
Sources

Brosnan, JT, Brosnan, ME. 2007. *Creatine: Endogenous, Metabolite, Dietary, and Therapeutic Supplement.* Ann. Rev. Nutr. 27: 241-261.

Chap. 12: Water—The Body's Inner Sea
Cited Sources

1. Almond, CSD et al. 2005. *Hyponatremia among Runners in the Boston Marathon.* New Eng. J. Med. 352:1550-1556.

Other Sources

Food and Nutrition Board, Institute of Medicine 2004. *Dietary Reference Intakes for Water, Potassium, Sodium, Chloride, and Sulfate.* National Academies Press, Wash DC. www.nap.edu

Food and Nutrition Board, Institute of Medicine. 2006. *Dietary Reference Intakes: The Essential Guide to Nutrient Requirements.* Editors: Otten, JJ et al. National Academies Press, Wash DC. www.nap.edu

Chap. 13: Some Practical Realities of Vitamins
Sources:

Food and Nutrition Board, Institute of Medicine. 2006. *Dietary Reference Intakes: The Essential Guide to Nutrient Requirements.* Editors: Otten, JJ et al. National Academies Press, Wash DC. www.nap.edu

Center for Food Safety and Applied Nutrition, Food and Drug Administration. 1995. *Dietary Supplements Health and Education Act of 1994.* www.cfsan.fda.gov/~dms/dietsupp.html

Chap. 14: Water-Soluble Vitamins
Cited Sources

1. Walter, R. 1974. *Anson's Voyage Round the World in the Years 1740-44.* Dover Publications, New York.

2. Carpenter, KJ. 1986. *The History of Scurvy arid Vitamin C.* Cambridge Univ. Press, p. 77.

Other Sources

Food and Nutrition Board, Institute of Medicine. 2000. *Dietary Reference Intakes for Vitamin C, Vitamin E, Selenium, and Carotenoids.* National Academies Press, Wash DC. www.nap.edu

Food and Nutrition Board, Institute of Medicine. 2000. *Dietary Reference Intakes for Thiamin, Riboflavin, Niacin, Vitamin B-6, Folate, Vitamin B-12, Pantothenic Acid, Biotin, and Choline.* National Academies Press, Wash DC. www.nap.edu

Food and Nutrition Board, Institute of Medicine. 1998. *Dietary Reference Intakes for Thiamin, Riboflavin, Niacin, Vitamin B-6, Folate, Vitamin B-12, Pantothenic Acid, Biotin, and Choline.* Wash DC, National Academies Press. www.nap.edu

Food and Nutrition Board, Institute of Medicine. 2006. *Dietary Reference Intakes: The Essential Guide to Nutrient Requirements.* Editors: Otten, JJ, Hellwig, JP, and LD Meyers. Wash DC, The National Academies Press. www.nap.edu

Chap. 15: Fat-Soluble Vitamins
Cited Sources

1. Allen, L et al. 2006. *Guidelines on Food Fortification with Micronutrients.* WHO (World Health Organization) Publications.

2. World Health Organization. 2007. *Vitamin A Deficiency.* www.who.int/nutrition/topics/vad/en/index.html (accessed 6/19/07)

3. ATBC (Alpha-Tocopherol, Beta Carotene) Cancer Prevention Study Group. 1994. *The effect of vitamin E and beta carotene on the incidence of lung cancer and other cancers in male smokers.* N Engl J Med 330:1029–1035.

4. Holick, M. 2007. *Vitamin D Deficiency.* New Engl J Med. 357:265-81.

Other Sources

Food and Nutrition Board, Institute of Medicine. 2000. *Dietary Reference Intakes for Vitamin A, Vitamin K, Arsenic, Boron, Chromium, Copper, Iodine, Iron, Manganese, Molybdenum, Nickel, Silicon, Vanadium, and Zinc.* National Academies Press, Wash DC.

Food and Nutrition Board, Institute of Medicine. 1997. *Dietary Reference Intakes for Calcium, Phosphorus, Magnesium, Vitamin D, and Fluoride.* National Academies Press, Wash DC. www.nap.edu

Food and Nutrition Board, Institute of Medicine. 2000. *Dietary Reference Intakes for Vitamin C, Vitamin E,*

Selenium, and Carotenoids. National Academies Press, Wash DC. www.nap.edu

Food and Nutrition Board, Institute of Medicine. 2006. *Dietary Reference Intakes: The Essential Guide to Nutrient Requirements.* Editors: Otten, JJ et al. National Academies Press, Wash DC. www.nap.edu

Chap. 16: Major Minerals
Cited Sources

1. Rossouw, JE, et al. 2002. *Risks and Benefits of Estrogen Plus Progestin in Healthy Postmenopausal Women: Principal Results from the Women's Health Initiative Randomized Controlled Trial.* JAMA 288:321-333.

2. Lambrinoudaki, I, et al. 2006. *Bisphosphonates.* Ann NY Acad Sci. 1092:397-402.

3. Strampel, W, et al. 2007. Safety Considerations with bisphosphonates for the Treatment of Osteoporosis. Drug Saf. 30:755-63.

4. Food and Nutrition Board, Institute of Medicine. 2004. *Dietary Reference Intakes for Water, Potassium, Sodium, Chloride, and Sulfate.* National Academies Press, Wash DC. www.nap.edu

5. Morrill, J, et al. 2003. *Are You Eating Right? Compare your diet to the official recommendations using the nutrient content of 5000+ foods.* Orange Grove Publ., Menlo Park, CA. www.orangegrovepub.com

6. Barinaga, M. *The Secret of Saltiness.* Science 254: 654, 1991.

Other Sources

Chapuy, MC et al. 1992. *Vitamin D3 and Calcium to Prevent Hip Fractures in Elderly Women.* New Engl J. Med. 327: 1637.

Food and Nutrition Board, Institute of Medicine. 1997. *Dietary Reference Intakes for Calcium, Phosphorus, Magnesium, Vitamin D, and Fluoride.* National Academies Press. Wash DC. www.nap.edu

Food and Nutrition Board, Institute of Medicine. 2006. *Dietary Reference Intakes: The Essential Guide to Nutrient Requirements.* Editors: Otten, JJ et al. National Academies Press, Wash DC. www.nap.edu

Surgeon General, Dept. of Health and Human Services. 2004. Bone Health and Osteoporosis: A Report of the Surgeon General. Wash DC. http://surgeongeneral.gov/library/bonehealth/content.html

Chap. 17: The Trace Minerals
Cited Sources

1. Dallman, RR. 1990. *Iron.* Present Knowledge in Nutrition, 6/e, International Life Sciences Institute—Nutrition Foundation, Wash DC.

2. Center for Disease Control. Sept. 12, 2003. *Surveillance for Elevated Blood Lead Levels Among Children—United States, 1997-2001.* Morbidity and Mortality Weekly Report. [www.cdc.gov/mmwr/PDF/ss/ss5210.pdf]

3. National Digestive Diseases Information Clearinghouse (NDDIC). April 2007. *Hemochromatosis.* http://digestive.niddk.nih.gov/ddiseases/pubs/hemochromatosis/index.htm (accessed 6/25/07)

4. Prasad, AS. 1974. *Trace Elements and Iron in Human*

Metabolism, Plenum Medical Book Co., New York, p. 253.

5. Kochupillai, N, Pandav, CS. June-July 1985. *Iodine Deficiency Disorders in China—Current Status, Control Measures, and Future Strategy.* UNICEF Consultants' Report. www.iqplusin.org/downloads/IDD_IN_CHINA.pdf

6. Yang, G et al. 1983. *Endemic Selenium Intoxication of Humans in China.* Am J. Clin. Nutr. 37: 872.

7. Center for Disease Control and Prevention, American Dental Association. 2006. *Water Fluoridation: Nature's Way to Prevent Tooth Decay.*

8. Anderson, R, Bryden, NA. 1983. *Concentration, Insulin Potentiation, and Absorption of Chromium in Beer.* J. Agric. Food Chem. 31: 308.

Other Sources

American Dental Association: www. ada.org

Food and Nutrition Board, Institute of Medicine. 2000. *Dietary Reference Intakes for Vitamin A, Vitamin K, Arsenic, Boron, Chromium, Copper, Iodine, Iron, Manganese, Molybdenum, Nickel, Silicon, Vanadium, and Zinc.* National Academies Press, Wash DC.

Food and Nutrition Board, Institute of Medicine. 2006. *Dietary Reference Intakes: The Essential Guide to Nutrient Requirements.* Editors: Otten, JJ et al. National Academies Press, Wash DC. www.nap.edu

Chap. 18: Between Food and Health
Cited Sources

1. British Nutrition Foundation. *Reference Nutrient Intakes for Vitamins and Minerals.*
(accessed 6/26/07)

2. U.S. Dept of Health and Human Services, U.S. Dept of Agriculture. 2005. *Dietary Guidelines for Americans.*

3. Kushi, LH et al. 2006. *American Cancer Society Guidelines on Nutrition and Physical Activity: Reducing the Risk of Cancer with Healthy Food Choices and Physical Activity.* CA Cancer J. Clin. 56: 254-281. http://caonline.amcancersoc.org/cgi/reprint/56/5/254

4. American Heart Association. 2006. *Our 2006 Diet and Lifestyle Recommendations.*
(accessed 8/8/07)

Other Sources

Nestle, M. 2007. *Eating Made Simple.* Scientific American 297(3): 60-69.

Harper, AE. 1990. *Dietary Standards and Dietary Guidelines,* in *Present Knowledge in Nutrition,* 6/e. Brown, ML ed. International Life Sciences Institute-Nutrition Foundation, Wash DC.

Chap. 19: Nutrition and the Life Cycle
Cited Sources

1. Food and Nutrition Board, Institute of Medicine. 2005. *Dietary Reference Intakes: The Essential Guide to Nutrient Requirements.* Editors: Otten, JJ et al. National Academies Press, Wash DC, p. 82. www.nap.edu

2. Food and Nutrition Board, Institute of Medicine. 2005. *Dietary Reference Intakes for Energy, Carbohydrates, Fat, Fatty Acids, Cholesterol, Protein, Amino Acids (Macronutrients)*. National Academies Press, Wash DC, p. 192. www.nap.edu

3. American Academy of Pediatrics. 2005. *Policy Statement on Breastfeeding and the Use of Human Milk*. Pediatrics 115:496-506.

4. Birch, LL. 1987. *The Role of Experience in Children's Food Acceptance Patterns*. J. Amer. Diet. Assoc. 87: S36-S40.

Other Sources

American Academy of Pediatrics, Committee on Nutrition. 2003. *Policy Statement: Prevention of Pediatric Overweight and Obesity*. Pediatrics 112:424-430.

Berman, C, Fromer, J. 2006. *Meals Without Squeals: Child Care Feeding Guide and Cookbook* (also available in Spanish). Bull Publishing, Boulder, CO.

Kimbro, RT, et al. 2007. Racial and Ethnic Differentials in Overweight and Obesity Among 3-Year-Old Children. Am J Public Health. 97:298-305.

Lorig, K et al. 2006. *Living a Healthy Life with Chronic Condition* (also available in Spanish). Bull Publishing, Boulder, CO.

Satter, E. 2000. *Child of Mine: Feeding with Love and Good Sense*. Bull Publishing, Boulder, CO.

Shanley, E, Thompson, C. 2001. *Fueling the Teen Machine*. Bull Publishing, Boulder, CO.

Speakman, JR, Hambly, C. 2007. *Starving for Life: What Animal Studies Can and Cannot Tell Us about the Use of Caloric Restriction to Prolong Human Lifespan*. J Nutr. 137:1078-1086.

Stewart, DD. 2006. *Baby & Me, The Essential Guide to Pregnancy* (also available in Spanish). Bull Publishing, Boulder, CO.

Thompson, C, Shanley, E. 2003. *Overcoming Childhood Obesity*. Bull Publishing, Boulder, CO.

Chap. 20: Agriculture—Realities of Leaf and Soil

Cited Sources

1. Moffat, AS. 1992. *Plants as Clean-up Artists*. Science 257: 1348.

2. Gough, P. 1975. *Natural Enemies Used to Fight Insect Ravages* in *That We May Eat,* The Yearbook of Agriculture, U.S. Dept. of Agriculture.

3. Ezzell, C. 1992. *Gene-spliced Rice Resists Stripe Virus*. Science News 142: 261.

4. Kang, IH, Gallo, M. 2007. *Cloning and characterization of a novel peanut allergen Ara h 3 isoform displaying potentially decreased allergenicity*. Plant Science 172(2): 345-353.

5. Ames, B, et al. 1987. *Ranking Possible Carcinogenic Hazards*. Science 236: 271.

6. Gold, LS, et al. 1992. *Rodent Carcinogens: Setting Priorities*. Science 258: 261.

7. Horsfall, JG. 1975. *The Fire Brigade Stops a Raging Corn Epidemic*. in *That We May Eat.* The Yearbook of Agriculture, U.S. Dept. of Agriculture.

8. Clysdesdale, FM, Francis, FJ. 1985. *Food Nutrition and Health*. Avi Publishing Co., Inc., Westport, CT. p. 216.

Other Sources

Bevan, DR. 1990. *Toxicants in Foods,*" in *Present Knowledge in Nutrition,* 6/e. Brown, ML ed., International Life Sciences Institute—Nutrition Foundation, Wash DC.

Kessler, DA et al. 1992. *The Safety of Foods Developed by Biotechnology*. Science 256: 1747.

Raney, T, Pingali, P. 2007. *Sowing a Gene Revolution*. Scientific American 297(3):104-111.

University of California. 1992 Annual Report, University of California Statewide IPM [Integrated Pest Management] Project.

U.S. Dept. of Agriculture, Economic Research Service. *Organic Agriculture*. www.ers.usda.gov/Briefing/ Organic/ (accessed 11/9/07).

Chap. 21: Food Processing and Food Safety

Cited Sources

1. Day, L. May 1985. *A Conversation with Bruce Ames*. California Monthly.

2. Linden, E. December 18, 1989. *Now Wait Just a Minute*. Time Magazine.

3. Gold, LS et al. 1992. *Rodent Carcinogens: Setting Priorities*. Science 258:261.

4. Arnon, SS et al. 1979. *Honey and Other Environmental Risk Factors for Infant Botulism*. J. Peds. 94: 331.

5. Coons, JM. 1974. *Natural Food Toxicants—A Perspective*. Nutr. Rev. 32: 321.

Other Sources

Fischetti, M. 2007. *Is Your Food Contaminated?* Scientific American 297(3):112-117.

Kauter, DA, Lynt, RK. 1973. *Botulism*. Nutr. Rev. 31: 265.

Popescu, CB. 1986. *Risk and Reason*, in *The Nutrition Debate*. Gussow, JD, Thomas, PB ed. Bull Publishing, Boulder, CO.

Chap. 22: Food Labeling

Cited Sources

1. www.cfsan.fda.gov/~dms/lab-ssa.html

2. Rader, JI, Schneeman, BO. 2006. *Prevalence of Neural Tube Defects, Folate Status, and Folate Fortification of Enriched Cereal-Grain Products in the United States*. Pediatrics 117: 1394-1399.

3. De Wals, P, et al. 2007. *Reduction in Neural-Tube Defects after Folic Acid Fortification in Canada*. New Engl J Med. 357:135-142

4. The National Organic Program, Agricultural Marketing Service, USDA, 2003. *Labeling Packaged Products*. www.ams.usda.gov/nop/ProdHandlers/labelTable.htm

Other Sources

Food and Drug Administration. December 10, 1992. *The New Food Label,* FDA Backgrounder.

Kessler, DA. 1989. *The Federal Regulation of Food Labeling—Promoting Foods to Prevent Disease*. New Eng. J. Med. 321: 717.

Porter, DV, Earl, RO ed. 1990. *Nutrition Labeling, Issues and Directions for the 1990s*, National Academy of Sciences, National Academies Press, Wash DC.

U

UL (Tolerable Upper Intake Value) 230, 231, 301
U.S. Department of Agriculture (USDA) 7, 108, 232, 258, 278, 296; and food grades 293; and labeling 295; organic seal 296
U.S. Dept. of Health and Human Services 108
U.S. Public Health Service; and pellagra 135
UL (Tolerable Upper Limit) 181
Ulcers 125; and anemia 220
Ultraviolet 179
Ultraviolet light; and vitamin D 9
Umami; definition 121
Umbilical cord 243
United Nations; and pesticides 262; and RDAs 231; report 268
Urea; and amino acids 143; and amonia 86
Uremia, Uremic toxicity 160
Ureter 159
Urinary tract infection 160
Urine 17, 45, 151, 160, 176, 215; and amonia 86; and glucose 56; and ketones 38; and urea 143; excreting vitamins 174
Urochrome 160
USDA (see US Dept. of Agriculture)
USP (United States Pharmacopeia) 208
Utah; and locusts 262
Uterus 242, 243

V

Valine 70
Vanadium 227
Vegans 77-78; and vitamin B-12 88, 186; and zinc 223; during pregnancy 244
Vegetable Group 233
Vegetable oil; and vitamin E 191
Vegetables; green leafy and vitamin K 191; solid food for babies 248
Vegetarian Diet (see also Vegans) 87; and proteins 74; and vitamin A 194
Vichysoisse 283
Vigor; and energy 19
Villi; in the small intestine 128
Vinblastine, Vincristine 265
Vinegar; acetic acid 142; as food additive 277; for microbe control 282
Virus(es) 264, 268; and diabetes 57 during pregnancy 242
Vitamin(s) 58; and energy 133; and metabolism 137 and urine color 160

deficiency 162; definition 162; different from medicine 163; fat-soluble (ADEK) 93, 189-204; myths 169; names 10; supplements 170; synthetic 169; water soluble 173-188
Vitamin A 92, 162, 169, 170, **190-195**; and birth defects 279; and blindness 5; and vision 5; deficiency worldwide 191; during pregnancy 194, 244; poisoning symptoms 194; RDA for infants 246 absorption 129; advised for the elderly 252; and vegan diets 77; in milk 87
Vitamin B-1 (see Thiamin)
Vitamin B-2 (see Riboflavin)
Vitamin B-6 164, 175, 179, **181-182** and amino acids 143 and protein synthesis 181; in infant formula 181; RDA 181, 301-302; toxic dose 164; UL 181
Vitamin B-12 5, 124, 167, 171, 175, **184-187,**188; and cobalt 261; and folate 185; and vegan 77; deficiency and nerve damage 185; discovery 184; during pregnancy 244; RDA 185
Vitamin B-15, B-17 10
Vitamin C 92, 164, 166, **174-176,** 273, 284; and common cold 164; and iron 221; and scurvy 174; deficiency 176; for smokers 166; natural vs. synthetic 169 RDA 176, 231, 301; RDA for infants 246, 302
Vitamin D 9, 162, 190, **195-198**; and blood calcium 207; and the kidneys 160; danger of excess 198; from cholesterol 101; RDA for infants 246, 302
Vitamin E 82, 190, **198-200**; as food additive 277; myths about 198; RDA 199, 301-302; toxicity 200
Vitamin K 92, 129, 190, **201-202**; and bacteria 9; shots for newborns 202
Vomiting 125, 152, 215, 284; and bulimia 41; and copper 219; and iron 219; and manganese 219
Vomitoria; Roman 118

W

Water 147-160; and athletic performance 154; and the structure of food 155; bottled 157-158; functions 159;

in food 155; intoxication 153; percent in foods 156; required intake 154
Water intoxication 153
Watermelon; and salt 122
Weed; control, and pests 262
Weight; and high blood pressure 107
Weight-loss schemes 23
Weight-reduction diets 36
Weight gain; during pregnancy 244
Weight loss; and water 16
Weight Watcher's diet plan 37
Wernicke-Korsakoff syndrome 178, 188
Whale; oil 92
Wheat 48, 49, 74; allergenicity 270; stone ground 72
Wheat germ 49, 274; source of zinc 219
Whisky 108; from corn 272
White blood cells 81; and zinc 219
White bread 274
Whole wheat; and fiber 275
Wiley, Harvey 278
Willow bark; and aspirin 265
Wilson's disease; and copper 226
Windpipe 122
Wine 108, 121; alcohol content 53; from sugar 53
Wine, red; source of chromium 219
Winter squash; and legumes 75
Women; and gallstones 128; and HDL 106
Women's Health Initiative 211
World Health Organization (WHO) 191
World War II 69, 272

X

Xerophthalmia, Xerox 191

Y

Yam; and legumes 75
Yeast 182, 187; and alcohol 53; growth limited by alcohol 53
Yersinia enterocolitica 284
Yew bark; and taxol 265
Yin, Yang; definition 3
Yo-yo dieting 36
Yogurt 130, 179, 252

Z

Zinc 219, **223**, 228, 275; and vegan diet 244; deficiency 223; for plants 261; toxicity 223
Zygote 242